SUSTAINABLE BIORESOURCE MANAGEMENT

Climate Change Mitigation and Natural Resource Conservation

SUSTAINABLE BIORESOURCE MANAGEMENT

Climate Change Mitigation and Natural Resource Conservation

Edited by

Ratikanta Maiti

Humberto González Rodriguez

Ch. Aruna Kumari

Debashis Mandal

Narayan Chandra Sarkar

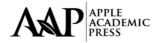

APPLE ACADEMIC PRESS

Apple Academic Press Inc.
4164 Lakeshore Road
Burlington ON L7L 1A4
Canada

Apple Academic Press, Inc.
1265 Goldenrod Circle NE
Palm Bay, Florida 32905
USA

ISBN 13: 978-1-77463-511-7 (pbk)
ISBN 13: 978-1-77188-815-8 (hbk)

Library and Archives Canada Cataloguing in Publication

Title: Sustainable bioresource management : climate change mitigation and natural resource
    conservation / edited by Ratikanta Maiti, Humberto González Rodriguez, Ch. Aruna Kumari,
    Debashis Mandal, Narayan Chandra Sarkar.
Names: Maiti, R. K., 1938- editor. | González Rodriguez, Humberto, 1959- editor. | Aruna Kumari, C. H.,
    1972- editor. | Mandal, Debashis, editor. | Sarkar, Narayan Chandra, 1976- editor.
Description: Includes bibliographical references and index.
Identifiers: Canadiana (print) 20190240903 | Canadiana (ebook) 2019024092X | ISBN 9781771888158
    (hardcover) | ISBN 9780429284229 (ebook)
Subjects: LCSH: Conservation of natural resources. | LCSH: Natural resources—Management. |
    LCSH: Natural resources—Environmental aspects. | LCSH: Climate change mitigation.
Classification: LCC S928 .S87 2020 | DDC 333.72—dc23

CIP data on file with US Library of Congress

About the Editors

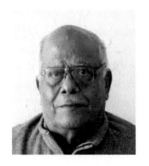

Ratikanta Maiti, PhD, DSc, was a world-renowned botanist and crop physiologist. He worked for nine years on jute and allied fibers at the former Jute Agricultural Research Institute (ICAR), India, and then he worked as a plant physiologist on sorghum and pearl millet at the International Crops Research Institute for the Semi-Arid Tropics for 10 years. After that he worked for more than 25 years as a professor and research scientist at three different universities in Mexico. He also worked for six years as a Research Adviser at Vibha Seeds, Hyderabad, India, and as Visiting Research Scientist for five years in the Forest Science Faculty, Autonomous University of Nuevo León, Mexico. He is the author of more than 40 books and about 500 research papers. He has won several international awards, including an Ethno-Botanist Award (USA) sponsored by Friends University, Wichita, Kansas; the United Nations Development Programme; a senior research scientist award offered by Consejo Nacional de Ciencia y Tecnología (CONNACYT), Mexico; and a gold medal from India in 2008, offered by ABI. He is Chairman of the Ratikanta Maiti Foundation and Chief Editor of three international journals. Dr. Maiti died in June 2019.

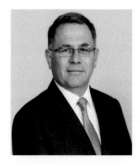

Humberto González Rodríguez, PhD, is a faculty member and Director of the Forest Science Faculty at Autonomous University of Nuevo León, Mexico. He is currently working on water relations and plant nutrition in native woody trees and shrubs, northeastern Mexico. In addition, his research includes nutrient deposition via throughfall, stemflow, and litterfall in different forest ecosystems. Dr. González teaches chemistry, plant physiology, and statistics. He has successfully guided 68 theses and has handled 10 research projects. Moreover, he has published 91 articles, five books, and 12 book chapters. He received his PhD in Plant Physiology from Texas A&M University under the guidance of Dr. Wayne R. Jordan and Dr. Malcolm C. Drew.

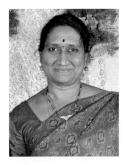

Ch. Aruna Kumari, PhD, is an Assistant Professor in the Department of Crop Physiology at Agricultural College, Jagtial, Professor Jaya Shankar Telangana State Agricultural University (PJTSAU), India. She has seven years of teaching experience at PJTSAU and seven years of research experience at varied ICAR institutes and at Vibha Seeds. She has received a CSIR fellowship during her doctoral studies and was awarded a Young Scientist Award for best thesis presentation on at the "National Seminar on Plant Physiology." She teaches courses on plant physiology and environmental science for BSc (Ag.) students. She has taught seed physiology and growth, yield, and modeling courses to MSc (Ag.) students. She also acted as a minor advisor to several MSc (Ag) students and guided them in their research work. She is the author of book chapters in four books. She is also one of the editors of the book *Glossary in Plant Physiology* and an editor of six international books, including *Advances in Bio-Resource and Stress Management; Applied Biology of Woody Plants; An Evocative Memoire: Living with Mexican Culture, Spirituality and Religion*; and *Gospel of Forests*. She has published over 50 research articles in national and international journals. Her field of specialization is seed dormancy of rice and sunflower.

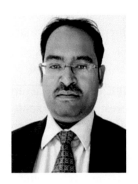

Debashis Mandal, PhD, is an Assistant Professor in the Department of Horticulture, Aromatic and Medicinal Plants at Mizoram University, Aizawl, India. He is a young academician and research fellow working in sustainable hill farming for past nine years. He was previously Assistant Professor at Sikkim University, India, and has published 35 research papers and book chapters in reputed journals and books. He has also published four books. He is currently chief editor for four volumes on fruits: production, processing, and marketing, and associate editor for four volumes on production, processing, and therapeutics of medicinal and aromatic plants. In addition, he is working as a member in the working group on Lychee and Other Sapindaceae Crops of the International Society for Horticultural Science, Belgium, and is also a member in the ISHS section on tropical-subtropical fruits and organic horticulture and the commission on quality and postharvest horticulture. Currently he is working as Editor-in-Lead (Horticulture) for the *International*

Journal of Bio Resources & Stress Management (IJBSM). He is also the founding Managing Editor for a new international publication *Chronicle of Bioresource Management.* Dr. Mandal is an editorial advisor for Horticulture Science to Cambridge Scholar Publishing, UK, and a regular reviewer of many journals. He is also a consultant horticulturist to the Department of Horticulture & Agriculture (Research & Extension), Govt. of Mizoram, India, and Himadri Specialty Chemicals Ltd. He also is handling externally funded research projects. He was the Convener for the International Symposium on Sustainable Horticulture, 2016, India; and Co-Convener, International Conference of Bio-Resource and Stress Management, 2017, Jaipur, India. He was a session moderator and keynote speaker at the ISHS Symposium on Litchi, India, 2016; on Post Harvest Technology, Vietnam, 2014 and at South Korea, 2017; and AFSA Conference, 2018, Cambodia. He has visited many countries for professional meetings, seminars, and symposia. His thrust areas of research are organic horticulture, pomology, postharvest technology, plant nutrition, and micro irrigation.

He did his PhD from BCKV, India, and was postdoctoral project scientist in IIT, Kharagpur.

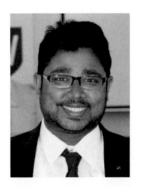

Narayan Chandra Sarkar, PhD, is a faculty member in the Department of Agronomy at the Institute of Agriculture, Visva-Bharati University, Sriniketan, West Bengal, India. Several past organizations with which he was affiliated include Vibha Seeds, Syngenta India Ltd., and Nagaland University. He has experience of conducting two international conferences as convener. He works as the managing editor of an international journal. His main area of research is nutrient management, and his a major focus is on the livelihood security of the farming community. Currently, he is deeply engaged with Western Sydney University under the Australia India Council funded research projects. Dr. Sarkar has guided 10 master students and four PhD students. He has published 28 research papers in national and international journals and has six books in his credit. He has received his MSc in Agronomy from G.B. Pant University of Agriculture & Technology, Pantnagar, India, and his PhD in Agronomy from India's premier institute, Indian Agricultural Research Institute, New Delhi. He has received a Junior Research Fellowship during his master's and institutional senior research fellowship during his PhD program.

Contents

Contributors

Eduardo Rangel Cortés
Escuela Superior de Apan-Universidad Autónoma del Estado de Hidalgo, Carretera Apan-Calpulalpan, Km 8, Chimalpa Tlalayote s/n, Colonia Chimalpa, 43900 Apan, Hidalgo, Mexico

Teresa Romero Cortes
Escuela Superior de Apan-Universidad Autónoma del Estado de Hidalgo, Carretera Apan-Calpulalpan, Km 8, Chimalpa Tlalayote s/n, Colonia Chimalpa, 43900 Apan, Hidalgo, Mexico

Jaime Alioscha Cuervo-Parra
Escuela Superior de Apan-Universidad Autónoma del Estado de Hidalgo, Carretera Apan-Calpulalpan, Km 8, Chimalpa Tlalayote s/n, Colonia Chimalpa, 43900 Apan, Hidalgo, Mexico

Anupam Das
Plant Biotechnology Laboratory, Department of Botany, Ramakrishna Mission Vivekananda Centenary College, Rahara, Kolkata 700118, India

Víctor Hugo Pérez España
Escuela Superior de Apan-Universidad Autónoma del Estado de Hidalgo, Carretera Apan-Calpulalpan, Km 8, Chimalpa Tlalayote s/n, Colonia Chimalpa, 43900 Apan, Hidalgo, Mexico

Cinzia Forni
Dipartimento di Biologia, Università di Roma Tor Vergata, Via della Ricerca Scientifica, 00133 Rome, Italy

Rahim Foroughbakhch
Facultad de Ciencias Biológicas, Departamento de Botánica, Universidad Autónoma de Nuevo León, Av. Universidad s/n Cd. Universitaria, San Nicolás de los Garza, C.P. 66451, Nuevo León, Mexico

Biswajit Ghosh
Plant Biotechnology Laboratory, Department of Botany, Ramakrishna Mission Vivekananda Centenary College, Rahara, Kolkata 700118, India

Tarun Halder
Plant Biotechnology Laboratory, Department of Botany, Ramakrishna Mission Vivekananda Centenary College, Rahara, Kolkata, India

Maginot Ngangyo Heya
Facultad de Ciencias Biológicas, Departamento de Botánica, Universidad Autónoma de Nuevo León, Av. Universidad s/n Cd. Universitaria, San Nicolás de los Garza, C.P. 66451, Nuevo León, Mexico

Michael J. H. Hickford
Marine Ecology Research Group, University of Canterbury, Christchurch, New Zealand

Valasia Iakovoglou
Department of Forestry and Natural Environment Management, Technologiko Ekpedeftiko Irdyma Anatolikis Makedonias and Thrakis (EMaTTech) Drama 66100, Greece

Natalya S. Ivanova
Botanical Garden of the Ural Branch of the Russian Academy of Sciences, 8th March Street, 202a, Yekaterinburg 620144, Russia
Ural State Forest Engineering University, Sibirskiy trakt, 37, Yekaterinburg 620100, Russia

S. M. Jalil
Former Chief Conservator of Forest and President, Forestry & Environment Forum, Dhaka, Bangladesh

Ahmed Ibrahim Jessim
Ministry of Higher Education, Scientific Research, Science and Technology, Treatment and Disposal of Chemical, Biological and Military Hazardous Wastes, Center of research and Development, Iraq

Pradeep Khanna
Former Chief Conservator of Forest, Gujarat, India

Ch. Aruna Kumari
Crop Physiology, Professor Jaya Shankar Telangana State Agricultural University, Agricultural College, Polasa, Jagtial 505529, India

Sujata Kumari
Department of Seed Science and Technology, University of Horticulture and Forestry, Nauni 173230, Solan, Himachal Pradesh, India

Subrata Kundu
Plant Biotechnology Laboratory, Department of Botany, Ramakrishna Mission Vivekananda Centenary College, Rahara, Kolkata 700118, India

R. C. Lalduhsangi
Department of Horticulture, Aromatic and Medicinal Plants, Mizoram University, Aizawl 796004, Mizoram, India

Roque Gonzalo Ramírez Lozano
Facultad de Ciencias Biológicas, Dpto. de Alimentos, Universidad Autónoma de Nuevo León

Marco Antonio Guzmán Lucio
Facultad de Ciencias Biológicas, Departamento de Botánica, Universidad Autónoma de Nuevo León, Av. Universidad s/n Cd. Universitaria, San Nicolás de los Garza, C.P. 66451, Nuevo León, Mexico

M. Madhavi
Department of Plant Pathology, Agricultural College, Professor Jayashanker Telangana State Agricultural University, Jagtial 505529, India

Ratikanta Maiti
Forest Science Faculty, Universidad de Nuevo Leon, Mexico
Universidad Autónoma de Nuevo León, Facultad de Ciencias Forestales, Carr. Nac. No. 85 Km. 45, Linares, Nuevo Leon 67700, México

Debashis Mandal
Department of Horticulture, Aromatic and Medicinal Plants, Mizoram University, Aizawl 796004, Mizoram, India

K. Manohar
Plant Pathologist, College of Agriculture, Rajendranagar, Hyderabad 500030, India

A. Navatha
Agricultural College, Professor Jayashanker Telangana State Agricultural University, Jagtial 505529, India

Shane Orchard
Waterways Centre for Freshwater Management, University of Canterbury and Lincoln University, Christchurch, New Zealand

Mario A. Morales Ovando
Universidad de Ciencias y Artes de Chiapas, Sede Acapetahua, Calle central norte s/n entre 4ª y 5ª norte, 30580. Acapetahua, Chiapas, Mexico

Mark Arango Owidhi
Department of Meteorology, University of Nairobi, Nairobi, Kenya

Artemio Carrillo Parra
Instituto de Silvicultura e Industria de la Madera, Universidad Juárez del Estado de Durango, Boulevard del Guadiana #501, Ciudad Universitaria, Torre de Investigación, C.P. 34120, Durango, Mexico

Pablo Antonio López Pérez
Escuela Superior de Apan-Universidad Autónoma del Estado de Hidalgo, Carretera Apan-Calpulalpan, Km 8, Chimalpa Tlalayote s/n, Colonia Chimalpa, 43900 Apan, Hidalgo, Mexico

B. Laxmi Prasanna
Department of Genetics and Plant Breeding, Agricultural College, Professor Jayashanker Telangana State Agricultural University, Jagtial 505529, India

Mario Ramírez-Lepe
Unidad de Investigación y Desarrollo en Alimentos, Instituto Tecnológico de Veracruz, Av. Miguel Ángel de Quevedo No. 2779, Colonia Formando Hogar, Veracruz, Ver, Mexico

V. Ram Reddy
Department of Genetics and Plant Breeding, Agricultural College, Professor Jayashanker Telangana State Agricultural University, Jagtial 505529, India

Catalina Rivas-Morales
Facultad de Ciencias Biológicas, Laboratorios de Fitoquímica y Química Analítica, Universidad Autónoma de Nuevo León, Av. Universidad s/n Cd. Universitaria, San Nicolás de los Garza, C.P. 66455, Nuevo León, Mexico

Humberto Gonzalez Rodriguez
Forest Science Faculty, Universidad de Nuevo Leon, Mexico
Facultad de Ciencias Forestales (School of Forest Sciences), Universidad Autonoma de Nuevo Leon, Linares, NL 67770, Mexico

Kamaljit K. Sangha
Research Fellow, Research Institute for the Environment and Livelihoods, Charles Darwin University, Darwin, Northern Territory 0810, Australia

Narayan Chandra Sarkar
Department of Agronomy, Palli Siksha Bhavan, Visva Bharati, Santiniketan, West Bengal, India

Israel Cantú Silva
Facultad de Ciencias Forestales (School of Forest Sciences), Universidad Autonoma de Nuevo Leon, Linares, NL 67770, Mexico

Ashok K. Thakur
Department of Seed Science and Technology, University of Horticulture and Forestry, Nauni 173230, Solan, Himachal Pradesh, India

Haydee Alejandra Dueñas Tijerina
Facultad de Ciencias Forestales (School of Forest Sciences), Universidad Autonoma de Nuevo Leon, Linares, NL 67770, Mexico

Marco Antonio Alvarado Vazquez
Facultad de Ciencias Biológicas, Departamento de Botánica, Universidad Autónoma de Nuevo León,
Av. Universidad s/n Cd. Universitaria, San Nicolás de los Garza, C.P. 66451, Nuevo León, Mexico

María Julia Verde-Star
Facultad de Ciencias Biológicas, Laboratorios de Fitoquímica y Química Analítica,
Universidad Autónoma de Nuevo León, Av. Universidad s/n Cd. Universitaria,
San Nicolás de los Garza, C.P. 66455, Nuevo León, Mexico

Abbreviations

ABA	abscisic acid
ACC	1-aminocyclopropane-1-carboxylate
AOO	area of occupancy
APX	ascorbate peroxidase
ASAL	arid and semiarid
ASDS	Agricultural Sector Development Strategy
BCAs	biocontrol agents
BR	brassinosteroid
CAT	catalase
CBLs	calcineurin B-like proteins
CK	cytokinins
DA	domoic acid
DCA	detrended correspondence analysis
DSP	diarrheic shellfish poisoning syndrome
DUS	distinctiveness, uniformity, and stability
ECe	electrical conductivity
EOO	extent of occurrence
ET	ethylene
FSI	Forest Survey of India
GDP	gross domestic product
GHGs	greenhouse gases
GOT	grow-out testing
HABs	harmful algal bloom
IMSCS	Indian Minimum Seed Certification Standards
IPBES	Intergovernmental Platform on Biodiversity and Ecosystem Services
JAs	jasmonates
MA	millennium ecosystem assessment
MFF	mangrove for future
MMGDA	molecular marker based genetic diversity analysis
MNP	Marine National Park
MOE_{dyn}	dynamic modulus of elasticity
NCCAP	National Climate Change Action Plan
NCCRS	National Climate Change Response Strategy

NNRs	nonrenewable natural resources
NPV	nuclear polyhedrosis virus
OECD	Organization for Economic Cooperation and Development
OR	osmotic stress-responsive
PAs	protected areas
PCR	polymerase chain reaction
PDA	potato dextrose agar
PGPB	plant growth growth-promoting bacteria
PGR	plant genetic resources
PSP	paralytic shellfish poisoning syndrome
QA	quality assurance
QC	quality control
QTL	quantitative trait locus
RAMPO	random amplified microsatellite polymorphism
RAPD	random amplified polymorphic DNA
RGP	root growth potential
RH	relative humidity
RL	reach lengths
RNRs	renewable natural resources
ROS	reactive oxygen species
RWC	relative water content
SA	salicylic acid
SDG	sustainable development goal
SESs	sites of ecological significance
SLA	specific leaf area
SNPs	single nucleotide polymorphisms
SOS	salt overly sensitive
STMS	sequence tagged microsatellite sites
TFs	transcription factors
USDA	United States Department of Agriculture
WHC	water holding capacity

Preface

Bioresources (plants, animals, and organisms) are the gifts of nature for our livelihood. They supply us with food, shelter, timber, medicinal plants, biofuels, bioenergy, and various domestic needs. Increasing global warming associated with increased emission of greenhouse gases (GHGs) and biotic and abiotic stresses is endangering the survival of these valuable bioresources. This urges a great necessity for efficient management, conservation, and sustainable uses of these bioresources.

Bioresource management in the recent past has drawn the attention of global participants. There is a need for sustainability of natural resources, which stands as a big challenge to overcome various stresses. Due to anthropogenic activities and human intervention in the changing surrounding environment, drastic quantitative and qualitative transformation is bound to happen. Increasing population pressure and habitual change in day-to-day life have paced the trend of ecological erosion in recent-past.

In this book, we have tried to emphasize the phenomenon change and provide an update in relation to bioresource management and the tools to manage stresses. It is the compilation and interpretation of the concrete scientific venture undertaken by specialists at the global level, with their extension services dedicated to the management of natural resources and controlling biotic and abiotic factors, making our mother earth vulnerable to these stresses. The book content gives an outline of the series of the development in the recent past on the bioresource and stress management.

This volume is widely focused on all types of bioresources on earth and their management at times of stress/crisis. There is need to focus on the documentation, validation, and recovery of ethnic indigenous knowledge and practices and native plant species, which could have great impact in stress management. Thus, the book acts as a platform for suggestions with possible solutions to make this earth a better place to live. The vulnerable earth needs utmost care that needs to be addressed cautiously in this progressive world.

The combined and interacting influences of over-exploitation, pollution, modification, destruction, or degradation of the native habitats amplify the vulnerability of bioresources. All these issues are really forcing natural biota to attain a smaller size with every passing day. Human interference for maintaining a balance to sustain the ecosystem can be attained with continued attempts to check the genetic erosion. Thus, this alarming situation needs multifaceted and diverse attempts in adapting and/or adopting an agenda for the management and conservation of bioresources.

Similarly, there is a need for an economically viable long-term solution to bioconservation of native species. Indiscriminate use of insecticides affects the quality of agricultural products and human health.

In addition, the most toxic pesticides and herbicides can pose a great risk to nontarget organisms. Biomagnification of chemicals is posing a sustained threat to living entities. Thus the anthropogenic activities and continuous change in the advancement of the daily life is bringing new issues of the stresses to the natural components. This book not only emphasizes the general conceptual approaches by different users but also presents methods of integrated conservation, utility, and importance of bioresources and also biotic and abiotic stresses affecting survival of these bioresources, essential for our livelihood.

This volume addresses the range of attributes, conservation, or management of resources and indicates, at the same time, the areas or topics where further research will be useful under the present scenario of climate change. The lucid presentation of the research highlights the wide range of themes for framing considerable management aspects. The book also provides an interesting overview of the current perspective to assess the level of depletion or exploitation on bioresources over the years.

The book also has covered aspects like genetics and breeding techniques directed toward sustainable management, biotechnological make-up, conservation of biota and abiotic components, natural resource management, climate change, etc. There is comprehensive call for inter- and intra-disciplinary research to save our earth. The content of the chapters has wide emphasis on future aptitude of research with multi-disciplinary approach.

Overall, the book will open the eyes of many research scientists, not only for current research, but also future strategies to combat such a sensitive agenda.

—**Ratikanta Maiti**
Humberto Gonzalez Rodríguez
Ch. Aruna Kumari
Debashis Mandal
Narayan Chandra Sarkar

PART I

Nature and Changing Climate Management, Adaptation, and Mitigation

CHAPTER 1

Understanding the Value of Natural Resources for Human Well-Being

KAMALJIT K. SANGHA*

Research Fellow, Research Institute for the Environment and Livelihoods, Charles Darwin University, Darwin, Northern Territory 0810, Australia

Corresponding author. E-mail: kamaljit.sangha@cdu.edu.au

ABSTRACT

This chapter focuses on the key benefits of managing nature's systems for people's well-being and, more broadly, for the modern economy and overall development. First, it explores a historical perspective of human connections with nature, and how nature has played a key role in shaping our ancient and modern civilizations. Second, it elaborates how natural resources are important for people's well-being, and outlines the consequences of mismanaging them in terms of social-economic repercussions in the present times. To understand and evaluate the role of natural resources toward human well-being for policy decision-making, this chapter outlines three main approaches: realizing our connections with nature; applying an integrated and inclusive approach to development; and an ethical approach to live in harmony with nature. It explains the need for, and how to, realize our connections with nature, and proposes an integrated development model that is focused on people's well-being, not the standard input and output measures, and accounts for the role of nature's services. Applying an ethical approach to lead a meaningful life that is in harmony with nature and embedding ethical principles in development, this chapter underscores the importance of natural systems in modern economy.

1.1   INTRODUCTION

Once the Dalai Lama (14th) was asked what surprises him about the humanity, he replied:

"Man. Because he sacrifices his health in order to make money. Then he
sacrifices money to recuperate his health. And then he is so anxious about
the future that he does not enjoy the present; the result being that he does
not live in the present or the future; he lives as if he is never going to die,
and then dies having never really lived."

In the modern world, one of our main goals in life is to accumulate
material wealth. For that, we work hard. In the process, we forgot where the
material wealth comes from, and we isolate ourselves from our mind and
the surroundings. We often mislead ourselves for what the main purpose of
life is, and fail to think about out how to lead a "balanced and meaningful
life" that is in harmony with ourselves, and with our social, economic, and
natural worlds. We spend too much time and efforts focusing on achieving
"material" opulence, which does not necessarily provide us satisfaction/
happiness nor helps us to lead a meaningful life. This quote from Mahatma
Gandhi (1869–1948) is most apposite here:

"A certain degree of physical harmony and comfort is necessary, but above
a certain level it becomes a hindrance instead of a help. Therefore, the ideal
of creating an unlimited number of wants and satisfying them seems to be
a delusion and a snare."

Irony is that in this cycle of material wealth, we even forget to realize the
importance of good air, water, and food, which are, indeed, the fundamental
needs for our living. So much so, nature's raw resources for producing our
material wealth, which is often assumed as a symbol of economic development, are either taken for guaranteed or remain overlooked.

A standard indicator to gauge development is the gross domestic product
(GDP), which is based on input and output (exchange) of materials in the
market. For the last 20 years, many researchers (Costanza, 1997, 2014;
Daly, 1996, 2013, 2015; Dasgupta, 2004, 2010 and others) have called for
modernizing development and the associated economic approaches. So far,
we have little success. The current utilitarian view of economy still prevails
with a strong focus on materials without considering the source of those
materials. Nature's goods and services and its capacity to absorb and process
the waste that we create, is completely overlooked in the state economies
input and output equations. Daly (2015) clearly outlines the importance of
nature's services/resources toward human welfare by contrasting an Empty
World model that existed in the past when nature's resources were in plenty
with a Full World model that exists at present with resources becoming
limited whereas the economy has expanded to its full capacity, as evident

from Figure 1.1. The paradox is that although our economy is becoming constrained by the limits of the natural world, we still continue to dismiss the role of nature toward our well-being and overall economic development.

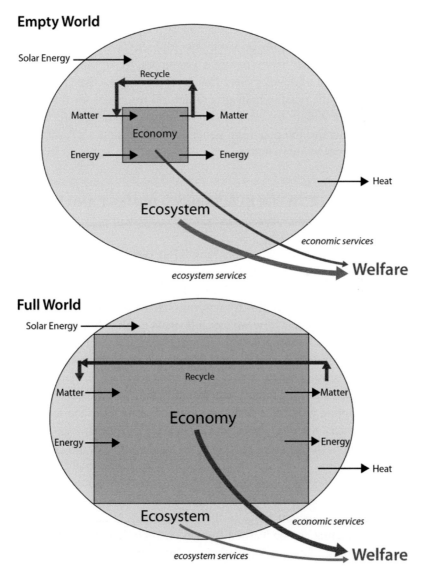

FIGURE 1.1 Limits to growth: An Empty World model when nature's resources were abundant in the past and a Full World model where those resources are becoming limited to contain the growth of modern economy.
Source: Reprinted from Daly (2015) with permission from **Great Transition Initiative**, Tellus Institute.)

Our continuous tendency to compromise natural resources to grow modern economies is rather scary and completely misleading. The key question is that how do we, as global citizens, realize the importance of nature toward our development so as to sustain on this planet?

This chapter explores this very question by providing historical evidence of resource use, and outlining how our development (well-being) is directly and indirectly derived from nature's resources by applying a broader holistic perspective of development that is well-being focused. It puts forth the argument for the need to manage our natural resources for future development—a topic widely covered in several other chapters of this book.

We or *us* refers to the people in general who use nature's resources and return little of real value to nature.

1.2 LINKAGES BETWEEN HUMAN DEVELOPMENT AND NATURE'S RESOURCES

At the 66th session, the United Nations (UN) General Assembly adopted a resolution on Harmony with Nature (A/RES/66/204). The UN General Assembly held a dialogue at their New York headquarters to examine how human activity has damaged Earth's natural systems and affected the planet's regenerative capacity, and how we can shift from a self (utilitarian)-centered to an Earth-centered approach. The dialogue emphasized that our success and wealth must be measured by the balance we create between ourselves and the world around us, that is, by our ability to live in harmony with nature. Rebalancing with nature, recognizing the role of Mother Earth in our socioeconomic fabric and reshaping the economy were the main points suggested to move nations forward with sustainable futures.

To apply an Earth-centered approach, we need to explore our connections with Mother Nature. A UN's report on "Sustainable Development—Harmony with Nature" (A/66/302) reflects on relationships humans have had with the Earth, as well as with their own existence, from various civilization, spanning from the ancient times to the 21st century. It also proposes some relevant lessons that can be learned from ancient civilizations for advancing our understanding of people's connections with nature:

1. Eastern traditions (Indian and other Asian countries) usually have no divide between the creator and his created animals. In Indian religions (Hinduism, Sikhism, Buddhism, and others), there is a focus on metaphysics and the belief that our bodies are made of

five elements: earth, water, air, fire, and the soul. There is strong emphasis on the concepts of *samsara* (reincarnation), *karma* (cosmic justice or the deeds we do), *moksha/mukti* (liberation from the cycle of existence), and *atma* (soul/inner ultimate reality). Promoting good deeds that include caring for Mother Nature and other living organisms created by God are central to this philosophy.

The Vedic philosophy of India has always emphasized the human connection with nature. Vedism shows a way of life which is in harmony with nature based on scriptures called Vedas/Aranyakas or "forest books," which were written by sages who lived in the forest. The Vedas, Upanishads, Puranas, and Smritis contain some of the earliest messages on ecological balance and suggest the need for humans' ethical treatment of nature. There are strong connections suggested between the stability in nature and human existence.

In Chinese traditions, external nature is never understood on its own terms. It is always intimately related to human life. Chinese culture believes that reality consists of countless manifestations of one unbroken continuum, the Tao. It has a cosmological myth in which the universe is viewed as an organic system of interdependent parts, thus representing a holistic perspective of life on Earth.

2. Ancient Egyptians worshiped a number of deities that involved their natural environment. They recognized the vital links between humans, nature, and the divine. The fact the Nile River served their lands to produce food was deeply embedded in their rituals and belief systems. With the Nile flowing to the north, the ancient Egyptians believed the sun rose on one side of the river and set on the other; and it passed through the underworld to begin the cycle again the next day. The bright star, Sirius, was believed to announce the annual floods, which supported irrigation and crop-enriching silt. This marker of time, crucial in the ancient calendar's development around 5000 years ago, provided a cyclical background to life rhythms of humans.

3. Among the African communities, natural phenomena were perceived as spiritual powers. The natural world that supplied food and shelter was respected. Certain trees were considered as God's trees, thus were sacred while the others were endowed with healing powers. Land belonged to clans which included the living, the dead, and even the unborn—a concept that enhanced the idea of sharing and caring for nature.

4. In the Andes, pre-Columbian cultures used the term "Pachamama" for Mother Earth. Pachamama means "fertile and fruitful mother." It symbolizes the symbiosis between humankind and nature.

5. In Western traditions, Romans had specific laws for the common use of air, water, and fish, as mentioned in the Justinian Code (A.D. 529). This code represents the first body of law related to the environment and asserted that the laws of nature pertain to all life forms.

Around the world, ancient civilizations have a rich history of understanding the symbiotic connection between human beings and nature. Ancient sites, many of which recognized by the United Nations Educational, Scientific and Cultural Organization (UNESCO) are part of the World Heritage. These have a key role to play in 21st century people's spiritual, cultural, and material lives.

1.3   A CASE STUDY OF MISUSE OF NATURE'S RESOURCES—THE DEMISE OF INDUS CIVILIZATION

The Indus region, from northeast Afghanistan to northwest India, flourished from ~9.5–3.3 ka BP (Fig. 1.2; Sarkar et al., 2016). The Indus people established a highly sophisticated urban culture, with their own "Dravidian" script, well-developed houses, public and private wells, wide roads, and underground drainage systems; proving to be one of the most extensive ancient civilization (Sarkar et al., 2016). Mohenjo-daro is currently listed as a UNESCO world heritage site.

The floodplains of the Indus ("Sindhu" river in Sanskrit or Hindi) and Ghaggar (used to be known as "Saraswati") rivers supported Indus civilization (Fig. 1.2). Both rivers and their channels offered fertile soils for agriculture, and people mastered the art of growing a variety of crops such as wheat, barley, cotton, mustard, and sesame. However, the waning of monsoons ~5–4 ka BP, coupled with large-scale droughts, led to changes in people's subsistence strategies. Particularly, these events caused reduced seed ubiquity and density of wheat and barley, which ultimately lessened food availability, and led to de-urbanization and the slow decline of this great civilization (Redman, 1999; Sarkar et al., 2016).

Although a number of factors including change in monsoon and river dynamics, trade decline with increased societal violence, and spread of infectious diseases are considered responsible for the demise of Indus civilization, the catastrophic floods and severe droughts that affected agricultural productivity, such as food resources, seem to be the key factors triggering sociopolitical turmoil (Sarkar et al., 2016; Weiss and Bradley, 2001). It is thought highly likely that reduced agricultural productivity disrupted the

Indus economy, making survival difficult for people; however, this requires further investigation (Ancient History Encyclopedia).

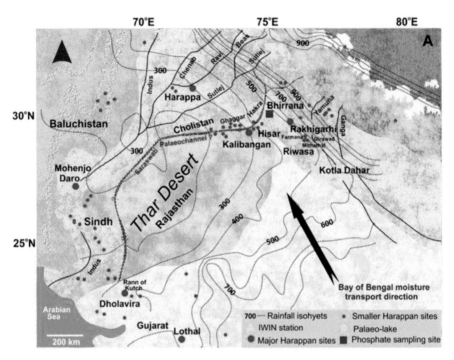

FIGURE 1.2   Map of northwest India and Pakistan indicating the location of main Harappan settlements (in pink circles). Black dotted lines suggest 100 mm rainfall isohyets.

Source: Reprinted with permission from Sarkar et al., 2016. http://creativecommons.org/licenses/by/4.0/

Analogous to the ancient Indus civilizations, our modern society equally faces the challenges of climate change, the uncertain and reduced availability of water and food resources due to droughts, floods, degradation of land, and their misuse, which further links to a myriad of social, economic, and health issues across the world.

1.4   CONTEMPORARY MISUSE OF RESOURCES AND CONSEQUENCES

Local, regional, and global assessments of natural systems, conducted by the MA (2005a-d) from 2000 to 2005 and Intergovernmental Platform on

Biodiversity and Ecosystem Services (IPBES) assessments in 2017 (the catalogue of assessments), clearly demonstrate their fast decline over the last century (shown in Fig. 1.3). More than 50% of the forestland has been converted for agriculture (MA, 2005e) (Fig. 1.3a). And, this conversion has instigated high rates of species extinction (Fig. 1.3b). Both terrestrial and marine systems are being overused in meeting human needs. Consequently, human activities have caused land degradation, pollution, loss of biodiversity, and changes to climate (MA, 2005e; The Economics of Land Degradation initiative 2015; IPCC, 2014; World Resources Institute (WRI), 2017; UN, 2016), resulting in multifold socioeconomic and ecological consequences, including increasing inequality both within and between the developed and developing world (UN, 2016).

There are a number of consequences of modern societies using and exploiting natural resources to develop and maximize economies. One of the main ones is the growing inequality among people in the developing and developed world over the past 20–30 years. So much so that we face social mayhem (Daly, 1996; Humphreys, 2003; Keeley, 2015; Organisation for Economic Cooperation and Development (OECD), 2008; 2017; Sen, 1989; Shiva, 2013, 2016). For example, economic inequality is on the rise in most developed (OECD) countries. It is even more evident in nearly every developing country (Keeley, 2015; OECD, 2017). As Keeley (2015) points out, "the gap between rich and poor is at its highest for the last 30 years, with the top 10% now earning 9.6 times more than the poorest 10%." Widening the income gap between the rich and poor, especially in the developing world, contributes to inequality in education, health, and other social services, setting up unjust and unfair social systems (Keeley, 2015; OECD, 2017 online database).

Our irony is that despite all the technological advances and extensive use of natural resources to support our material-based development over the last century, we still fail to meet the basic need for food for the millions of the world's population who are undernourished (MA, 2005e; Human Development Report (HDR), 2016; UN, 2016).

1.5   HOW DO WE MANAGE OUR NATURAL RESOURCES—THE BASIS OF OUR LIVING—TO CONTINUE BENEFITING FROM NATURE AND TO LEAD A MEANINGFUL LIFE

To lead a life that is ecologically sustainable and aligns with our economic aspirations, can be a difficult proposition. However, it is perfectly possible

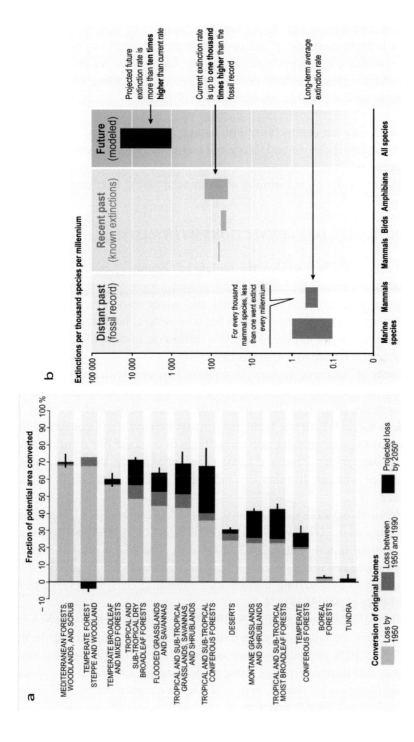

FIGURE 1.3 Decline of natural systems: (a) conversion of terrestrial systems for cultivation systems; (b) extinctions of species.

Source: Reprinted with permission from Millennium Ecosystem Assessment, 2005e. © 2005 World Resources Institute. https://www.millenniumassessment.org/documents/document.356.aspx.pdf

to match our economic and ecological aspirations. For this, we all need to explore a holistic meaning of life coupled with a diligent consideration of nature's resources, which underpin our living, but how do we do it?

This chapter proposes three possible pathways to achieve development that is sustainable and enhances our quality of life as:

1. Realizing our connections with nature;
2. Applying inclusive and integrated economic approaches to development;
3. Practicing living in harmony with nature applying an ethical approach.

1.5.1   *REALIZING OUR CONNECTIONS WITH NATURE*

From an ecological perspective, the feeling of "oneness" and "relatedness" to land or nature among the local and indigenous people helps them to follow customs and practices that sustain land and water resources. This ethical approach seems to be the main reason for why several local and indigenous communities have not exploited nature's resources; instead they integrated themselves with nature to coexist as one entity.

The view of "oneness" fosters the sense of harmony with nature, particularly when we realize the basic needs for our living are directly derived from natural systems (Fig. 1.4). It is something we are desperately missing in the modern world where our focus remains on materials and consumerism, using nature to produce more and more items to enhance our comforts. We often consider various aspects of human life, for example, the social, health or economics without deeming the linkages that exist between them and with nature.

The Millennium Ecosystem Assessment (MA) Programme, a UN's initiative commenced in 2000, was the first global effort of its kind and produced several seminal reports (MA, 2003, 2005 a-e). The MA work has significantly advanced our understanding of connections with the natural systems by proposing an overarching framework connecting ecosystem services to the well-being of people (Fig. 1.5).

Another UN initiative, an IPBES, 2017, now follows on from the MA for connecting science with policy. To date, 127 nations are signatories to the IPBES. The IPBES particularly emphasizes including the role of nature and its resources in to public policy through developing targeted policy documents and frameworks, thus showing the way to enhance human well-being for developing sustainable economies.

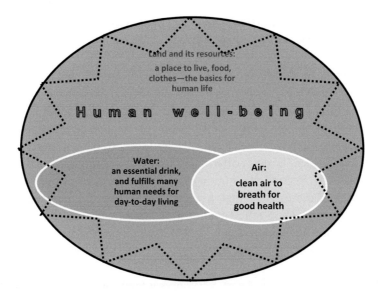

FIGURE 1.4 Dependence of human well-being on natural resources.
Source: Adapted from Sangha, 2015.

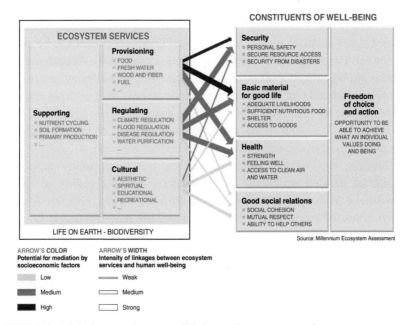

FIGURE 1.5 Links between human well-being and ecosystem services.

Source: Reprinted with permission from Millennium Ecosystem Assessment, 2005e. © 2005 World Resources Institute. https://www.millenniumassessment.org/documents/document.356.aspx.pdf

1.5.2   APPLYING INCLUSIVE AND INTEGRATED ECONOMIC APPROACHES TO DEVELOPMENT

An integrated, modernized concept of *development*—focusing on people's well-being enabling them to lead their lives as they want—is essential (Costanza et al., 2014; Sen, 1999a,b). To facilitate this, some key reforms are required. First, we need a new vision for *development* that focuses on enabling people, that is, enhancing capabilities, freedoms and rights, and better social justice, through offering appropriate opportunities, as suggested by Sen (1999a). Second, the notion of *development* needs to be linked with the supplier of the fundamental services that support human living, that is, nature, by incorporating efficient allocation, sustainable scale, and fair distribution of nature's resources (Daly, 1996). Blending *development* and natural resources at a sustainable scale can help us develop the ideal integrated framework to improve both human well-being and the state of nature's resources.

A simple integrated model of *development* focusing on people's well-being and nature is illustrated in Figure 1.6. Nature is shown as the basis for supporting the socioeconomic and cultural fabric of households and businesses. The model shows the importance of continual flows (goods and services) from nature to human well-being. To sustain these flows, the waste (the throughput including recycled materials that also require energy and resources) needs to be matched with the carrying capacity of nature's systems (Daly, 1996). At each individual business and household level, a balanced uptake from, and throughput to, nature becomes an integral part of the total economic activity, that is, input and output in order to operate at a sustainable, efficient, equitable scale to enhance human well-being. To do so, this model emphasizes integrating ethical principles with the economic activity to achieve *development* that we want.

However, this kind of *development* requires wise policy support and recognition. It also needs the policy makers and the public to think of *development* as supporting people's capabilities, rights, and freedoms and opportunities for employment, beyond simply the material needs, while still valuing, caring, and accounting for the natural environment.

1.5.3   PRACTICING LIVING IN HARMONY WITH NATURE APPLYING AN ETHICAL APPROACH

We need to find the ways to limit our material needs which are currently beyond the necessities. By limiting our needs, we will exert less pressure on natural resources that are already in declining state.

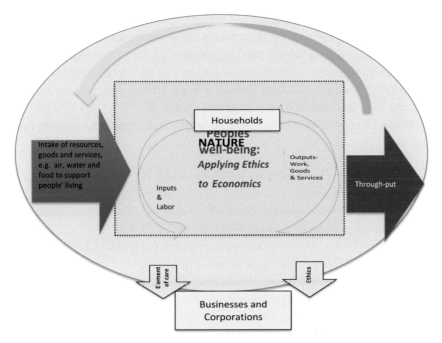

FIGURE 1.6   An integrated model for well-being focused *development*.

One of the ways to think what materials we need and how to value the resources producing those materials is to cogitate on the greater meaning of our lives. Doing so will help us focus on the main aspects in life and will help us limiting our needs for materials.

Spirituality is an important part and parcel of human life that allows us to explore and improve ourselves. Spirituality cannot exist without nature. Thus, nature is a fundamental part of our spiritual experiences whether one believes in religion or not. This service by nature is irreplaceable, and it is beyond any price.

Our ancient scriptures guide us to explore the meaning of human life and to apply right ethics in day-to-day life. A prayer from the *Atharva Veda*, one of Hinduism's most sacred texts, suggests worshipping natural elements such as fire (agni), Earth (dharti; as mother), and water (pani) and asking for peace on Earth and peace for all the living organisms including plants and animals:

"Supreme Lord, let there be peace in the sky and in the atmosphere. Let there be peace in the plant world and in the forests. Let the cosmic powers be peaceful. Let the Brahman, the true essence and source of life, be peaceful. Let there be undiluted and fulfilling peace everywhere."

In Hinduism, many mantras and preachings link us directly with Mother Earth, water, air, and fire; these elements are worshipped at many occasions. There are four Vedas which are large bodies of text in ancient India, and these connect human existence with nature and ultimately with God. Four Vedas and Upanishads indeed present a huge knowledge base for mankind that can help us connect with the natural elements.

Other examples of Hindu mantras, which link people to Mother Earth, include:

1. *Om, that (Divine power) which pervades the BhuLoka (Earth as the Physical Plane),*
    BhuvarLoka (outside Earth/sky AntarikshaLoka) and SuvarLoka (Swarga Loka or heaven or the Celestial Plane),
    That Savitr (Divine Illumination) which is the Most Adorable,
    On that Divine Radiance we meditate,
    May that enlighten our intellect and awaken our spiritual wisdom.
2. *Om, may there be peace in heaven,*
    May there be peace in the sky,
    May there be peace on Earth,
    May there be peace in the water,
    May there be peace in the plants,
    May there be peace in the trees,
    May there be peace in the gods in the various worlds,
    May there be peace in Brahman,
    May there be peace in all,
    May there be peace indeed within peace,
    Giving me the peace which grows within me, Om, peace, peace, peace.

Similarly, Buddhism, Jainism, Sikhism, Islam, and Christianity preach to practice right ethos to be compassionate for all the components of nature as well as to fellow human beings.

1.6 CONCLUSION

Over the last century, exploitation and misuse of resources by people have caused significant environmental impacts in terms of climate change, land degradation, and loss of biodiversity to name a few that we all face today. However, to prevent further losses requires urgent action if we really want to continue benefiting from nature. This chapter explores the main pathways for how to reduce our usage of nature's resources and how to better manage them especially when we are experiencing seriously limited supply and/or the consequences. Transforming our ways of living, reducing material needs and usages, thinking of holistic development, and valuing and mainstreaming nature's services into policy decision-making are the key elements to bring in this much needed change for maintaining and preserving nature's resources.

As outlined and argued in this chapter, an integrated approach to modernize economies, which is focused on improving peoples' well-being, is required at a local, regional, and global scale. Moreover, there is a need to commence a public awareness movement to understand the value of nature and the nature of value to collectively proceed toward sustainable development that is focused on human well-being. As Shiva (2016) says, "it is time to create a new economy and new democracy with life and people's freedom at the centre of the human enterprise."

KEYWORDS

- **human well-being**
- **value of nature's services**
- **ecosystem services**
- **modern economy**
- **integrated development model**
- **ethical approaches to economics and nature**

REFERENCES

Anónimo. *Human Development Report. Work for Human Development*; United Nations Development Programme, United Nations, 2015.

Anónimo. *Human Development Report, Human Development for Everyone*. The United Nations Development Programme (UNDP), 2016.

Costanza, R.; d' Arge, R.; de Groot, R.; Farber, S.; Grasso, M.; Hannon, B.; Limburg, K.; Naeem, S.; O'Neill, R. V.; Paruelo, J.; Raskin, R.G.; Sutton, P; van den Belt, M. The Value of the World's Ecosystem Services and Natural Capital. *Nature* **1997,** *387*, 253–260.

Costanza, R.; Kubiszewski, I.; Giovannini, E.; Lovins, H.; Mc Glade, J.; Pickett, K.E.; Ragnarsdóttir, K.V.; Roberts, D.; Vogli, R.D.; Wilkinson, R. Development: Time to Leave GDP Behind. *Nature*. **2014,** *505*, 283–285.

Daly, H. E. Beyond Growth: The Economics of Sustainable Development; Beacon Press: Boston, Massachusetts, 1996.

Daly, H. A Further Critique of Growth Economics. *Ecol. Econ.* **2013,** *88*, 20–24.

Daly, H. E. Economics for a Full World, Great Transition Initiative 2015 (June 2015).

Dasgupta, P. Human Well Being and the Natural Environment, 2nd ed.; Oxford University Press: UK, 2004.

Dasgupta P. Nature's Role in Sustaining Economic Development. *Philos. Trans. R. Soc. B. Biol. Sci.* **2010,** *365*, 5–11.

Humphreys, M. Economics and Violent Conflict. 2003. http://www.preventconflict.org/portal/economics, p 31 (accessed May 14, 2017).

Intergovernmental Panel on Climate Change (IPCC). Climate Change 2014: Synthesis Report. Contribution of Working Groups I, II and III to the Fifth Assessment Report of the Intergovernmental Panel on Climate Change. IPCC, Geneva, Switzerland.

IPBES (Intergovernmental Platform on Biodiversity and Ecosystem Services), 2017. IPBES Conceptual Framework. http://www.ipbes.net (accessed June 1, 2017).

Keeley, B. Income Inequality: The Gap between Rich and Poor; OECD Insights, 2015.

Millennium Ecosystem Assessment. *Ecosystems and Human Well-being: A Framework for Assessment*; Island Press: Washington, D.C., 2003.

Millennium Ecosystem Assessment. *Ecosystems and Human well-being: Current State and Trends*. Hussan, R., Scholes, R., Ash, N., Eds.; Island Press: Washington, D.C., 2005;Vol. 1, p 917.

Millennium Ecosystem Assessment. In *Ecosystems and Human Well-Being: Scenarios*: Carpenter, S. R., Pingali, P. L., Bennett, E. M., Zurek, M. B., Eds.; Island Press: Washington, D.C., 2005; Vol. 2, p 560.

Millennium Ecosystem Assessment. In *Ecosystems and Human Well-Being: Policy Responses*. Chopra, K., Leemans, R., Kumar, P., Simons, H., Eds.; Island Press: Washington, D.C., 2005, p 621.

Millennium Ecosystem Assessment. In *Ecosystems and Human Well-Being: Multiple Assessments*; Capistrano, D., Samper, K. C., Lee, M. J., Raudsepp-Hearne, C., Eds.; Island Press: Washington, D.C., 2005; Vol. 4, p 388.

Millennium Ecosystem Assessment. *Ecosystems and Human Well-Being: Synthesis.* Island press, Washington, DC. 2005.

OECD (Organisation for Economic Cooperation and Development). Growing Unequal?: Income Distribution and Poverty in OECD Countries. 2008. DOI: http://dx.doi.org/10.1787/9789264044197-en. OECD Publishing, Paris.

OECD (Organisation for Economic Co-operation and Development). Income Inequality. 2017. https://data.oecd.org/inequality/income-inequality.htm. OECD. *Human Impact on Ancient Environment*; Redman, C. L., Ed: University of Arizona Press: Tuscon , 1999 (accessed on May 16, 2017).

Sangha, K. K. *Ways to Live in Harmony with Nature*; JoJo Publishing, Classic Author and Publishing Services Pty Ltd: Docklands VIC 3008, 2015.

Sarkar, A.; Mukherjee, A. D.; Bera, M. K.; Das, B.; Juyal, N.; Morthekai, P.; Deshpande, R. D.; Shinde, V. S.; Rao, L. S. *Oxygen Isotope in Archaeological Bioapatites from India: Implications to Climate Change and Decline of Bronze Age Harappan Civilization.* 2016, Vol 6, p 26555.

Sen, A. *On Ethics and Economics*; Wiley-Blackwell Publishers, US, 1989.

Sen, A. *Commodities and Capabilities*; Oxford University Press, UK, 1999.

Sen, A. *Development as Freedom*; Oxford University Press, UK, 1999.

Shiva, V. *Making Peace with The Earth*; Pluto Press, London, 2013.

Shiva, V. *Earth Democracy: Justice, Sustainability and Peace*; ZED Books Ltd.: London, UK.

The Economics of Land Degradation (ELD) Initiative, 2015. The Value of Land: Prosperous Lands and Positive Rewards Through Sustainable Land Management. ELD Secretariat, Bonn, Germany. www.eld-initiative.org (2016) (accessed May 16, 2017).

United Nations. *Sustainable Development—Harmony with Nature*; UN General Assembly Report (A/66/302). UN, General Assembly 2011, 66th Session.

United Nations. *The Sustainable Development Goals Report.* United Nations: New York, USA, 2016.

Weiss, H.; Bradley, R.S. What Drives Societal Collapse? *Science* **2001,** *291,* 609–610.

World Resources 2000–2001, 2000. *A Guide to World Resources 2000–2001: People and Ecosystems: The Fraying Web of Life*; World Resources Institute: Washington.

World Resources Institute (WRI), 2017. Various Reports and Projects on Ecosystem Services. http://www.wri.org (accessed July 1, 2017).

CHAPTER 2

Climate Change and Agriculture in Kenya

MARK ARANGO OWIDHI[*]

Department of Meteorology, University of Nairobi, Nairobi, Kenya

[*]*Corresponding author. E-mail: arango.mark@gmail.com*

ABSTRACT

The economic growth of Kenya has been greatly contributed by the agricultural sector. Approximately, a fifth of Kenya's Gross Domestic Product (GDP) is as a result of agricultural sector. Besides, the agricultural sector adds to the foreign exchange earning of Kenya by about 50%. A greater percentage of people living in Kenya have agriculture as the main livelihood source. However, the agricultural industry significantly depends on rainfall.

Dependency on rainfall makes the agricultural industry extremely susceptible to the changing climate. This is due to the changing patterns of rainfall, extreme weather events, and increasing temperatures. Changing climate is real in Kenya and the harmful impacts are evident. The increased occurrences of pests and diseases have affected crop and livestock production. Besides, the frequent occurrence of drought in Kenya has led to death of many livestock in arid and semi-arid (ASAL) areas and hence, interfering with the livelihoods of the communities living in ASAL regions. Therefore, climate change effects levy a great risk to the agricultural sectors and also the future livings for most Kenyans especially those living in the rural regions.

This chapter has put more attention on the effects of changing climate on farming in Kenya. In addition, this chapter also looked at some adaptation measures as well as mitigation measures that have been put in place by both the government and NGOs with purpose of ensuring there is proper adaptation to the impacts of changing climate by the communities. This chapter has also focused on the policies at the national level as well as international level that are geared toward addressing adaptation measures and mitigation measures on agriculture.

2.1 INTRODUCTION

Agriculture is a critical sector for the Kenyan government because agriculture helps in achieving food security, poverty alleviation, and rural livelihoods. This implies that the agricultural sector is the backbone of the Giller economy of Kenya (IITA, 2009). The agricultural sector in Kenya constitutes both crops and livestock. The agricultural industry in Kenya provides about 70% of occupation for rural people (Kabubo, 2008). In 2011, agricultural output constituted about 22% of the Kenyan GDP. Agriculture has been given the first priority in line with the Kenyan Vision 2030. The Vision 2030 focuses on achieving commercially oriented, an innovative, modern agricultural sector, and this will be achieved through increased productivity, increased market access, institutional reforms, and land use transformation (Cairns et al., 2013). This will be done in the ASAL parts of Kenya. In line with the economic pillar of Vision 2030, attaining annual growth of the economy by approximately 10% will be greatly driven by the sector of agriculture. This will be achieved through plans that have been set out under Agricultural Sector Development Strategy (ASDS) 2010–2020 (GoK, 2010).

In Kenya, historically the growth of the economy has been associated with the growth and development of agricultural sector. Trend analysis has shown that the growth of the agricultural sector has been increasing annually by an average of about 2.4% increase annually in the year 2000 up to the year 2008 where it was affected by postelection violence. A greater percentage of farming in Kenya is small scale and about 75% of the agricultural output being produced depends on rainfall. About 16% of the total land area in Kenya is said to be from medium to high agricultural potential and this support about 80% of the Kenyan population. The remaining 84% of Kenya's land area is ASAL and this supports the remaining 20% of the population of Kenya. With the changing climate, this will impact the food security status of the government of Kenya.

The changing climate is greatly distressing the agricultural sector and therefore, this makes the sector to be highly vulnerable. Over the last decades, Kenya has been experiencing variability in drought and floods and this is anticipated to increase as the climate is changing. Depletion of nutrient and also soil erosion is becoming a major concern due to the changing climate (Cai et al., 2014). This implies that food security is under threat. Use of poor farming technologies and techniques, and also cultivating the low potential land is causing the agricultural system to be unsustainable now and in the future (Adger et al., 2009). Therefore, this chapter will review some of the changing climate impacts on the agriculture and also address some of the adaptation and mitigation measures put in place by the government of Kenya toward combating the effects of climate Kenya.

2.2 CLIMATE CHANGE RISKS AND EFFECTS ON AGRICULTURE

In Kenya, the agricultural industry is highly vulnerable to climate change and therefore, there is a need for establishing adaptation measures that will ensure that there is food security. The change in rainfall patterns has resulted in great impact for both the livestock farmers and crop farmers. There is an increase in the occurrence of drought conditions in parts of Kenya and this has affected the agricultural harvest (Cooper et al., 2008). This increase in the occurrence in drought condition is attributed to reduced precipitation being received in every rainfall season in Kenya. Kenya has two seasons that most farmers depend on to enable them to carry on with their agricultural activities. The seasons are MAM (March to May) and OND (October to December). The MAM season is a long rainy period and OND is the short rain season. Trend analysis shows that the two seasons are shrinking, and this implies that little rainfall is received during these two seasons as compared to the past decades. The change is attributed to the changing climate.

The livestock division has also been affected by the changing climate condition over the last few years. A research carried out by Bryan et al. (2013) indicates that drought conditions in Kenya are resulting in mortality and morbidity of livestock. Many pastoralists have recorded huge losses as a result of drought conditions. Drought conditions affect the availability of grassland (pasture) and water for livestock consumption, and this forces many pastoralists to walk a long distance in pursuit of water and pasture. The increase in cases of droughts in part of Kenya, especially the ASAL areas is a result of the changing climate.

Climate change has caused great impact on the crop yield in Kenya especially food crops. Kenya has maize as its staple food, and therefore, impacts of climate change have caused a great reduction in the yield of maize in Kenya. This has led the country in a food insecurity situation. The reduction in the rainfall amount has led to reduced planting season and this implies that crops will not be able to reach maturity as a result of reduced water availability, which is essential for the growth of plants (Bryan et al., 2013). However, there are some regions in Kenya that are expected to have an increase in crop yield. This is due to the changing climate that is causing some regions to have a favorable climate for growing some crops.

The projected increase in an annual evaporation rate and annual temperature will have an impact on the water available for crops. This will also have an impact on livestock as the increase in annual temperature and evaporation will lead to a reduction in water and pasture for livestock. This implies that agricultural production will go down leading to a reduction in revenue earned from exporting agricultural products (Cairns et al., 2012). At present, the ASAL regions of Kenya are experiencing drought frequently and this has led to a great loss in the livestock sector since those regions are occupied by the pastoralists (IFPRI, 2010; KARI, 2010).

In the year 2014, there was a reduction in the agricultural yield in Kenya and this was as a result of unreliable and low long rains and short rains. The reduction in agricultural yield resulted in the low rate of agricultural GDP. Besides, in the year 2013, there was a reduction of about 2.9% of the value-added agricultural GDP (World Bank, 2014).

In Kenya, the agricultural sector is viewed in three subsectors and these include fisheries, livestock, and crops. These three agricultural subsectors contribute to the agricultural GDP by about 2%, 20%, and 78%, respectively (FAO, 2012). However, the reduction in the amount of rainfall received coupled with an increasing temperature and evaporation rate has led to a reduction in the agricultural yield in three agricultural subsectors. For example, in the year 2011, about 3.5 million Kenyans were said to be food insecure, and this was as a result of the reduced rainfall amount during the long rainy season (FAO, 2012). The reduction of maize production was evident in the year 2013 which was about 38.9 million bags as compared to 39.7 million bags in the year 2012. Furthermore, drastic fall in maize production was evident in the 2013/2014 season where the amount of bags received were 28.9 million bags compared to the projected amount of bags that was 43.4 million bags of maize. This reduction in maize production and also other crops is attributed to the constant decrease in the amount of rainfall received every season. Similar impact has been felt in the livestock sector where there has been a fluctuation in the amount of livestock like sheep, cattle, and goats (IFPRI, 2010; KARI, 2010). Therefore, according to FAO (2012), climate change is triggering great impact on agriculture and especially the livestock sector. This means that measures should be put into action to ensure that future livestock production is maintained and well secured in order to protect the livelihoods of the people.

These graphs clearly show that climate change is causing great impact on agriculture and especially the livestock sector. This means that measures should be put into action to ensure that future livestock production is maintained and well secured.

2.3 MITIGATION MEASURES AND ADAPTATION MEASURES ON CLIMATE CHANGE

The agricultural sector under the Ministry of Agriculture, Livestock and Fisheries has taken some measures toward responding to the climate change effects. This has resulted in the assimilation of climate change effects into projects and programs in agriculture under the ministry. The integration has been done in line with low-carbon objectives and climate resilience to guarantee that climate change matters are applicable to the sector of agriculture. This implies that projects and programs being carried out are geared toward reducing climate vulnerability and also reducing emissions (Wegary et al., 2012). This will ensure that there is improved potential in agricultural production in Kenya. Most of the adaptation measures carried out is linked to the improvement of the livelihoods of many people staying in rural areas and in the ASAL parts of Kenya. The adaptation measures are community-based and also location-based since the climate change impacts affect locations and people differently. The adaptation measures in Kenya are always rolled out with a purpose of ensuring the communities are resilient to climate disaster and climate variability and as a result, this reduces the susceptibility to climate change effects at the community level.

The government of Kenya has rolled out some adaptation programs to help boost the agricultural sector. These programs are carried out to help both the small- and large-scale farmers to cope with the adverse weather events which are linked with climate change. For example, the government of Kenya has ensured there is water harvesting to improve water availability during the dry seasons (Walubengo, 2007). The government has dug dams in areas that are frequently affected by droughts. Besides, the government has promoted integrated management of soil fertility, the distribution of drought-resistant or tolerant crops, and development of strategic food reserves (Tambo and Abdoulaye, 2012). The government has also promoted insurance schemes and price stabilization schemes for farmers living in ASAL regions in Kenya. This has helped many livestock farmers who are at present feeling the impacts of the changing climate like droughts and floods. Another adaptation measure taken by the Kenyan government is incorporating climate change into extension services of agriculture and these services are delivered through the help of agricultural officers.

Mitigation measures have also been put in place to ensure there is a reduction in the emission level in the atmosphere. The government of Kenya has developed an improved grazing management system to enable control of pasture land and access to water by the pastoralists (Jaetzold et al., 2009).

There is also livestock breeding to improve the capability of livestock to cope with the changing climate and to produce lower emissions of methane (Herrero et al., 2010). There is also the promotion of livestock diversification by the government. Other mitigation measures include management of the dairy herd by improving feeds and also the breeding system to enable farmers to cope with the changing climatic conditions. There is the management of manure through the use of biogas technology to help in reducing the emission of methane into the atmosphere from the manure. Besides, the Ministry of Agriculture, Livestock and Fisheries have ensured that there is conservation, management, and rehabilitation of rangeland pasture. These measures have ensured the different communities in different locations have the ability to adapt to the shifting climatic circumstances (Okoba et al., 2010). Besides, these are of great importance for societies living in the ASAL parts of Kenya.

2.4   CLIMATE CHANGE POLICY MEASURES

The government has established policies and acts to help streamline the climate change agenda within the country. These policies and acts help in decreasing the susceptibility of agricultural sector to the changing climate. Through the Kenyan parliament, the legislature came up with climate change Act 2016 to give guidelines on climate change issues in Kenya. The Act was established in line with international agreements such as the Paris Agreement.

The Kenyan parliament enacted the Crops Act 2013. The act was to ensure that agricultural production is carried out in a way that is environmentally friendly and sustainable. The act also gave the county government the responsibility to ensure that they implement other national laws and policies such as those that ensure that water and soil are conserved. This act has helped in ensuring that all agricultural lands are used in a productive and economical manner.

There is also the development National Climate Change Action Plan (NCCAP) that was mandated with the implantation of National Climate Change Response Strategy (NCCRS). The NCCAP activities benefit the climate change mitigation and adaptation objectives (GoK, 2010). There are also other rules that help in ensuring the agricultural sector is effective. These include land preservation rules, farm forestry rules, and rules of basic land usage. The farm forestry rules help in ensuring that farmers maintain and establish farm forestry and this should cover about 10% of agricultural land holding. The rules on basic land usage give guidelines on the use of land that is sloping in order to reduce the cases of soil erosion.

2.5   CONCLUSION

Climate change has a great influence on the agricultural industry since the sector is most vulnerable to the changing climatic conditions. Therefore, there is a need for coordination within the sector of agriculture to ensure there is food security within the country and also to build resilience among different communities. Projects and programs should be initiated to boost the agricultural sector. Adaptation measures should also be put in place to build the community resilient by reducing the vulnerability to climate change. The government should also work closely with the communities when carrying out the adaptation programs and projects. Working closely with the community members will improve the ability of the projects and programs being successful. Besides, full implementation of policies will help in reducing the emission rate from the agricultural activities carried out in the farm such as poor disposal of animal wastes.

KEYWORDS

- **climate change**
- **agriculture**
- **kenya**
- **crop yield**
- **adaptation and mitigation**
- **policy measures**

REFERENCES

Adger, W. N.; Dessai, S.; Goulden, M.; Hulme, M.; Lorenzoni, I.; Nelson, D. R.; Wreford, A. Are there Social Limits to Adaptation to Climate Change? *Climatic Change.* **2009,** *93,* 335–354.

Bryan, E.; Ringler, C.; Okoba, B.; Roncoli, C.; Silvestri, S.; Herrero, M. Adapting Agriculture to Climate Change in Kenya: Household Strategies and Determinants. *J. Environ. Manag.* **2013,** *114,* 26–35.

Cai, W.; Borlace, S.; Lengaigne, M.; Van Rensch, P.; Collins, M.; Vecchi, G.; England, M. H. Increasing Frequency of Extreme El Niño Events Due to Greenhouse Warming. *Nat. Climate Change.* **2014,** *4,* 111–116.

Cairns, J. E.; Hellin, J.; Sonder, K.; Araus, J. L.; MacRobert, J. F.; Thierfelder, C.; Prasanna, B. M. Adapting Maize Production to Climate Change in Sub-Saharan Africa. *Food Secur.* **2013,** *5*, 345–360.

Cairns, J. E.; Sonder, K.; Zaidi, P. H.; Verhulst, N.; Mahuk, G.; Babu, R.; Rashid, Z. 1 Maize Production in a Changing Climate: Impacts, Adaptation, and Mitigation Strategies. *Adv. Agronomy.* **2012,** *114*, 1.

Cooper, P. J. M.; Dimes, J.; Rao, K. P. C.; Shapiro, B.; Shiferaw, B.; Twomlow, S. Coping Better with Current Climatic Variability in the Rain-Fed Farming Systems of Sub-Saharan Africa: An Essential First Step in Adapting to Future Climate Change? *Agric. Ecosyst. Environ.* **2008,** *126*, 24–35.

FAO 2012. Maize Production Data for Kenya. http://faostat.fao.org/site/567/DesktopDefault. aspx?PageID=567#ancor (accessed Aug 28, 2017).

Giller, K. E.; Tittonell, P.; Rufino, M. C.; Van Wijk, M. T.; Zingore, S.; Mapfumo, P.; Rowe, E. C. Communicating Complexity: Integrated Assessment of Trade-Offs Concerning Soil Fertility Management Within African Farming Systems to Support Innovation and Development. *Agric. Syst.* **2011,** *104*, 191–203.

GoK (2010). Agricultural Sector Development Strategy 2010–2020. http://www.ascu.go.ke/ DOCS/ASDS%20Final.pdf (accessed Aug 25, 2017).

Herrero, M.; Thornton, P. K.; Nouala, S.; Notenbaert, A. M. O.; Ericksen, P.; Leeuw, J. D. Coping with Drought and Climate Change in the Pastoral Sector in Sub-Saharan Africa: Policy Considerations. In Proceedings of the 8th Meeting of Ministers responsible for Animal Resources in Africa, Entebbe, Uganda,10-11 May 2010.

IFPRI (2010). Aflatoxins in Kenya: An Overview. August 24, 2017. http://www.ifpri.org/ sites/default/files/publications/aflacontrolpn01.pdf.

IITA (2009). Maize Production. May 6, 2014. http://www.iita.org/maize.

Jaetzold, R.; Schmidt, H.; Hornetz, B.; Shisanya, C. Farm Management Handbook of Kenya Vol. II. In *Natural Conditions and Farm Management Information-ANNEX: Atlas of Agro-Ecological Zones, Soils and Fertilising by Group of Districts. Subpart B1a: Southern Rift Valley Province*; Nairobi: Ministry of Agriculture, Kenya and Cooperation with the German Agency for Technical Cooperation (GTZ), 2009.

Kabubo, M. J. Climate Change Adaptation and Livestock Activity Choices in Kenya: An Economic Analysis. In *Natural Resources Forum.* 2008; 32, pp 131–141. https://doi. org/10.1111/j.1477-8947.2008.00178.x

Roncoli, C.; Okoba, B.; Gathaara, V.; Ngugi, J.; Nganga, T. R. Adaptation to Climate Change for Smallholder Agriculture in Kenya. 2010. International Food Policy Research Institute-Project Note, Washington DC, USA.

Tambo, J. A.; Abdoulaye, T. Climate Change and Agricultural Technology Adoption: The Case of Drought Tolerant Maize in Rural Nigeria. *Mitig. Adapt. Strategies Global Change.* **2012,** *17*, 277–292.

Walubengo, D. Community-Led Action to Use Forestry in Building Resilience to Climate Change: A Kenyan Case Study Njoro Division, Nakuru District, Kenya. Forest Action. International Institute for Environment and Development: London, United Kingdom. 2007.

Wegary, D.; Labuschagne, M.; Vivek, B. The Influence of Water Stress on Yield and Related Characteristics in Inbred Quality Protein Maize Lines and Their Hybrid Progeny. In *Water Stress.* IntechOpen: London, UK, 2012. DOI: 10.5772/30213.

CHAPTER 3

Impact of Climate Changes, Timber Harvesting, and Fires on Boreal Forests (Example of the Ural Mountains, Russia)

NATALYA S. IVANOVA*

Botanical Garden of the Ural Branch of the Russian Academy of Sciences, 8th March Street, 202a, Yekaterinburg 620144, Russia

Ural State Forest Engineering University, Sibirskiy trakt, 37, Yekaterinburg 620100, Russia

Corresponding author. E-mail: i.n.s@bk.ru

ABSTRACT

Climatic changes, timber harvesting, and fires are the main factors that determine the structure, functions, and dynamics of forest ecosystems all around the world. Long time development of the Ural Mountains contributed to the wealth and diversity of natural complexes. The Ural Mountains have a unique location. This mountain system is located in the center of Eurasia. These mountains are distinguished by high biodiversity, the preservation of which is extremely important for the biosphere. The geographical location, large extent, great age of the Ural Mountains and the heterogeneity of landscapes make the Ural Mountains a unique object for studying the effects of climate change, timber harvesting, and fire on vegetation. The objective of the research is to study the effects of climate change, logging and fires on boreal forests in order to predict their dynamics. We conducted our study in Zauralsky (Trans-Ural) hilly piedmont province (Russia, the Middle Urals): coordinates 57°00′–57°10′ N and 60°10′–60°30′E. The district is subdivided into foothills formed by alternating meridional low mountains and ridges with wide, intermountain elongated low lands, in which are marked large lakes surrounded by moors. The mountains have altitudes of

180–450 m a.s.l. The climate is continental and humid. Frostless periods last 90–115 days, the mean annual temperature does not exceed 1°C, and usual snow cover is not less than 45 cm. All major mountain habitats are included in our study. We visited the most-capped mountains. The steep and gentle slopes of the northern, southern, eastern, and western exposure were investigated by us. Swamp forests and marshes were not left unattended by us. All forest types were investigated. It is diverse of light coniferous and dark coniferous forests. The number of trees on the plot was not less than 200. The age by the annual rings was identified. Tapes 4×20 m were laid for the study of young generations of woody plants. A total of 10–20 accounting sites with the size of 1 m^2 were used to study the productivity of the herbaceous layer. It has been established that climatic and topographic conditions are significant factors determining the composition and productivity of forest communities. The influence of climate leads to a shift in the range of forest types and the replacement of one forest community by another, which is more in tune with new climatic conditions. Forests growing on the border of its spread of habitat are the most vulnerable. Harvesting and fires are superimposed on climate change. The forest dynamics becomes extremely difficult. Timber harvesting leads to the emergence of many plant communities within the same growing conditions (climax forest). Over time, differences between these ecosystems persist. The differences relate to both the dominant species in the tree stand and the grassy layer, development trends and succession rates. Therefore, the management of such ecosystems should have its own specifics. The results of the research reflect the modern evolution of forest vegetation as an adaptation to clear cutting and other impacts in a continuously changing climate.

3.1 INTRODUCTION

The huge scale of economic use of the forests of the Northern Hemisphere, fires and windfalls led to serious changes in their structure, functions, and trends in dynamics (Zobel, 2016). A widespread intensive decrease in the area of forests and the deterioration of their condition will be the cause of a decrease in their ecosystem functions and the depletion of biodiversity on all continents (Pavlov et al., 2010). In the recent past, environmental crises were only local in nature. However, in the near future, the global consequences of the violations of the biosphere are predicted (Maiti et al., 2016). Climate change is recognized as the most pressing problem of our time from the decision of which the future of human existence depends

(Global Biodiversity Outlook, 2006). The changing climate provokes the occurrence of dangerous dry periods, which lead to the spread of wild fires and enormous economic damage (Battisti and Naylor, 2009; Maiti et al., 2016).

Forests grow on 52% of the land (Boisvenue and Running, 2006), of which 5% belongs to forest plantations (Siri et al., 2005). Forests maintained the climate and water resources throughout its preanthropogenic history (Korotkov, 2017). Boreal forest ecosystem services are important not only at the regional level but also globally (Global Forest Resources Assessment, 2006). It is generally recognized that climate change, timber harvesting, and fires are causes of the transformation of the structure and function of forest ecosystems. Growing worldwide timber harvesting and fires are becoming a root of global problems (Maiti et al., 2016). The need to manage these processes is very acute. To solve this problem, additional detailed and comprehensive information is required on mechanisms to maintain sustainability and trends in climate and restoration shifts (Maiti et al., 2016; Kellomäki, 2016). Therefore, research in these areas receives great attention in all countries and on all continents.

3.2 REVIEW OF MODERN RESEARCH

3.2.1 IMPACT OF CLIMATE CHANGES ON BOREAL FORESTS

Currently, human activity is recognized as an important factor in recent climate change, which is often called global warming (Anderegg et al., 2010; Climate Change, 2014; Haunschild et al., 2016). Most researchers believe that advancing climate change can significantly affect the forest ecosystem biomass and species composition (Kellomäki, 2016; Schaphoffa et al., 2016; Ochuodho, 2016; Murray et al., 2017). Many researchers use anthropogenic impact scenarios to describe and predict climate change (Casajus et al., 2016). This leads to a rapid increase in the number of publications on this topic; every 5–6 years of publication becomes two times more (Grieneisen and Zhang, 2011; Haunschild et al., 2016). The most numerous are the studies devoted to the problem of bioproductivity. Climate change modeling is second in the publication rate. The search for adaptation mechanisms is a new and rapidly developing scientific field, the publications of which are actively read and quoted (Haunschild et al., 2016). Climate change management is an extraordinarily challenging task that is being addressed by researchers from various countries (Kellomäki, 2016).

The general approach of determination of productivity (Net Primary Prodcutivity, NPP) relies on the use of land cover maps in combination with bioproductivity based on GIS technologies (Jiang et al., 1999). LAI index (the ratio of leaf area to the area occupied by plantation) is a highly informative characterization of forest canopy associated with its energy and mass transfer, and is evaluated with satellite sensors with high resolution in wide areas (Running et al., 1986).

It is introduced in the model as the main independent variable for calculating the processes of light interception of the canopy, transpiration, photosynthesis, growth, and carbon sequestration. However, large databases make it difficult to use generally accepted methods of statistical analysis. Lankin and Ivanova (2015) propose to use dynamic neural networks, which are extremely flexible and efficient tool for data analysis. High flexibility, precision, and high simulation efficiency are important features of neural networks which allow solving wide range of tasks using the same mathematical algorithms (Lankin et al., 2012). Modeling and forecasting using artificial neural networks is based on samples of the source data required for training neural networks. There are examples that show a good ratio of empirical and theoretical data (Lankin et al., 2012).

Kellomäki (2016) explores the carbon cycle and he comes to the conclusion that the patterns found will help in solving the problem of climate change mitigation. His studies unite experimental and modeling approaches to discuss how to use climate change to one's advantage and optimize forest management in the boreal zone.

Ecological studies are focused on the analysis of plant habitats and transformation of growing conditions, which are initiated by factors of a changing climate (Lawler, 2013). However, various researchers obtained conflicting results using different methods (Thuiller, 2004). Therefore, new approaches are being tested to solve this problem. Chai et al. (2016) use a synthesis of traditional risk assessments with habitat suitability modeling to disseminate and introduce new species. The proposed approach is promising to use for the analysis of ecological niche species and the transformation of the species structure.

Murray et al. (2017) use large-scale environmental niche models. They found that climatic factors have a significant impact on the distribution and growth of most species in North America.

D'Orangeville et al. (2016) predict the effects of climate warming on natural complexes in North America. The study of the annual growth of trees allowed researchers to identify habitats in which current climate change will favorably affect the growth of woody plants.

3.2.2 IMPACT OF TIMBER HARVESTING AND FIRES ON BOREAL FORESTS

Currently, most boreal forests are used to produce wood. The sustainability of ecosystems is on the verge of disaster (Gauthier et al., 2015). Wildfires are of particular concern and can cause enormous economic damage (Rodriguez-Baca et al., 2016). In boreal forests, fire is a force that can influence forest succession and structure (Li et al., 2013). Forecast and observations warn that the number of wildfires will increase with climate warming (Krawchuk et al., 2009). These forecasts are valid for both Russia and Canada (Flannigan et al., 2005). Therefore, a lot of publications are devoted to the development of sustainable forestry, forest protection from fires, and reforestation (Gunn, 2007; Li et al., 2013; Kuuluvainen, 2016).

The greatest difficulties in the organization of sustainable forestry are complicated by the problem of uncertainty (Rodriguez-Baca et al., 2016). The use of risk and uncertainty accounting methods is a good basis for decision-making concerning natural resource management (Hildebrandt and Knoke, 2011). Therefore, further development of risk assessment methods in forestry is extremely important and should be strengthened in the near future (Yousefpour et al., 2012; Rodriguez-Baca et al., 2016).

A. Komarov and his colleagues developed system of forest ecosystems models EFIMOD (Komarov et al., 2003). The model allows you to calculate the growth of a single tree with the help of maximum net biological productivity per unit mass of photosynthetic organs. Further, the potential growth is reduced depending on the shading of the tree and availability of soil nitrogen. Annual growth of biomass is allocated to organs of the tree (trunk, branches, and roots). Researchers are focused on interactions between trees like competition for light and competition for available nitrogen in the soil, which allows simulating various reforestation and logging.

The next achievement was the program the EFIMOD 2 that described and predicted the growth not only of individual woody plants, but also of the whole planting as a whole. Further, it led to the opportunity to analyze the circulation of elements in the plants (Komarov et al., 2003). The model can work with the following wood species: *Pinus sylvestris* L., *Picea abies* L. Karst, and *Betula pendula* L. The structure and biodiversity of modern boreal forests in Eurasia is the result of long-term economic use (Kalyakin et al., 2016; Korotkov, 2017).

3.2.3 MODERN FOREST RESEARCH IN THE URAL MOUNTAINS (RUSSIA)

Ural Mountains (Russia) are located in the center of Eurasia (Fig. 3.1) (Komar and Chikushev, 1968).

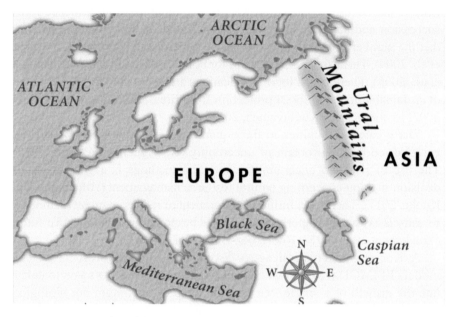

FIGURE 3.1 Location of the Ural Mountains.

The Ural Mountains are among the oldest mountains. Their history is long and complex. It begins in the Proterozoic era with the breach of the crust. This period lasted 2 billion years. At this time, on the site of the mountains settled the ocean. The formation of the Ural Mountains began 300 million years ago (Komar and Chikushev, 1968).

Now the Ural Mountains are a whole system of mountain ridges, which extend parallel to one another in the meridional direction. The Ural Mountains are represented by low ridges of great length. The highest of them have a height of 1200–1640 m above sea level. The height of the Middle Ural Mountains is not more than 600–650 m above sea level (Komar and Chikushev, 1968).

The long time of formation is contributed to the increase in the diversity of natural complexes. Forests are the most common type of vegetation. The forests stretch along the mountain slopes of the Ural Mountains continuous strip. Dark coniferous forests prevail on the western slopes. Spruce forests and fir forests are dominant ecosystems. Pine forests prevail on the eastern slopes. The geographical location, a large distance from north to south, extreme heterogeneity of landscapes, and long-term intensive economic activities make the Ural Mountains a unique object for studying forest dynamics (Komar and Chikushev, 1968).

The dynamics of vegetation due to climate is most clearly seen in the mountains at the upper limit of the distribution of woody plants. This problem has been studied for many years by Russian researchers (Shiyatov, 1995; Mazepa, 2005; Kapralov et al., 2006; Hagedorn et al., 2014). A survey of highland areas revealed the emergence of abundant undergrowth of conifers above the forest boundary. The cause of this phenomenon is climate warming. Long-term studies in the Polar Urals have established the beginning of the active invasion of woody vegetation into the mountain tundra. This process actively proceeds about 100 years. Probably, this tendency speaks of mitigating the factors limiting the distribution of woody plants. Stepana Shiyatov proposed a unique method for monitoring the state of vegetation. This method consists in photographing landscapes from one point, but after many years and decades. He received several thousands of landscape photos. He compared the photos which are taken at different times in the Southern, North, Subpolar, and Polar Urals. His study found that forest boundary rose to 4–8 m in all four regions over the past decade, and the forests became more dense (Hagedorn et al., 2014).

Typological studies of forests are of particular importance for scientific research and silviculture, since on their basis continual vegetation cover is divided into discrete units with which to work. The large-scale anthropogenic destruction of climax forests and the invasion of dynamic secondary plant communities necessitated the reflection of this process in forest classification schemes. Kolesnikov et al. (1973) have done a great deal of research on forest dynamics. The most detailed forest type schemes are the result of their hard work of many years. However, detailed quantitative characteristics of the structure of vegetation were not enough in these schemes until recently. Therefore, E. S. Zolotova and N. S. Ivanova (Ivanova and Zolotova, 2013) conducted a comprehensive study of the characteristics of plants and soils from 12 types of forest and 11 species of cuttings in the Urals. A database was created with data on plant structure and physical and chemical characteristics of natural forests and clear fellings within a unified topoecological profile. The scientists have found that each forest type and cutting type has its unique vegetation structure and dynamics, as well as unique patterns of soil evolution within soil profiles (Zolotova, 2013).

Forest syntaxonomy develops parallel to forest typology (Mirkin et al., 2009, 2014; Mirkin, Ermakov, 2010). Initially, this scientific direction was intended to study the diversity of plant communities (Mirkin et al., 2014). Currently, forest syntaxonomy has been tested to compare climax forests with secondary communities (Mirkin et al., 2015). Ural researchers attempted to analyze successions using the floristic approach methodology (Martynenko et al., 2014).

Research on the biomass of the Ural forests has received close attention for many years. Many years of research by Usoltsev (2007) are of interest from the point of view of the collected databases, unique techniques, and thoughtful in-depth analysis. He focused on the uncertainties that lead to risks in forestry. The formation of the most complete database, which includes almost all available information on the biomass of woody plants, can be considered an outstanding achievement of this researcher (Usoltsev, 2001). Identifying dependencies based on multiple regression is a second important result. Conduct drawing detailed maps of the carbon pool of the Ural Federal district is another valuable direction of research.

Thus, despite the huge number of publications that have been made within the framework of this scientific direction, satisfactory solutions have not been obtained at present. The effects of various natural and human factors are interrelated very often. Their actions overlap and reinforce the final effect, which is likely to lead to even greater environmental problems. Therefore, the study of adaptive strategies of woody plants is extremely important (Schaphoffa et al., 2016).

A comprehensive analysis that includes all plant species can be extremely useful for objectively assessing the extent of climate change (Murray et al., 2017). Understanding these processes is critical to developing a strategy for sustainable management of resources (Lankin and Ivanova, 2015; Murray et al., 2017).

Research objective: study of the patterns of the impact of climate change, timber harvesting, and fires on boreal forests with a view to predicting their natural and anthropogenic dynamics.

3.3   RESEARCH METHODOLOGY

3.3.1   RESEARCH AREA

We conducted our study in Zauralsky (Trans-Ural) hilly piedmont province (Russia, the Middle Urals): between 57°00′–57°10′N and 60°10′–60°30′E.

This province includes foothills, which consist of alternating meridional low mountains and ridges with wide, intermountain elongated low lands, in which there are large lakes surrounded by moors (Kolesnikov et al., 1973). The mountains have altitudes of 200–500 m a.s.l. The mountains have soft contours, blunt and broad peaks, while the slopes are long and flat. The climate is moderately cold and humid. The main factors of soil formation in the Urals are mountainous terrain, continental climate, both for ancient and young forming soils, which, combined with a great diversity of vegetation, alters soil characteristics. Mountain soils are characterized by relatively small depth, light mechanical composition (dominated by light and medium loam), different degrees of skeleton (skeletal soil), going up with decreasing soil depth. In the soil distribution of Zauralsky (Trans-Ural) hilly piedmont province of the Middle Urals the dependence on the terrain is clearly visible. The tops and upper thirds of steeper slopes, where the thickness of alluvial soil deposits is least of all, are occupied by shallow, underdeveloped soil with a high degree of skeleton and relatively light texture. Brown nonpodzolized and podzolized soils are confined to the middle and lower thirds of the gentle slopes. Flat-topped low ridges, gentle slopes, and well-drained downward slopes are occupied with sod-pale-yellow-podzolic soil, which differs in thickness of the soil profile and the degree of podzolization. The soil of smoother slopes, intermountain depressions, and the lows are often characterized by greater depth and moderate skeleton (Ivanova et al., 2000; Ivanova and Zolotova, 2011, 2013).

3.3.2 RESEARCH OBJECTS

All major mountain habitats are included in our study. We climbed to the most-capped mountains. The steep and gentle slopes of the northern, southern, eastern and western exposure were investigated by us. Swamp forests and marshes were not left unattended by us. All forest types were investigated. It is diverse pine and spruce forests.

3.3.3 SAMPLING PROCEDURES

The number of trees on the plot was not less than 200 (Forest Communities Study Methods, 2002). All the trees on the sampling plot were counted; their diameter and height were also measured. The age by the annual rings was identified. Tapes 4 × 20 m were laid for the study of young generations of woody plants. For characteristic shrubs, the projective cover was defined. A total of 10–20 accounting sites with the size of 1 m² were used to study the productivity of the herbaceous layer. The herbs were cut with scissors near the soil itself and were separated by species, then we dried the samples in a drying cabinet at 105° C to constant weight (absolutely dry). Dried samples were weighed to an accuracy of 0.01 g. We used the calculation method to estimate the biomass of woody plants (Iziumsky, 1972; Usoltsev, 1997). The biomass of needles and leaves is calculated using regression equations, which are obtained taking into account the physiology (pipe model) (Usoltsev, 1997).

3.3.4   DATA ANALYSIS

Ordination charts are constructed using detrended correspondence analysis (DCA). For the numerical analysis of community data, R package vegan [version 2.15.1 (2012-06-22)] (Oksanen, 2006) was used.

3.4   RESULTS AND DISCUSSION

3.4.1   IMPACT OF CLIMATIC FACTORS ON FOREST VEGETATION OF URAL MOUNTAINS

3.4.1.1   IMPACT OF CLIMATIC FACTORS ON FOREST BIODIVERSITY

As a result of multiple studies, we described the vegetation of the study area. The data obtained characterize all the main forest types and reflect the diversity of plant communities. Geographic-genetic forest typology was used as the basis for the classification of the obtained descriptions of vegetation (Ivanova and Zolotova, 2014). The analysis showed that the greatest differences in the species structure of forests are associated with a change in the edificator. Two large groups (pine forest and spruce forest) are clearly seen in Figure 3.2.

Various dark coniferous forests are located in Figure 3.2. Forest type No.11 is waterlogged spruce forests with Siberian pine. This type of forest is spread around lakes, rivers, and swamps. Soil waterlogging can be considered a common occurrence throughout the growing season. The abundance of sphagnum moss is considered a diagnostic feature of this type of dark coniferous forest. The increased diversity of swamp species also distinguishes these forests.

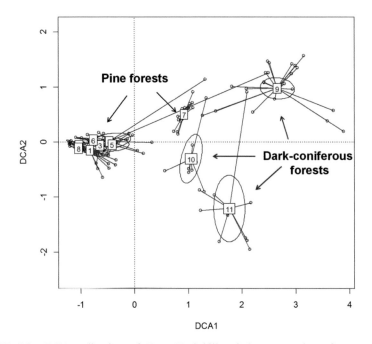

FIGURE 3.2 DCA ordination of Trans-Ural hilly piedmont province forests of Ural Mountains: 1–11, number of forest types.

Dark coniferous forests with a strongly developed grassy layer (forest type number 10) grow in close proximity to the marshes on powerful well-watered soils. Soil is waterlogged at the beginning of the growing season. Herbs form an intensely developed closed tier.

Spruce forests with *Oxalis acetosella* (forest type number 9) are found at the foot of the mountains, where the slopes are long and very gentle. Deep loamy soils are a characteristic feature of these spruce forests. Moisture conditions can be considered close to optimal; only after melting snow a brief overmoistening is noted.

Pine forests with multispecies herbaceous layer (forest type number 7) grow on the deep and rich soils. A total of 25–30 species of herbs is 1 m².

Marked 1–6 and 8 forest types formed one group (Fig. 3.2). These forest types are confined to the slopes of different exposure and steepness. The grassy tier under their canopy has a small number of species, the tier is rarely dense and its biomass is much less than in the forest types discussed above.

We conducted a special research to answer the question: what caused the formation of so many different forest communities. The analysis included the study of climatic and soil factors. E. Zolotova (Zolotova, 2013; Ivanova and Zolotova, 2015) has identified factor values on environmental scales (Fig. 3.3). We can judge the strength of a particular factor by its length. According to Figure 3.3, soil factors (nitrogen content) are associated with the axis 1 DCA. The second axis DCA is associated with the climate. Factors listed below are of great importance in the formation of forests. These factors can be interpreted as the main factor determining the type of vegetation.

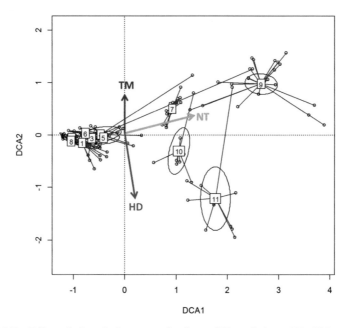

FIGURE 3.3   Effect of climatic factors on the forest differentiation of Ural Mountains: the numbers—number of forest types, HD—moistening, TM—temperature, NT—nitrogen.

3.4.1.2   CHANGE OF VEGETATION IN THE HOLOCENE

To understand the modern dynamics of vegetation, it is useful to consider changes in the Holocene. In former times, the climate of the Urals experienced repeated cyclical fluctuations, sometimes it was much cooler (which led to glaciation), sometimes it was much warmer than at present. These fluctuations were the reasons for serious changes in the species composition and appearance of plant communities (Panova, 2001; Panova et al., 2003; Antipina et al., 2014). The three periods that are the least similar to each other are described in detail for the Ural Mountains (Panova and Antipina, 2016).

3.4.2   IMPACT OF TIMBER HARVESTING AND FIRES ON FOREST VEGETATION OF URAL MOUNTAINS

3.4.2.1   PATTERNS OF REFORESTATION AFTER TIMBER HARVESTING AND FIRES

We studied the natural reforestation in open habitats. The intensity of reforestation has features depending on the disturbance and habitats. We have noticed that the renewal of pine proceeds better on forest burns (Fig. 3.4). However, the intensity of the renewal of *Pinus sylvestris* decreases rapidly with increasing soil thickness, both after harvest and after fires. Optimal environmental conditions for the emergence of new generations of pines are marked on soils with a thickness of 10–30 cm. About 100–300 thousand copies per hectare are counted in these conditions after fires. The abundance of new generations of pine on deep soils is small both after harvest and after fires.

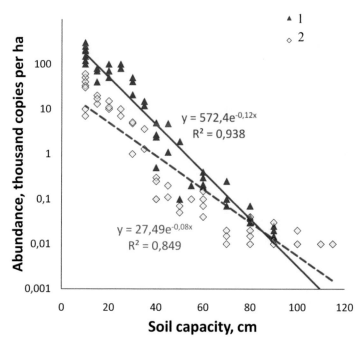

FIGURE 3.4   Effect of soil capacity on the abundance of young growth of *Pinus sylvestris* in the Ural Mountains: (1) abundance of young growth of *Pinus sylvestris* after fires, (2) abundance of young growth of *Pinus sylvestris* after harvesting.

It is also interesting to consider the relationship between different woody species after harvesting and wildfires. Birch is the main competitor for pine. Pine renews better than birch after wildfires. Young growth of *Pinus sylvestris* after fires prevails over the young growth of birch on shallow soil (Fig. 3.5). The critical soil capacity (when the number of pine and birch equal) is 65–70 cm. The predominance of young growth of *Pinus sylvestris* after the harvest is possible only in very shallow soils. The critical thickness of soils is 10–20 cm (Fig. 3.6). Therefore, the reforestation after harvesting and wildfires occur differently in different habitats (forest types). Pine forests are restored well both after fires and after felling only on mountain peaks and steep slopes with small gravelly soils. The middle parts of the slopes with gravelly soils of medium capacity are favorable for the restoration of coniferous forests after wildfires. However, harvesting contributes to the spread of secondary birch forests. A rapidly growing birch depresses juvenile pine trees under these habitats on clear cutting. The natural restoration of coniferous forests in the lower parts of slopes with deep soils is difficult. Artificial reforestation is necessary in these growing conditions.

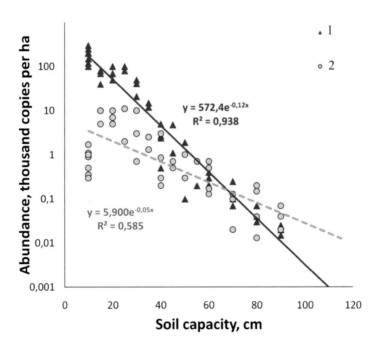

FIGURE 3.5   Effect of soil capacity on the abundance of young growth of pine and birch after wildfires in the Ural Mountains: (1) abundance of young growth of *Pinus sylvestris*, (2) abundance of young growth of *Betula pubescens* Ehrh. and *B. pendula* Roth.

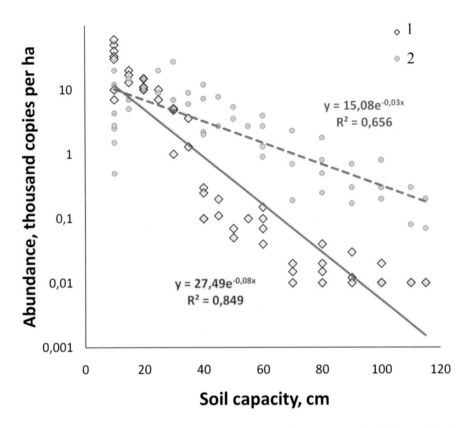

FIGURE 3.6 Effect of soil capacity on the abundance of young growth of pine and birch after harvesting in the Ural Mountains: (1) abundance of young growth of *Pinus sylvestris*, (2) abundance of young growth of *Betula pubescens* Ehrh. and *B. pendula* Roth.

3.4.2.2   COMPARISON OF PRODUCTIVITY AND DIVERSITY OF HERBACEOUS SPECIES IN FORESTS AND CLEAR CUTTING

The lower parts of the slopes with deep soils, which provide a stable regime of moisture supply, are characterized by a complex and diverse vegetation dynamics. Forests dominated by Siberian spruce are recognized as indigenous ecosystems in the area (Fig. 3.7). The fire centers practically do not meet in these conditions. However, harvesting leads to an extreme variety of derived ecosystems. Great changes affect all tiers of forest vegetation. The grassy layer reacts first to external disturbances. The exploration included the dark coniferous forest and two variants of birch forests (with thick spruce undergrowth and rare spruce undergrowth). Also studied was the meadow hayfields. The forest was cut down 67 years ago.

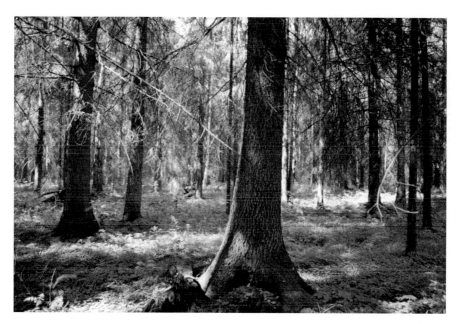

FIGURE 3.7   Ural dark coniferous forest, under the canopy of which is dominated by a continuous cover of *Oxalis acetosella*.

The main data on the structure of the studied communities are given in Table 3.1. The forest disturbances studied changed to a greater degree the productivity of plant species. Changes of each species are specific (Table 3.2).

The plant species that dominated the climax spruce were most severely affected after the disturbances. The opposite trend was revealed for some plant species that were found in the spruce forest in small quantities (Table 3.2).

In order to understand the mechanisms of change, we investigated the age structure of the Siberian spruce populations. Studies have shown that a generation over 67 years old prevailed. Thus, a new generation of Siberian spruce appeared in the dark coniferous forest and young trees were able to survive during the felling. The study of the vitality of the renewal of Siberian spruce showed that almost all young specimens have a good vertical growth. Thus, the younger generations of coniferous plants, which were preserved in the process of logging, determined the direction of reforestation.

TABLE 3.1   Studied Plant Communities Formed After Clear Cutting in One Type of Climax Forest.

Sign	Dark coniferous forest	Spruce-birch forest	Birch forest	Forest meadow
Characteristics of the tree layer				
Average, maximum age of trees, years	180, 220	65, 67	65, 67	–
Average height, m	26.3	24.2	20.4	–
Characteristics of the soil				
Litter thickness, cm	3.9	2.1	2.2	1.9
Average soil depth, cm	120–130	93–97	145–155	93–105
Yung generations of *Picea obovata*				
Number, thousand copies/ha	+	4.02	0.51	+
Predominant height, m	0.12–0.49	4.7–9.9	1.9–6.9	–
Yung generations of *Pinus sylvestris*				
Number, thousand copies/ha	–	–	–	+
Predominant height, m	–	–	–	0.09–0.33
Characteristics of herb				
Diversity	24	22	45	57
Average height, cm	6.9	6.9	48.5	60.1
Aboveground biomass (g/m² in absolutely dry state)/ Variation coefficient, %	17.7 33.23	4.4 66.21	100.9 7.03	280.6 7.72

To summarize, logging leads to the emergence of a multitude of plant communities within one climax forest. Recovery shifts come at varying speeds. The convergence of the structure of secondary and climax ecosystems occurs slowly. The results of this research are fundamental to understanding the evolution of modern ecosystems under anthropogenic impact and climate change.

3.5   CONCLUSION

Climate change, fires, and harvesting are recognized as urgent problems of modern science. Contrary to the fact that a lot of research is devoted to this problem, there are no complete solutions for today. Natural factors affecting boreal forest overlap with other environmental and social changes. It leads to increased effects and complication of environmental problems. We carried

TABLE 3.2 Biomass of the Most Dynamic Species of Herbaceous Layer in Indigenous Dark Coniferous Forests and Secondary Plant Communities in the Ural Mountains.

Species	Dark coniferous forest		Spruce-birch forest		Birch forest		Forest meadow	
	A	B	A	B	A	B	A	B
Oxalis acetosella L.	8.07	54	1.7	83.0	0.28	84.3	–	–
Calamagrostis arundinacea (L.) Roth	1.16	123.7	0.41	176.6	55.18	18.4	–	–
Gymnocarpium dryopteris (L.) Newm.	1.65	226.0	0.04	264.6	–	–	–	–
Fragaria vesca L.	0.42	142.2	0.38	212.9	0.51	95.2	–	–
Asarum europaeum L.	0.72	174.7	0.08	115.4	0.33	153.2	–	–
Rubus saxatilis L.	0.53	240.7	–	–	–	–	0.03	173.2
Athyrium filix-femina (L.) Roth	0.75	216.1	–	–	0.6	244.9	–	–
Linnaea borealis L.	0.16	206.4	–	–	0.55	120.5	0.22	153.7
Maianthemum bifolium (L.) F. W. Schmidt	0.45	94.3	0.24	218.3	0.48	83.9	0.1	173.2
Aegopodium podagraria L.	0.31	161.9	–	–	6.78	56.9	–	–
Viola selkirkii	0.62	144.8	–	–	0.02	118.3	–	–
Equisetum sylvaticum L.	0.33	148.3	–	–	–	–	–	–
Cerastium pauciflorum Stev. ex Ser.	0.59	118.8	0.4	124.2	1.17	60.8	–	–
Dryopteris expansa L.	0.17	294.0	0.12	246.9	–	–	–	–
Luzula pilosa (L.) Willd.	0.11	192.0	0.26	101.7	0.03	244.9	0.8	162.5
Pyrola rotundifolia L.	0.06	479.6	0.47	237.7	0.02	244.9	–	–
Stellaria holostea L.	0.23	188.2	0.11	244.6	2.1	68.1	–	–
Aconitum septentrionale Koelle	–	–	–	–	4.67	132.6	–	–
Cirsium heterophyllum (L.) Hill	–	–	–	–	0.88	125.3	39.43	78.29
Thalictrum minus L.	0.05	479.6	–	–	3.13	114.7	–	–

TABLE 3.2 *(Continued)*

Species	Dark coniferous forest		Spruce-birch forest		Birch forest		Forest meadow	
	A	B	A	B	A	B	A	B
Geranium sylvaticum L.	0.15	226.0	–	–	5.67	67.8	11.77	119.6
Pulmonaria mollis Wulf.	0.05	479.6	0.03	170.8	3.09	87.4	–	–
Carex nigra (L.) Reichard	0.23	200.1	0.01	264.6	9.47	74.6	0.03	86.6
Lathyrus vernus (L.) Bernh.	0.04	248.4	0.04	196.6	1.28	91.1	0.02	173.2
Vicia sepium L.	–	–	–	–	1.0	110.6	0.83	91.7
Senecio nemorensis L.	–	–	–	–	1.37	144.1	–	–
Deschampsia cespitosa (L.) Beauv.	0.04	479.6	–	–	–	–	23.97	12.8
Bistorta carnea (C. Koch) Kom.	–	–	–	–	–	–	30.97	73.4
Carex pallescens L.	–	–	–	–	–	–	21.97	41.8
Carex leporina L.	–	–	–	–	–	–	9.73	120.1
Agrostis tenuis SIBTH.	–	–	–	–	–	–	34.03	36.8
Alchemilla vulgaris L.	–	–	–	–	–	–	19.67	33.3
Filipendula ulmaria (L.) Maxim.	–	–	–	–	–	–	29.8	159.2
Trollius europaeus L.	0.01	479.6	–	–	–	–	8.70	71.7
Ranunculus auricomus L.	–	–	–	–	–	–	12.37	34.3
Myosotis L.	–	–	–	–	–	–	6.60	53.9

[A]average aboveground biomass (g/m² in absolutely dry state).

[B]Variation coefficient (%), "—"—species is not found.

out such an analysis for the plant communities of the Ural region. All major mountain habitats were investigated by us. The study found that the structure of vegetation is influenced primarily by climatic and edaphic influences. The influence of climate is manifested in the shift of areas of distribution of forest types in space. To some extent, the association of forest types with landscape elements changes. The plant communities that grow on the forest boundary turn out to be the most sensitive to the action of external factors. One of the manifestations of anthropogenic impact is the repeated increase in the influence of climatic factors. The forest dynamics becomes extremely difficult. Timber harvesting leads to the emergence of many plant communities within one the same growing conditions (climax forest). Over time, differences between these ecosystems persist. The differences relate to both the dominant species in the tree stand and the grassy layer, development trends and succession rates. Therefore, the management of such ecosystems should have its own specifics. The results of the research reflect the modern evolution of forest vegetation as an adaptation to clear cutting and other impacts in a continuously changing climate.

KEYWORDS

- **boreal forest**
- **biodiversity**
- **climate changes**
- **timber harvesting**
- **wildfires**

REFERENCES

Anderegg, W. R. L.; Prall, J. W.; Harold, J.; Schneider, S. H. *Expert Credibility in Climate Change*, Proceedings of the National Academy of Sciences of the United States of America, 2010, 107, 12107–12109.

Antipina, T. G.; Panova, N. K.; Korona, O. M. The Holocene Dynamics of Vegetation and Environmental Conditions on the Eastern Slope of the Northern Urals. *Russ. J. Ecol.* **2014,** *45,* 351–358.

Battisti, D. S.; Naylor, R. L. Historical Warnings of Future Food Insecurity with Unprecedented Seasonal Heat. *Science* **2009,** *323,* 240–244.

Boisvenue, C.; Running, S. W. Impacts of Climate Change on Natural Forest Productivity— Evidence Since the Middle of the 20th Century. *Global Change Biol.* **2006,** *12*, 862–882.

Casajus, N.; Périé, C.; Logan, T.; Lambert, M-C; de Blois, S.; Berteaux, D. An Objective Approach to Select Climate Scenarios when Projecting Species Distribution under Climate Change. *PLoS ONE.* **2016,** *11*(3), e0152495.

Chai, S-L.; Zhang, J.; Nixon, A.; Nielsen, S. Using Risk Assessment and Habitat Suitability Models to Prioritise Invasive Species for Management in a Changing Climate. *PLoS ONE.* **2016,** *11*(10), e0165292.

Climate Change. IPCC Synthesis Report. Summary for policymakers 2014. https://www.ipcc.ch/pdf/assessment-report/ar5/syr/AR5_SYR_FINAL_SPM.pdf (accessed Sep 18, 2017).

Flannigan, M. D.; Logan, K. A., Amiro, B. D.; Skinner, W. R.; Stocks, B. J. Future Area Burned in Canada. *Climatic Change* **2005,** *72*, 1–16.

Foley, J. A.; DeFries, R.; Asner, G. P.; Barford, C.; Bonan, C.; Carpenter, S. C.; Coe, M. T.; Daily, G. C.; Gibbs, H. K.; Helkowski, J. H.; Holloway, T.; Howard, E. A.; Kucharik, C. J.; Monfreda, C.; Patz, J. A.; Prentice, C.; Ramankutty, N.; Snyder, P. C. Global Consequences of Land Use. *Science.* **2005,** *309*, 570–574.

Forest Communities Study Methods, St. Petersburg: Chemistry R&D Institute of St. Petersburg State University, 240, 2002.

Gauthier, S.; Bernier, P.; Kuuluvainen, T.; Shvidenko, A. Z.; Schepaschenko, D. G. Boreal Forest Health and Global Change. *Science.* **2015,** *349*, (6250), 819–822.

Global Forest Resources Assessment, 2005: Progress Towards Sustainable Forest Management. 2006. FAO Forestry 147.

Grieneisen, M. L.; Zhang, M. The Current Status of Climate Change Research. *Nat. Clim. Change.* **2011,** *1,* 72–73. http://www.nature.com/nclimate/journal/v1/n2/abs/nclimate1093.html#supplementary-information (accessed Sep 22, 2017).

Gunn, E. A. Models for Strategic Forest Management. In *Handbook of Operations Research in Natural Resources*; Weintraub, A., Romero, C., Bjørndal, T., Epstein, R., Eds.; Springer: New York, 2007; pp 317–341.

Hagedorn, F.; Shiyatov, S. G.; Mazepa, V. S.; Devi, N. M.; Grigor'ev, A. A.; Bartysh, A. A.; Fomin, V. V.; Kapralov, D. S.; Terent'ev M.; Bugman, H.; Rigling, A.; Moiseev, P. A. Treeline Advances Along the Urals Mountain Range—Driven by Improved Winter Conditions? *Global Change Biol.* **2014,** *20*, 3530–3543.

Haunschild, R.; Bornmann, L.; Marx, W. Climate Change Research in View of Bibliometrics. *PLoS ONE.* **2016,** *11*.

Hildebrandt, P.; Knoke, T. Investment Decisions Under Uncertainty—A Methodological Review on Forest Science Studies. *For. Policy Econ.* **2011,** *13*, 1–15.

Ivanova, N. S.; Novogorodova, G. G.; Chetkina, E. S. Tendencies of Anthropogenic Dynamics of Vegetation and Soil in Montaineous Dark-Coniferous Forests of the Ural region. Biodiversity and Dynamics of Ecosystems in North Euraia. *Forest and Soil Ecosystems of North Eurasia*, Vol. 4; Russian Academy of Scieces Siberian Branch: Novosibirsk, 2000; pp 58–60.

Ivanova, N. S.; Zolotova, E. S. Vegetation and Soil Differentiation Within the Limits of Ecotope on the Middle Ural region. *Eur. J. Nat. Hist.* **2011,** *1*, 44–46.

Ivanova, N. S.; Zolotova, E. S. Biodiversity of the Natural Forests in the Zauralsky Hilly Piedmont Province. Modern Problems of Education and Science (Sovremenniye problemy nauki i obrazovanija). 2013.

Ivanova, N. S.; Zolotova E. S. Development of Forest Typology in Russia. *Int. J. Bio-resour. Stress Manag.* **2014,** *5*, 298–303.

Ivanova, N. S.; Zolotova, E. S. Ecological Space of Forest Type in the Montains of Middle Urals. Modern Problems of Education and Science (Sovremenniye problemy nauki i obrazovanija). 2015.

Iziumsky, P. P. *Valuation of the Thin Wood,* Forest Industry; Moscow, 1972; p 88.

Jiang, H.; Apps, M. J.; Zhang, Y.; Peng, C.; Woodard, P. M. Modelling the Spatial Pattern of Net Primary Productivity in Chinese Forests. *Ecol. Model.* **1999,** *122,* 275–288.

Kalyakin V. N.; Turubanova S. A; Smirnova O. V. The Origin and Development of the East European Taiga in Late Cenozoic. *Russ. J. Ecosyst. Ecol.* **2016,** *1,* 1-26. (DOI: 10.21685/2500-0578-2016-1-2).

Kapralov, D. S.; Shiyatov, S. G.; Moiseev, P. A.; Fomin, V. V. Changes in the Composition, Structure, and Altitudinal Distribution of Low Forests at the Upper Limit of their Growth in the North Ural Mountains. *Russ. J. Ecol.* **2006,** *37* (6), 367–372.

Kellomäki, S. *Managing Boreal Forests in the Context of Climate Change: Impacts, Adaptation and Climate Change Mitigation*; CRC Press, 2016; p 365.

Kolesnikov, B. P.; Zubareva, R. S.; Smolonogov, E. P. *Forest Vegetation Conditions and Forest Types of the Sverdlovsk Region*; UNTS of Academy of science of the USSR: Sverdlovsk, 1973; p 176.

Komar, I. V.; Chikushev, A. G. 1968. *Introduction Urals.* Nauka: Moscow, 1973; pp 7–16.

Komarov, A.; Chertov, O.; Zudin, S.; Nadporozhskaya, M.; Mikhailov, A.; Bykhovets, S.; Zudina, E.; Zoubkova, E. EFIMOD 2—a Model of Growth and Cycling of Elements in Boreal Forest Ecosystems. *Ecol. Model.* **2003,** *170,* 373–392.

Korotkov, V. N. Basic Concepts and Metods of Restoration of Natural Forests in Eastern Europe. *Russ. J. Ecosyst. Ecol.* **2017,** *2,* 1–18.

Krawchuk, M.; Cumming, S.; Flannigan, M. Predicted Changes in Fire Weather Suggest Increases in Lightning Fire Initiation and Future Area Burned in the Mixedwood Boreal Forest. *Clim. Change.* **2009,** *92,* 83–97.

Kuuluvainen, T. *Ecosystem Management of the Boreal Forest*. Oxford Research Encyclopedias. 2016.

Lankin, Y. P.; Mokogon, D. A.; Tereshin, S. V. Adaptive Modeling of Planetary Processes on the Basis of Satellite Data. Modern Problems of Science and Education. 2012, *6.* https://science-education.ru/en/article/view?id=7136 (accessed Sep 19, 2017).

Lankin, Y. P.; Ivanova, N. S. Methodological Problems in the Modeling of Ecosystems and Ways of Solutions. *Int. J. Bio-resour. Stress Manag.* **2015,** *6,* 631–638.

Lawler, J. J.; Ruesch, A. S.; Olden, J. D.; McRae, B. H. Projected Climate-Driven Faunal Movement Routes. *Ecol. Lett.* **2013,** *16,* 1014–1022.

Li, X.; He, H. S.; Wu, Z.; Liang, Y.; Schneiderman, J. E. Comparing Effects of Climate Warming, Fire, and Timber Harvesting on a Boreal Forest Landscape in Northeastern China. *PLoS ONE.* **2013,** *8,* e59747. (DOI:10.1371/journal.pone.0059747).

Maiti, R.; Rodriguez, H. G.; Kumari, Ch. A. *Applied Biology of Woody Plants USA*; American Academic Press, Salt Lake City, USA. 2016; p 367.

Maiti, R.; Rodriguez, H. G.; Ivanova, N. S. *Autoecology and Ecophysiology of Woody Shrubs and Trees: Concepts and Applications*; John Wiley & Sons: New Jersey, USA, 2016; p 352.

Martynenko, V. B.; Shirokikh, P. S.; Mirkin, B. M.; Naumova, L. G. Syntaxonomic Analysis of Restorative Successions After Cutting Down Light Coniferous Forests of South Ural Region. *Biol. Bulletin Rev.* **2014,** *75,* 478–490.

Mazepa, V. S. Stand Density in the Last Millennium at the Upper Tree-Line Ecotone in the Polar Ural Mountains. *Can. J. For. Res.* **2005,** *35,* 2082–2091.

Mirkin, B. M.; Martynenko, V. B.; Yamalov, S. M.; Naumova, L. G. The Theory and Practice in Making Decisions on Classic and Non-Classic Syntaxonomical Analysis. *Veg. Russ. (Rastitel'nost' Rossii).* **2009,** *14,* 142–151.

Mirkin, B.; Ermakov, N. The History of the Braun-Blanquet Approach Application and the Modern State of Syntaxonomy in Russia. *Braun-Blanquetia.* **2010,** *46,* 47–54.

Mirkin, B. M.; Martynenko, V. B.; Naumova, L. G. Assessment of Vegetation β-Diversity on the Basis of Syntaxonomy. *Russ. J. Ecol.* **2014,** *45,* 103–106.

Mirkin, B. M.; Martynenko, V. B.; Shirokikh, P. S.; Naumova, L. G. Contribution of the Braun-Blanquet Syntaxonomy to Research on Successions of Plant Communities. *Russ. J. Ecol.* **2015,** *46,* 303–308.

Murray, D. L.; Peer, M. J. L.; Majchrzak, Y. N.; Wehtje, M.; Ferreira, C.; Pickles, R. S. A. Continental Divide: Predicting Climate-Mediated Fragmentation and Biodiversity Loss in the Boreal Forest. *PLoS ONE.* **2017,** 12.

Ochuodho, T. O.; Lantz, V. A.; Olale, E. Economic Impacts of Climate Change Considering Individual, Additive, and Simultaneous changes in Forest and Agriculture Sectors in Canada: A Dynamic, Multi-regional CGE Model Analysis. *For. Policy Econ.* **2016,** *63,* 43–51.

Oksanen, J. *Multivariate Analysis of Ecological Communities in R: Vegan Tutorial,* 2006. (https://www.researchgate.net/profile/Andrew_Monks/publication/260638399_Denitrification_in_a_Laurentian_Great_Lakes_coastal_wetland_invaded_by_hybrid_cattail_Typha_glauca/links/5641012708aebaaea1f6d1b7.pdf) (accessed Nov 19, 2019).

D'Orangeville, L.; Duchesne, L.; Houle, D.; Kneeshaw, D.; Côté, B.; Pederson, N. Northeastern North America as a Potential Refugium for Boreal Forests in a Warming Climate. *Science.* **2016,** *352,* 1452–1455.

Panova, N. K. The History of Lakes and Vegetation in the Central Part of the Middle Trans-Urals During Late Glacial and Post Glacial Time. *Yekaterinburg: Rescue Archaeol. Res. Middle Urals.* **2001,** *4,* 48–59.

Panova, N. K.; Jankovska, V.; Korona, O. M.; Zinov'ev, E. V. The Holocene Dynamics of Vegetation and Ecological Conditions in the Polar Urals. *Russ. J. Ecol.* **2003,** *34,* 219–230.

Panova, N. K.; Antipina, T. G. Late Glacial and Holocene Environmental History on the Eastern Slope of the Middle Ural Mountains, Russia. *Quat. Int.* **2016,** 420, 76–89. (DOI:https://doi.org/10.1016/j.quaint.2015.10.035).

Pavlov, D. S.; Striganova, B. R.; Bukvareva, E. N. An Environment-Oriented Concept of Nature Use. *Her. Russ. Acad. Sci.* **2010,** *80,* 74–82.

Rodriguez-Baca, G.; Raulie, F.; Leduc, A. Rating a Wildfire Mitigation Strategy with an Insurance Premium: A Boreal Forest Case Study. *Forests.* **2016,** *7,* 107.

Running, S. W.; Peterson, D. L.; Spanner, M. A.; Teuber, K. B. Remote Sensing of Coniferous Forest Leaf Area. *Ecology.* **1986,** *67,* 273–276.

Shiyatov, S. G. *Reconstruction of Climate and the Upper Timberline Dynamics Since AD 745 by Tree-Ring Data in the Polar Ural Mountains,* International Conference on Past, Present and Future Climate; Henkinheimo, P., Ed.; Painatuskeskus, Publication of the Academy of Finland: Finland, 1995, 6, 144–147.

Schaphoffa, S.; Reyera, Ch. P. O.; Schepaschenkob, D.; Gertena, D.; Shvidenko, A. Tamm Review: Observed and Projected Climate Change Impacts on Russia's Forests and its Carbon Balance. *For. Ecol. Manag.* **2016,** *361,* 432–444.

Siry, J. P.; Cubbage, F. W.; Ahmed, M. R. Sustainable Forest Management: Global Trends and Opportunities. *For. Policy Econ.* **2005,** *7,* 551–561.

Thuiller, W. Patterns and Uncertainties of Species' Range Shifts under Climate Change. *Global Change Biol.* **2004,** *10,* 2020–2027.

Usoltsev, V. A. *Bioecological Aspects of Valuation of Trees Phytomass*; Ural Branch of the
Russian Academy of Sciences: Yekaterinburg, 1997; p 216.

Usoltsev, V. A. *Forest Biomass of Northern Eurasia: Database and Geography*; Ural Branch
of the Russian Academy of Sciences: Yekaterinburg, 2001; p 541.

Usoltsev, V. A. *Biological Productivity of Northern Eurasia's Forests: Methods, Datasets,
Applications*; Ural Branch of the Russian Academy of Sciences: Yekaterinburg, 2007; p 637.

Yousefpour, R.; Jacobsen, J. B.; Thorsen, B. J.; Meilby H.; Hanewinkel, M.; Oehler, K. A.
Review of Decision-Making Approaches to Handle Uncertainty and Risk in Adaptive
Forest Management under Climate Change. *Ann. For. Sci.* **2012,** *69*, 1–15.

Zobel, M. The Species Pool Concept as a Framework for Studying Patterns of Plant Diversity.
J. Veg. Sci. **2016,** *27*, 8–18.

Zolotova E. S. Forest Typological Features of Vegetation and Soils in Zauralsky Hilly Piedmont
Province. Dissertation of Candidate of Biology: 06.03.02, Yekaterinburg, 2013. 208.

CHAPTER 4

Climate Change and Horticulture: An Indian Perspective

DEBASHIS MANDAL* and R. C. LALDUHSANGI

Department of Horticulture, Aromatic and Medicinal Plants, Mizoram University, Aizawl 796004, Mizoram, India

Corresponding author. E-mail: debashismandal1982@gmail.com

ABSTRACT

Climate change and global warming are the greatest concerns of contemporary time. Due to its impact, commercial cultivation of horticultural crops like fruits, vegetables, flowers and ornamentals, spices and plantation crops, and medicinal plants will perform poorly. On one hand melting ice of Himalayas will impact the chilling requirement of temperate crops; on the other hand extremes of temperature will be vulnerable for crop cultivation in open field condition. Besides, pollination will also be hampered because of its effect on pollinators and thus will have significant impact of fruit set and yield. Flowering, crop growth and development, pest and disease infestation will also be influenced due to changing climate. Hence, a sustainable approach is needed to address and mitigate the problem. Conservation, use of renewable energy, reforestation, cultivation of location specific crops suitable in changed climate, resistant and tolerant crops to biotic and abiotic stresses; and hi-tech horticulture involving green houses, shade nets, fertigation, and so on will be crucial for having climate resilient horticulture. Breeding and biotechnological approach for evolving more suitable varieties for stress situations should definitely have to be a thrust area for research.

4.1   INTRODUCTION

Global horticulture has numerous challenges and opportunities in present day condition. Climate change indeed is a new challenge as faced by horticulturists worldwide. Climate change is undoubtedly one of the serious issues today. Its impact has become a major concern on the global level because it affects every forms of life. Most importantly, it has direct influence on agriculture and horticulture crops. It has become a serious issue which is discussed more frequently globally. The year 2015 was the hottest year yet recorded which crossed the average temperature across global land and ocean surface, 1.62°F (0.90°C) above the 20th century average, the same year when United Nations Climate Change Conference also known as COP 21 or CMP 11 was held in Paris. Every nation is facing this problem and hence highly commits them in combating this environmental issue.

India is bestowed with different soil and climatic conditions under several agroecological regions which provides great scope to grow a wide variety of horticultural crops, that is, fruits, vegetables, flowers, medicinal aromatics plants, spices, plantation crops, and so on. Horticultural crops form the most important component of human diet to meet the demands of vitamins, minerals, fibers, and so on of the body and also to prevent numerous diseases and value to life. Its importance and value in terms of nutrition, income and employment generation, contribution to GDP of the country, and wellness of physical and mental health are well recognized. The rich land of the country including the Northeast Himalayan region is endowed with diversity of nutritious and highly valued fruits, vegetables, medicinal and aromatic plants, spices and rare flowers. The Indian agroecosystem has contributed in the overall prosperity of the country and still offers a huge scope and potential for resource tapping and development.

Climate change may be defined as the weather changing in a certain manner during the course of the year which includes temperature, atmospheric humidity, rainfall and wind, and so on. Prediction is made to have an increase in average air temperature between 1.4°C to 5.8°C and also to have increase in atmospheric CO_2 concentration and difference in rainfall pattern (Houghton et al., 2001). It was further reported that climate change is impacting four major contributors to economy, that is, agriculture, water, ecosystems and biodiversity, and health in major climate sensitive regions like Himalayas, Western Ghats, Coastal areas, and Northeast region (Datta, 2013). Global climate change, water scarcity, soil and water pollution, and urbanization are the add-on problems. In one hand temperature is increasing with deceasing rainfall and thus causing scarcity in irrigation water and enhanced evapotranspiration which leads to severe crop water stress conditions (Datta, 2013).

The world average temperature of the Earth's surface has been increasing for the past 100 years. In simple words, climate change is the change in climate for an uncomparable and infinite time. It has its huge impact directly or indirectly on all forms of life. It can lead to an erratic or unpredictable rainfall pattern, drying up of local lakes and springs, migration of species to higher elevation, change in the period of sowing and harvesting plants, vulnerability and rapid extinctions of flora and fauna. Ozone depletion is one of the major causes of global warming. Major greenhouse gases like carbon dioxide, methane, nitrous oxide, and so on are increasing in the atmosphere through industrial processes, deforestation, burning of fossil fuels, and land degradation.

India, like any other country also felt the impact of climate change tremendously, mainly because of its developing urbanization and agriculture-based economy. Developing countries are more vulnerable to such climate change owing to factors like less technological advancement, lack of resources to mitigate the adversities on agriculture, and so on. Moreover, a greater dependence on agriculture for livelihood of larger proportion of population can further aggravate the situation (Nath and Behera, 2011). India which ranked second in the production of wheat, rice, and sorghum in 2014 was adversely affected due to climate change and also witnessed loss of production in mustard, tomatoes, onions, vegetables, and food crops. As per the recent IPCC report, projection was made to have 10–40% loss in crop production due global warming in India by 2080–2100 (Chadha, 2015).

4.2 EFFECT OF CLIMATE CHANGE ON FRUITS

The extreme weather events of hot and cold wave conditions have been reported to cause considerable damage to many fruits. Temperature has a big influence on fruit growth, a large number of fruits crops production timing will change due to rise in temperature like mango, citrus, banana, and guava crops will develop more rapidly and mature earlier due to rise in temperature (Malhotra, 2017). Strawberries will produce more runners at the expense of fruits (Datta, 2013). Leaf scorching and twig dying are common symptoms of heat stroke in bearing and nonbearing mango plants (Rajan et al., 2011). Elevated temperature with moisture deficit cause cracking and sun burning in apple (Rai et al., 2015) and increase in high temperature during the maturity stage will cause cracking in litchi (Kumar and Kumar, 2007). Dry spell during flower emergence and fruit sheds can reduce the crop duration of banana (Chadha, 2015). Pest and diseases prevalence, for example, fruit fly infestation in guava increased due to hot and humid weather conditions (Malhotra, 2017). The crop likes peach, plum, which require low chilling temperature are also showing sign of decline in productivity (Hazarika, 2015). Erratic rainfall coupled with increasing temperature, less chilling hours is affecting the hill agriculture and food security (Datta, 2013). Apple faced poor fruit set, decrease in productivity when temperature drastically reduced along with rains during end of April. Besides, occurrence of high temperature caused 15 days early flowering in apple. Frost in winter and severe dry heat in summer resulted in poor fruit growth and cracking in litchi. High temperature and high velocity wind during fruit development caused heavy fruit drop in guava. In citrus increase in 1–2°C temperature beyond 25–30°C promotes vegetative flushes instead of flowers, while untimed winter rain affects flower initiation and increase Psylla incidence in citrus (Malhotra, 2017). Low temperature (4–11°C), high humidity (80%), and cloudy weather during the month of January caused delayed panicle emergence in mango. Strong wind and cyclone during mango fruit season reduced yield by shedding of fruits and also affects the fruit size and quality (Chadha, 2015).

4.3   EFFECT OF CLIMATE CHANGE ON VEGETABLE

India is the second largest producer of vegetable in the world. Environmental stress is the major cause of crop losses worldwide reducing average yield for most of the major crops by more than 50% (Bray et al., 2000). Vegetables being succulent are generally sensitive to environmental extremes and high temperature, limited and excess moisture stresses are the major causes of loss in yields and causes reduction of marketable grade of tomato, potato, and so on (Malhotra, 2017). Most of the vegetable crops are highly sensitive to flooding and genetic variation with respect to its characters. Many vegetable crops namely tomato, watermelon, potato, soybeans, peas, carrot, turnip, and so on are more likely to be damaged by air pollution. Vegetable yields can be reduced by 5–15% when ozone concentration reaches to greater than 50 ppb (Narayan, 2009). Flooding caused accumulation of endogenous ethylene and under high temperature caused rapid wilting which damaged tomato plants (Drew, 1979; Kuo et al., 1982). High temperature caused failure of fruit set mediated by bud drop, abnormal flower development, poor pollen production, ovule abortion, poor viability in tomato and pepper (Hazra et al., 2007; Hazarika, 2015; Erickson and Markhart, 2002). Again, water stress in tomatoes when accompanied by high temperature (above 28°C) caused significant (30–45%) flower drop (Rao, 1995). High temperature (above 40°C) impacted yield to onion by poor bulb size (Lawande, 2010; Daymond et al., 1997) and result shortening of crop duration (Wheeler et al., 1996).

Temperature variation had marked influence on growth and development of vegetable crops. Temperature below 17°C resulted with no seed germination in okra while night temperature below 13°C hampered fruit set in tomatoes. High temperature caused premature bolting in cabbage and sturdy roots in carrot and bitterness in lettuce. Very high temperature impacted low tuber formation in potato and lycopene degradation in tomatoes. However, low temperature also marked effect on sex expression of cucumber by providing more female flower, instead in high temperature it was more male flower production (Hazarika, 2015).

4.4 EFFECT OF CLIMATE CHANGE ON SPICES AND PLANTATION CROPS

Due to decrease in annual rainfall and fluctuation in day temperature, there is decreasing trend in most of the spices crop such as in cardamom, seed spices, and black pepper growing areas (Datta, 2013; Muthusami et al., 2012). Indian pepper production has been declining rapidly in the past 10 years due to effect of climate change (Malhotra, 2017). Vagaries in rain caused tremendous problem in saffron production in Kashmir. Its production got 40% reduction due to erratic rain as it is mainly a rain fed crop. Chilling and frost was found quite detrimental for successful seed spices production. Fennel, fenugreek, cumin, ajowan, nigella, and so on were getting huge crop loss as to more prone to frost injury. In Cashew nut, high temperature above 34°C with low relative humidity (below 20%) caused drying of flowers and resulted in yield reduction (Datta, 2013; Malhotra, 2017). Cashew is mainly grown in rain-fed condition, therefore change in climate and drought or shifts in rainfall pattern caused crop loss (Yadukumar et al., 2010). It was reported that drought and cyclonic weather affect the nut yield of coconut (Laxman et al., 2010).

4.5 EFFECT OF CLIMATE CHANGE ON FLOWERS, MEDICINAL AND AROMATIC PLANTS

Changing climate has marked an impact on commercial flower crops in particular which use to grow in open field condition. Extremes of temperature caused poor flowering, improper floral development, and color. When temperature falls below 15°C, tropical orchids failed to flower, while in Jasmine caused reduction in flower size (Datta, 2013). Climate change which is impacting the ice cover of Himalayas is influencing the chilling requirement for many temperate flower crops like Rhododendrons, Orchids, Tulips, Magnolias, Alstromerea, and so on (Hazarika, 2015).

Medicinal and aromatic plants are not exception to the situation of having climate change effect. Secondary metabolites and related other compounds which are key components behind its medicinal properties can have serious influence because of temperature stress. Disrupted seasonal events, extreme weather, drought, warming of temperatures, and other human activities and natural hazards have serious impact on medicinal and aromatic plants. The World Health Organization recommends the use of rotation to minimize problems with pests and plant diseases. Care is required to obtain satisfactory yields.

4.6   INFLUENCE OF CLIMATE CHANGE ON POLLINATION, PHENOLOGY, AND MATURITY OF PLANTS

Climate change is an emerging global phenomenon which has the potential to affect every forms of life mainly agricultural ecosystem. Rise in temperature leads to increase in soil salinity which in turn results in toxicity of plants like stunted plant growth, small leaves, and distortion of fruits. Low temperature and rainy spring may pose a threat in pollination. On the other hand cold temperature reduces the speed of pollen tube growth and shortens the life of pollination period. Flowers are fast losing their capacity to produce fragrance due to global warming and this is affecting the process of pollination. Climate change, will impact bees at various levels including their pollinating efficiency (Reddy et al., 2012).

According to Ameglio et al. (2000), lack of chilling as in the mild winter conditions result in abnormal pattern of budbreak and development in temperate fruit trees. When chilling requirements are not completely fulfilled, trees display irregular and temporally spread out flowering, leading to anomalous growth and in homogeneous crop development (Petri and Leite, 2004). It is predicted that reduction in the winter regime (chilling duration) may affect pollination in some plants owing to early and frequent flower and fruit drop, anthocyanin production may be affected in apples and capsicum, tuber initiation process in vegetables like potato may be delayed, tip burn and blossom end rot may result in decreased tomato production, and so on. Sunburn and cracking and cracking in apple, apricot, cherries, and litchi have been reported owing to high temperature and moisture stress. Such morphological, physiological, and phonological changes like malformations in plant structures, sterility, yield reduction, delay or advancement in maturity affecting the reproductive phase of the plant, increase in vegetative growth, and so on have been reported due to the variable climatic conditions experienced by the crop plants (Naorem and Thongatabam, 2015).

There can be no fertilization if the temperature is either very low or high. If there is no fertilization, the fruit set can be damaged. It was evident from the reports of the previous studies that population abundance, pollination activities, and geographic range of important pollinators like bees, butterflies, moths, and so on are declining with climate change (FAO, 2008). Ozone injures plants by damaging the stomata in the leaf surface and can result in suppressed photosynthesis, decreased growth, lower yields, lowering of nutritive values in plants. Past phenological studies explained that temperature has marked influence on flower induction. For instance, in temperate fruits low temperature has great influence on blossoming (Rai et al., 2015). High humidity, cloudy weather, and low temperature can delay panicle emergence and can reduce the quality of some crops and plants. However, excessively high temperature results in delay of fruit maturation, reduces the quality and nutritional values of fruits and decreasing color. The effect of temperature can be different on different crops simultaneously.

4.7 INFLUENCE OF CLIMATE CHANGE ON POSTHARVEST MANAGEMENT OF CROPS

The production and quality of fresh horticulture and vegetable crops can be directly and indirectly affected by the hot and cold wave of temperature, rise in global temperature can affect crop photosynthesis, causing alterations in sugar content, peel color and firmness, organic acid and antioxidant activity. Increase in temperature can reduce yield in fruit crop by lowering photosynthesis, increasing respiration, and causing reproductive failure. Potato when grown under carbon dioxide accumulation in the atmosphere has direct affect on tuber malformation and change in reducing sugar content (Rai et al., 2015).

4.8 STRATEGIES AND MITIGATING OPTIONS

Climate change cause a lot of hindrances in all forms of life which lead to the need of changing in several cultural traditions and practices in food growing and resource management. Impact of climate change has to be analyzed and understood at regional levels for providing effective solutions through better innovation, technology evaluation, and refinement. It is appropriate to utilize modeling tools for impact analysis for various horticultural crops. Impact of climate change depends both on climate and system's ability to adapt to change. To sustain productivity, crop-based adaptation strategies need to be developed based on the vulnerability of the crop to a specific agro-eco region and growing season. Agro technologies for crop management and production in high temperature and other stress conditions are already being worked out which has to be utilized properly. Resistant root stocks and varieties for various food crops tolerant to stresses have been identified and being used to combat climate change. Several institutions have evolved hybrids and varieties, which are tolerant to heat and drought stress conditions, which have potential to combat impact of climate change (Malhotra, 2017).

There are good numbers of rootstocks developed by researchers to address the biotic and abiotic stresses which can be a weapon in handling the climate change impact in fruit production industry. Arka Sahan, *Ziziphus numularia*, Rangpur Lime, Dogridge, *Psidium molle X Psidium guajava*, *Punica granatum* (Var. Ruby), Khirni, Deanna and Excel, and so on are the drought tolerant rootstocks for Anona, ber, citrus, grape, guava, pomegranate, and sapota and fig, respectively (Singh et al., 2009; Singh 2010; Malhotra, 2017). Duke, and its progeny, Duke 7, Barr-Duke, D9 and Thomas are the Phytophthora root rot tolerant rootstocks for avocado; whereas, Rangpur lime for citrus. Dogridge, 110R, SO-4; Rangpur Lime and Cleopatra mandarin; Kurakkan, Nileshwar dwarf, Bappakai; *Ficus glomerata* are the salinity tolerant rootstocks for grape, lime, mango, and fig (Bose and Mitra, 1996). *Psidium friedrichsthalianum* (Chinese guava), *P. alata* are the wilt resistant rootstock for guava and passion fruit *and P. edulis f. Flavicarpa* are *Fusarium* collar rot, nematode tolerant rootstock for passion fruit can be used to handle the abiotic and biotic stress conditions. There are lemon varieties like Pramalini, Sai Sarbati, PKM-1 which are tolerant to bacterial canker and tristeza virus (Chadha, 2015).

In case of vegetable crops, scientists have developed suitable varieties/ lines for addressing the problem of biotic and abiotic stresses, which can pave the way to mitigate the counter effect of climate change in vegetable cultivation. Advance lines like RF-4A, MST-42, and 46, IIHR Sel.-132 for tomato, onion, and chilli and varieties like Arka Vikas, Arka Kalyan, and Arka Lohit are drought/rainfall tolerant varieties for tomato, onion, and chilli (Datta, 2013; Hazarika, 2015). Arka Jay, Arka Vijay, Arka Sambram, Arka Amogh, Arka Soumya and Arka Garima, Arka Suman, Arka Samrudhi are the photo insensitive varieties for Dolichos bean and cowpea. IIHR Sel.-3, IIHR-19-1, IIHR-1&8, IIHR 316-1 and 37-1 are the high temperature tolerant lines developed by IIHR Bangalore for capsicum, French bean, peas and cauliflower, respectively (Hazra and Som, 1999; Rai and Yadav, 2005). Similarly, IARI; New Delhi has developed varieties tolerant to cold stress in radish (Pusa Himani) and tomato (Pusa Sheetal) (Chadha, 2015).

Further, information on land situation specific crop suggestions is also available which can be helpful in tackling effect of climate change in crop cultivation. For waterlogged areas, crops like *Makhana* and lotus can be cultivated, whereas, aonla, guava, turmeric can be options in rain-fed areas with poor soil fertility. Japanese mint, vegetables, marigold can be crops for flood affected areas while bael, mahua, karonda, phalsa, citronella in saline patches and kair, khejri and karonda, and so on in ravenous areas (Chadha, 2015). Sandy waste land can suitably be used for cultivation of fruits like guava, tamarind, khejri; vegetables like chilli, cowpea, garlic and onion; medicinal plants like *Aloe vera*, aswagandha, and *Vitex regundo*. Aonal, bael, ber, and so on fruits; beet, carrot, chilli, okra, methi, spinach, drumstick, and so on vegetables and *Calotropis,* fennel, *Lawsonia inermis* (Henna) can be cultivated in wastelands with high salt concentrations. Khejri, *Phoenix* sp.; chilli, cluster bean, cowpea, and dolichos bean; *Ailanthus excelsa, Boswellia serrata, Bursera panicillata, Cassia fistula*, Kusum, Sheesham, and so on are potential crops for gullied and riverine lands. For undulating land situations fruits like ber, guava, olive, and peach; vegetables like cluster bean, cucumber, French bean, water melon, musk melon, and pointed gourd; medicinal plants like Henna and Chirayta can be cultivated; whereas lotus, jamun, tamarind, water chestnut, khas khas in waterlogged areas and karonda, jamun, ber, neem, *Simarouba glauca* in strip lands can be cultivated (Chadha, 2015).

In Hills, farm mechanization is extremely difficult due to the sloppy land and shallow depth of soil is another major contributing factor toward soil erosion. Development of new varieties which has higher yield potential and tolerance to drought, heat, and salinity is highly needed. Selection of appropriate horticulture crops based on land, soil, and climatic suitability for maximizing overall increase in production of horticultural crops is very crucial. Integrated nutrient management strategies for difficult horticultural crops and amelioration of multinutrient deficiency should be standardized and practiced. Rainwater harvesting is a need for farmers especially in hilly areas. Therefore, water harvesting in different forms like watershed approach, Jalkund (micro rain water harvesting structure for hills), roof water harvesting for life saving irrigation, and so on should be adopted to meet the future water requirement and combat drought. To mitigate the effects of higher temperature, there are number of tools that can be adopted. Mulching is one of the best and common method, plastic film to white polythene color can be used for summer production and black mulch or radiation blocks can reduce heat effect by reflecting away solar radiation. Shading is another strategy commonly shade cloth or netting is used. Shading is applied during the hottest period when the plant is most sensitive to heat.

Processing can reduce the incidence of food borne disease and is less susceptible to early spoilage than fresh fruit and it helps to alleviate shortages and improve the overall nutrition of produce fruit crops. This increases delicate perishable and good quality fruits across long distances and makes food safe to eat by deactivating spoilage and pathogenic microorganism.

Ecosystem services like carbon sequestration and storage, hydrological services, and biodiversity are to be enhanced for climate change adaptation and mitigation. Soil management practices like manuring, less tillage, farm residue incorporation, improvement of soil biodiversity, mulching can play important roles in carbon sequestration in soil (Wassmann and Pathak, 2007).

Collection, characterization, conservation, and evaluation of lesser-known underutilized crops are of utmost importance. Further development of package of practices for cultivation of these diverse indigenous crops is much needed. For sustainable horticulture in changing climate, judicious use of natural resources, more use of green house and hi-tech horticulture along with usage of heat tolerant, pest-disease resistant, and short duration crop species and varieties are of immense importance.

4.9 CONCLUSION

In review and emphasis on changing climate and its impact on all forms of life shows us the need for saving horticulture. We can conclude that development of new crops which are tolerant to high temperature, resistance to pest and diseases, and high yielding varieties will probably prevent losses due to increase in temperature. Water conservation, reforestation, reduction in the emission of green house gases, green house technology, and adoption of more developed technology and management of land resources are the main strategies to combat the negative impact of changing climate. Human beings, as a whole have a very significant role to play and more awareness regarding this issue is the need of time.

KEYWORDS

- **climate change**
- **horticulture**
- **resilient**
- **biotic**
- **abiotic**
- **stress**

REFERENCES

Ameglio, T.; Alves, G.; Bonhomme, M.; Cochard, H; Ewres, F. Winter Functioning of Walnut: Involvement in Branching Processes. In *L'Arbre, Biologieet Development*; Isabelle Qentin: Montreal, Canada, 2000; pp 230–238.

Bose, T. K.; Mitra, S. K. *Fruits: Tropical and Subtropical*; Nayaprakash: Kolkata, India, 1996.

Bray, E. A.; Bailey-Serres, J.; Weretilnyk, E. Responses to Abiotic Stresses. In *Biochemistry and Molecular Biology of Plants;* Gruissem, W., Buchannan, B., Jones, R., Eds.; ASPP: Rockville, MD, 2000; pp 1158–1249.

Chadha, K. L. Global Climate Change and Indian Horticulture. In *Climate Dynamics in Horticultural Science*, Vol. 2: Impact, Adaptation, and Mitigation; Choudhary, M. L., Patel, V. B., Mohammed Wasim Siddiqui, Verma, R. B., Eds.; CRC Press: USA, 2015; pp 1–26.

Datta, S. Impact of Climate Change in Indian Horticulture—A Review. *Int. J. Sci. Environ. Technol.* **2013,** *2*, 661–671.

Daymond, A. J.; Wheeler, T. R.; Hadley, P.; Ellis, R. H.; Morison, J. L. Effects of Temperature, CO2 and their Interaction on the Growth, Development and Yield of Two Varieties of Onion (Allium cepa L.). *J. Exp. Bot.* **1997,** *30*, 108–118.

Drew, M. C. Plant Responses to Anaerobic Conditions in Soil and Solution Culture. *Curr. Adv. Plant Sci.* **1979,** *36*, 1–14.

Erickson, A. N.; Markhart, A. H. Flower Development Stage and Organ Sensitivity of Bell Pepper (Capsicum annuum L.) to Elevated Temperature. *Plant Cell Environ.* **2002,** *25*, 123–130.

Hazarika, T. K. Climate Change and Indian Horticulture: Opportunities for Adaptation and Mitigation Strategies. In *Climate Change and Socio-Ecological Transformation*; Sati, V. P., Eds.; Today and Tomorrow's Printers and Publishers: New Delhi, India, 2015; pp 313–325.

Hazra, P.; Som, M. G. *Technology for Vegetbale Prodcution and Improvement*; Naya Prokash: Kolkata, India, 1999.

Hazra, P.; Samsul, H. A.; Sikder, D.; Peter, K. V. Breeding Tomato (*Lycopersicon esculentum* Mill) Resistant to High Temperature Stress. *Int. J. Plant Breed.* **2007,** *1*, 31–40.

Houghton, J.; Ding, Y.; Griggs, D.; Noguer, M; Van der Linden, P. *Climate Change 2001: The Scientific Basis. Intergovernmental Panel on Climate Change*; Cambridge University Press: Cambridge, UK, 2001, p 881.

Kumar, R.; Kumar, K. K. Managing Physiological Disorders in Litchi. *Indian Hortic.* **2007,** *52,* 22–24.

Kuo, D. G.; Tsay, J. S.; Chen, B. W.; Lin, P. Y. Screening for Flooding Tolerance in Genus Lycopersicon. *Hort. Sci.* **1982,** *17,* 6–78.

Lawande, K. E. Impact of Climate Change on Onion and Garlic Production. In *Challenges of Climate Change in Indian Horticulture*; Singh H. P., Singh, J. P., Lal, S. S., Eds.; Westville Publication House: New Delhi, 2010; pp 100–103.

Laxman, R. H.; Shivasham Bora, K. S.; Srinivasa Rao, N. K. An Assessment of Potential Impacts of Climate Change on Fruit Crops. In *Challenges of Climate Change in Indian Horticulture*; Singh, H. P., Singh, J. P., Lal, S. S., Eds.; Westville Publishing House: New Delhi, 2010; pp 23–30.

Malhotra, S. K. Horticultural Crops and Climate Change: A Review. *Indian J. Agric. Sci.* **2017,** *87,* 12–22.

Murugan, M.; Shetty, P. K.; Ravi, R.; Anandhi, A.; Rajkumar, A. J. Climate Change and Crop Yields in the Indian Cardamom Hills, 1978–2007 CE. *Clim. Ch.* **2012,** *110,* 737–753.

Naorem, A. S.; Thongatabam, B. In *Climate Change: A Threat to Agriculture in India*, Proceedings of the National Conference on Climate Change: Impacts, Adaptation, Mitigation Scenario & Future Challenges in Indian Perspective, New Delhi, 2015; pp 99–103.

Narayan R. In *Air Pollution—A Threat in Vegetable Production*, Proceedings of International Conference on Horticulture (ICH-2009) Horticulture for Livelihood Security and Economic Growth; Eds. Sulladmath, U. V., Swamy, K. R. M., Eds; 2009; pp 158–159

Nath, P. K.; Behara, B. A Critical Review of Impact and Adaptation to Climate Change in Developed and Developing Countries. *Environ. Dev. Sustain.* **2011,** 141–162.

Petri, J. L.; Leite, G. B. Consequences of Insufficient Winter Chilling on Apple Tree Bud-Break. *Acta Hortic.* **2004,** *662,* 53–60.

Rai, N.; Yadav, D. S. *Advances in Vegetable Production*; Researchco Book Centre: New Delhi, India, 2005.

Rai, R.; Joshi, S.; Roy, S.; Singh, O.; Samir, M.; Chandra, A. Implication of Changing Climate on Productivity of Temperate Fruit Crops with Special Reference to Apple. *J. Hortic.* **2015,** *2,* 1–6.

Rajan, S.; Tiwari, D.; Singh, V. K.; Saxena, P.; Singh, S.; Reddy, Y. T. N.; Upreti, K. K.; Burondkar, M. M.; Bhagwan, A.; Kennedy, R. Application of Extended BBCH Scale for Phenological Studies in Mango (Mangifera indica L.). *J. Appl. Hortic.* **2011,** *13,* 108–114.

Reddy, R. P. V.; Verghese, A.; Rajan, V. V. Potential Impact of Climate Change on Honeybess (Apis spp.) and their Pollination Services. *Pest Manag. Hortic. Ecosyst.* **2012,** *18,* 121–127.

Singh, H. P.; Shukla, S.; Malhotra, S. K. Ensuring Quality Planting Material in Horticulture Crops. In *A Book of Lead Papers 9th Agricultural Science Congress, held from 22–24 June, 2009 at SKUA&T*; Kashmir, Srinagar, 2009; pp 469–484.

Singh, H. P. Impact of Climate Change on Horticultural Crops. In *Challenges of Climate Change in Indian Horticulture*; Singh, H. P., Singh, J. P., Lal, S. S., Eds.; Westville Publishing House: New Delhi, 2010; pp 1–8.

Srinivasa Rao, N. K. Management of Heat Moisture and Other Physical Stress Factors in Tomato and Chilli in India. In *Collaborative Vegetable Research in South Asia*, Proceedings of the SAVERNET Midterm Review Workshop, AVRDC, Taiwan, 1995.

Wassmann, R.; Pathak, H. Introducing Greenhouse Gas Mitigation as a Development Objective in Rice-Based Agriculture: II. Cost-Benefit Assessment for Different Technologies, Regions and Scales. *Agric. Syst.* **2007,** *94,* 826–840.

Wheeler, T. R.; Ellis, R. H.; Hadley, P.; Morison, J. I. L.; Batts, G. R.; Daymond, A. J. Assessing the Effects of Climate Change on Field Crop Production Aspects. *Appl. Biol.* **1996,** *45*, 49–54.

Yadaukumar, N.; Raniprasad, T. N.; Bhat, M. G. Effect of Climate Change on Yield and Insect Pests Incidence on Cashew. In *Challenges of Climate Change in Indian Horticulture*; Singh, H. P., Singh, J. P., Lal, S.S, Eds.; Westville Publishing House: New Delhi, 2010; pp 49–54.

PART II
Forest Resources Management

CHAPTER 5

Ecological Structure and Wood Volume of *Prosopis* Species (Mesquite) Communities in Northeast of Mexico

RAHIM FOROUGHBAKHCH[1*], MAGINOT NGANGYO HEYA[1],
ARTEMIO CARRILLO PARRA[2], MARCO ANTONIO GUZMÁN LUCIO[1],
and MARCO ANTONIO ALVARADO VAZQUEZ[1]

[1]*Facultad de Ciencias Biológicas, Departamento de Botánica, Universidad Autónoma de Nuevo León, Av. Universidad s/n Cd. Universitaria, San Nicolás de los Garza, C.P. 66451, Nuevo León, Mexico*

[2]*Instituto de Silvicultura e Industria de la Madera, Universidad Juárez del Estado de Durango, Boulevard del Guadiana #501, Ciudad Universitaria, Torre de Investigación, C.P. 34120, Durango, Dgo. Mexico*

Corresponding author. E-mail: rahimforo@hotmail.com

ABSTRACT

The Mexican Gulf coast is characterized by dry regions with high variations in climatic conditions, rich in drought-tolerant or subhumid species, and including multipurpose trees (MPTs) and shrubs, which have more than one substantial contribution such as products or service functions to the land-use systems in which they are grown.

This chapter aims to introduce the lecturer with ecological characterization and forest productivity of the mesquite scrub and woodland, their diverse uses as MPTs and shrubs of tropical and subtropical areas of semi-arid zones of northeastern Mexico.

In three physiographic zones, 30 sampling sites were randomly selected, based on cartographic material and digital ortophotos where mesquite was the dominant species.

All mesquite individuals were registered, measuring their height, crown projection, and wood volume. The canopy density, frequency, and importance value (IV) were determined, as well as basal diameter (BD), length of the main stem and in branches with diameters greater than 5 cm, the inferior and superior diameter and corresponding length.

The physiognomy of the studied sites was dominated by shrub and arboreal plants, where the most outstanding vegetation was *Prosopis glandulosa*. The total floral diversity found were 160 taxa belonging to 59 families, of which Poaceae, Asteraceae, Cactaceae, Fabaceae, and Euphorbiaceae presented the greater number of taxa. The average density of shrubs was of 6575 individuals/ha. The accumulated average cover per site taking in consideration the three layers was 203.20%, being the shrub layer the greatest vegetative cover (85.6%). The shrub and arboreal layers presented greatest IVs (80.31%) of *P. glandulosa*. The timber volume was significantly greater in arboreal layers (64.675 m^3/ha) than shrub layers (26.563 m^3/ha). The wood volume had a strong relationship with the variables of BD and crown projection.

The relative values of vegetative cover, frequency, density, and IV of *P. glandulosa* varied significantly by site. In the arboreal layer, *P. glandulosa* reached the greater percentage in all the parameters, dominating completely the stratum. In most of the sites, the mesquite population was integrated by young individuals with short vegetative development, BDs smaller than 20 cm, height average of 4.86 m, cover average of 23.03 m^2, and total density of 554.87 individuals/ha in the shrub and arboreal layers.

5.1   INTRODUCTION

It has been estimated that there are currently more than 50,000 plant species worldwide. The largest number of native tree species found in a single country is 7880 in Brazil. Astonishingly, only about 1000 different tree species are utilized globally (Sutton, 1999; FAO, 2006). Thus, thousands of tree species are either not utilized, underutilized, or used inappropriately. The present human population has wood consumption needs ranging from 0.3 to 0.6 m^3/year/habitant (Aktuell, 2007). As a result, the annual wood and wood-based products consumption have been calculated to be around 3.5 billion m^3 approximately, 66% of which are hardwoods used mainly as fuel; the rest are softwoods used principally in industry (Youngquist and Hamilton, 1999).

In order to satisfy wood needs, the forestry research has been focused on increasing wood production by improving forestry management. Plantations provide another option. In areas of Venezuela and Brazil, 5–90,000 m³/ha/year of *Pinus caribea* and *Eucalyptus grandis* are produced, respectively (FAO, 2006); however, the material obtained from these plantations is "different" qualitywise in comparison to wood coming from natural forests (Zamudio et al., 2010).

In a particular case, the Gulf of Mexican coastal plain is vegetated with a woodland shrub community dominated by small trees and shrubs, referred as "Tamaulipas thorny scrub" (Rzedowsky, 1978; INE, 2005). The Tamaulipan shrubland occurs extending from the coastal plain of the Mexican Gulf to the southern rim of Texas State, United States. In these arid and semiarid zones of northeastern Mexico, a great variability in climatic and edaphic conditions causes extremely diverse shrublands in terms of species composition, height, density, and plant associations. The various species occurring in this region can be categorized in several groups based on their ecological adaptations and forestry use, such as the production of timber, posts, firewood, food, medicines, handicrafts, forage, and so on (Bainbridge et al., 1990; Felker, 1996).

One of the tasks of wood and nonwood products must be to concentrate on increasing research to ensure a better utilization of lesser-known tree species from around the world. This should particularly be applied to trees grown on arid and semiarid land which have shown desirable characteristics like genera *Prosopis, Helietta, Condalia,* and some *Acacia* species. *Prosopis glandulosa* (honey mesquite) and *P. laevigate* make a good alternative for a variety of wood and nonwood products (Pasiecznik et al., 2001; Estrada et al., 2004).

For the reasons mentioned above, the present study was made to know the growth characteristics and the population structure of mesquite trees in natural conditions as a contribution to build up the basis for the implementation of a management program of this plant resource with the purpose to guarantee its sustainable exploitation.

5.1.1 DISTRIBUTION AND IMPORTANCE OF PROSOPIS SPP.

Mesquite is widely distributed in the dry regions of America, constituting frequently the only arboreal element of the vegetation. Of the 42 species reported for the American continent, 9 of them are distributed in the arid and semiarid zones of Mexico and south of Texas, United States. Its distribution in Mexico is estimated to take place over 7,000,000 ha, concentrated mainly in the north and center of the country, being *P. laevigata* and *P. glandulosa* the species of greater occurrence in the north of Mexico.

P. glandulosa in the northeast of the country is reported in the states of Coahuila, Tamaulipas, and Nuevo León (Pasiecznik et al., 2001). On the other hand, *P. laevigata* distributes from the northeast toward the Great Plain and center of the country, occurring in the same areas where *P. glandulosa* and its two varieties are distributed. It is reported that in certain areas of their distribution, the species *P. laevigata* and *P. glandulosa* coexist with the presence of individuals that present intermediate characters. Rzedowsky (1988) considers that the original distribution of these two species has been modified by human intervention, which caused an intense introgression.

In the vegetal communities of north and northeast of Mexico, the mesquite species are distributed in the Tamaulipan thornscrub (Fig. 5.1) where more than 70% of the species integrating this type of vegetation are thorny deciduous. In this vegetation, mesquite is associated with the species *Acacia rigidula, Cercidium macrum, Leucophyllum frutescens, Condalia hookerii,* and *Castela tortuosa*, in the arboreal and shrub layer, whereas the herbaceous layer are represented by Cactaceous like *Ferocactus hamatacanthus, Echinocactus texensis*, and *Echinocereus enneacanthus*, as well as species of the Compositae family: *Circium texanum, Eupatorium coelestinum*, and *Gymnosperma glutinosum* among others (Alanís et al., 1996; INEGI, 2002).

The *Prosopis* genus comprises about 44 species of trees and shrubs; the number could be as high as 77 since similar species are now included in other genus like *Acacia* (USDA, 2007). The taxonomy is very complex; the species have been divided into five sections, distributed in North America, Central/ South America, Africa, and Asia (Pasiecznic et al., 2001). The species from the *Prosopis* section are native to Asia and North Africa; the *Anonychium* section is composed of a single species *P. africana*, which is found on arid lands of North Africa. The species from the *Strombocarpa, Monilicarpa,* and *Algarobia* sections are indigenous to Central and South America where the largest *Prosopis* forests are also found (Lopez et al., 2006).

Tropical Africa could be where *Prosopis* originated. As all species are closely related to *Adenanthera* L. and *Pseudoprosopis* Harms, all species may have evolved from these two genera. The name *Prosopis* comes from the ancient Greek word "*Prosopis,*" which means "bark used for tanning sheep skins" (Rodríguez and Maldonado, 1996).

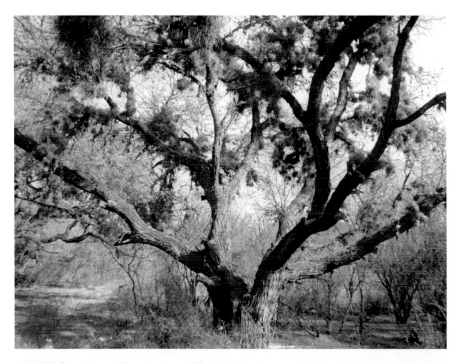

FIGURE 5.1 Tamaulipan scrub modified by disturbance alterations in the semiarid land of northeastern Mexico.

The importance of *Prosopis* trees have been confirmed in many ecosystems around the world. These species have the capacity to positively influence soils, thus improving the environmental conditions for themselves as well for other plants and animal species. For that reason, they have been grown on plantations in a number of habitats. Even though there are no exact records about the distribution of *Prosopis*, the common belief is that the first travelers across America used the sweet pods during their journeys. They could have also been spread indirectly by domestic animals consuming the sweet pods. In the last 200 years, the *Prosopis* species have been introduced or reintroduced in certain areas of Argentina, Chile, Peru, Mexico, and the United States (Pasiecznic et al., 2001), as well as in some regions of Asia, Africa, India, and Australia.

There are contradicting opinions regarding the use of some species in reforestation programs. As a result of their fast colonizing behavior, they have been considered as problematic trees. In fact, some users consider these tree species to be amongst the worst invasive weeds. *Prosopis* have already infested areas of Africa, Australia, Brazil, and Hawaii, where large amounts of money have been spent on eradication by mechanical, chemical, or biocontrol means (Richardson, 1998; Hughes, 2001). In the United States, an eradication program lasting more than 50 years has been employed to remove *Prosopis* from grasslands; however, neither herbicides nor mechanical means have proved successful. After a period of time the *Prosopis* has always returned (Pasiecznik, 2002).

Natural *Prosopis* stands have been use as fodder for domestic animals, for example, cows and goats. In 1965, approximately 40,000 metric tons of *Prosopis* pods were used to feed cattle, sheep, goats, horses, donkeys, and mules (Felker, 1996).

It is also possible to produce flour for human consumption and due to its sugar content even an alcoholic brew. *Prosopis* flour absorbs 185% of its weight in water, which is quite similar to the results obtained for *Phaseolus sp.* (Barba de la Rosa et al., 2006).

As *Prosopis* trees produce an abundance of blossoms, they play an important role in quality honey production (Pasiecznik et al., 2004). Gums are also produced in large amounts from wounds to the bark; which is mainly used as an emulsion stabilizer, colloid protector, and flavor encapsulating agent in the food, cosmetic, pharmaceutical, and petrochemical industries (Beristain et al., 1996; Gérardin et al., 2004).

Mexico's charcoal exports increased from 2000 to 20,000 mt from 1982 to 1992 (Meraz et al., 1998) with the United States being its main buyer. Five cubic meters of wood are needed to produce a metric ton of charcoal, which means that 100,000 m^3 of wood were used in only 1 year. In two traditional *Prosopis* harvesting municipalities of northwest Mexico, the logging of only approximately 50,000 m^3 was authorized from 1990 to 1997 (León-Luz et al., 2005; Somoza, 2014). The official statistics regarding nationwide *Prosopis* harvesting do not reflect the actual harvest, since this wood is grouped together with other species such as *Populus sp., Liquidambar sp., Fraxinus sp.,* and *Juglans sp.* Records for these show an overall wood production of 135,563 m^3 in 2003 (SEMARNAT, 2007a).

5.2   MATERIALS AND METHODS

5.2.1   STUDY AREA

The study was carried out in Nuevo Leon State, at the Northeast Mexico, located within the coordinates 23° 10'27" and 27° 46'06" of North latitude,

98° 26'24" and 101° 13'55" West longitude, with a territorial extension of 65,103 km^2. The Tropic of Cancer line is located in the parallel 23° 27' N crossing the State in the south. It is politically divided in 52 municipalities and has a population of 3,834,141 inhabitants. The analysis was made within the *Rio Grande* river hydrological basin (39,661.014 km^2), San Fernando-Soto *La Marina* area (11,521.683 km^2), and *El Salado* area (12,373.772 km^2).

Based on thematic maps of land use and vegetation, scale 1:50,000 and digital ortophotos published by the INEGI (2002), stands with vegetation including mesquite were delimited, numbered in progressive form, and selected at random in order to determine the minimum size of the parcel using the method of the species/area curve (Franco et al., 2001). The study area was visited for the correct localization of the selected sites and the recognition of the communities with mesquite using a Global Positioning System (GPS) receiver to register the geographical coordinates of latitude, longitude, and elevation above sea level of each one of the study sites selected (Table 5.1 and Fig. 5.2).

5.2.2   CLIMATE AND SOILS

The climate of northeast Mexico (Nuevo León State) is in extreme contrast. The hot and dry climate predominates and it is associated to "B" dry climate, "Bw" arid or very dry, and "Bs" semiarid or semidry of the Kopen classification. Most of the year it is very hot, mainly in the plains, since at the mountain regions the altitude attenuates the warm temperatures. In these areas the months from November to January are cold.

Other types of climates are also present at a lesser extent, as the semicalid (A)C and the temperate subhumid C(W). The high climatic contrast is also verified in the top of the mountain range with an alpine climate Project Management Organization Energy, Technology, Sustainability (ETN) is loacted at Forschungszentrum Jülich.

The mean annual temperature is 22.3°C with a large difference between winter and summer (−2.3 to 41.1°C). Hail and frosts usually occur every year even after the beginning of the growing season in March. The long-term mean annual precipitation values vary from 380 mm (arid zones) to 749 mm (semiarid zones) with two peaks in late May and July–September and drought periods in June and winter. The water budget is unbalanced. The ratio of precipitation to free evaporation is 0.48 and precipitation to potential evaporation is 0.62 (Navar et al., 2004).

TABLE 5.1 Sampling Sites in the State of Nuevo León, Mexico and its Geographic Location.

Physiographic province	Site/municipality	UTM X	UTM Y	Altitude
Great Plain of North America	2: Ejido Colorados de Arriba, Vallecillo	400906	2927506	239
	4: La Barretosa, Los Herreras	451990	2858539	166
	5: Ejido Emiliano Zapata, Parás	431651	2937498	164
	6: Puente del Río Salado, Anáhuac	413460	2982484	146
	7: Loma Larga, General Treviño	448858	2904109	147
	9: Ejido El Álamo, Vallecillo	421068	2929095	195
	24: El Nogal, Anáhuac	399125	3005741	177
	25: Comun. Regantes 26, Anáhuac	367140	3024331	228
	26: Rancho La Ceja, Los Aldama	476956	2883426	112
Mountain ranges and plains of Coahuila	1: Plan del Orégano, Melchor Ocampo	457694	2883106	152
	3: El Llano, Los Ramones	437024	2854589	193
	13: Los Pajaritos, Doctor González	408854	2863751	423
	17: El Resumidero, Salinas Victoria	373712	2882558	451
	18: El Puente, Salinas Victoria	372252	2872246	424
	19: Rancho Gomas, Salinas Victoria	353164	2895485	568
	23: Ejido Las Presas, Lampazos	348405	2982066	341
	27: El cuchillo, China	474439	2845014	138
Coastal plain of the North Gulf	8: Los Ébanos, Los Ramones	453517	2824931	196
	10: Dulces Nombres, Pesquería	394236	2844953	351
	11: Hacienda San Pedro, Gral. Zuazua	384066	2867217	369
	12: Higueras, Higueras	398119	2872672	503
	14: Rancho El Recuerdo, Gral. Terán	427656	2806597	285
	15: Loma La Parada, Marín	401847	2856144	323
	16: El Bajío, Marín	402122	2858136	342
	20: Kilómetro 80, Los Ramones	446057	2837409	191
	21: Rancho La Bonanza, Gral. Terán	467187	2787506	217
	22: Rancho Nuevo, Gral. Terán	452841	2790393	259
	28: San Pedro de los Escobedo Linares	462356	2760631	261
	29: San Ignacio de Texas, Galeana	379092	2690496	1684
	30: Ejido Puentes, Aramberri	390606	2670446	1581

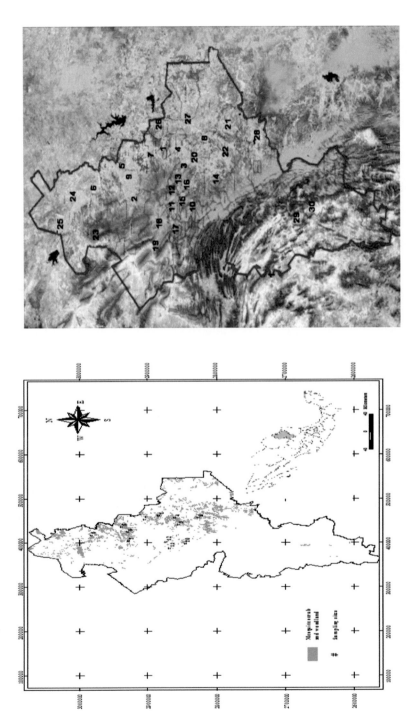

FIGURE 5.2 Distribution of mesquite scrub and woodland covered areas in northeast Mexico and sampling sites.

The soils of the region are basically stony of Upper Cretaceous siltstone, with pH 7.5–8.5 and abundant limestone. In the FAO (2006) classification, these soils are classified as rendzine, vertisoils, feozem, and castañozem with low organic matter content and low levels of phosphorus and nitrogen. Underground water is hard but not saline.

The Nuevo Leon State presents five morphological zones well defined which correspond to the physiographical provinces. These morphological units are demonstrated in the Figure 5.3.

Once the sites were located in each geographic zone, the minimum area in each one of them was considered with the purpose to obtain a represented vegetal composition employing the technique of the nested sample according to Salvador and Alvarez (2004). The species occurring in each subsample were registered and the minimum area of sampling was determined as the surface where at least 95% of the species of the vegetal community were contained.

Permanent 10 × 10 m quadrant sampling along each study zones and site was made at random. The average distance among the plots varied according to the vegetative composition and the heterogeneity degree.

In each quadrate, all the arboreal and shrub species were identified. The following measurements were made.

5.2.3   ESTIMATION OF FOREST PRODUCTION OF THORN SCRUB

The forest potential was evaluated by determining the volume of each species per hectare, taking into account of total height, BD, and diameter at breast height (DBH) of all the individuals, also including shoots.

These variables were selected to determine the developmental behavior of individuals, since the proportions between height and diameter, between tree crown size and diameter, between biomass and diameter, usually respond to a general rule, which is the same for all trees that develop under the same environmental conditions, being considered from the smallest to the largest (Archibald and Bond, 2003; Bohlman and O'Brien, 2006; Dietze et al., 2008).

5.2.3.1   DIAMETER AND HEIGHT

The measurement of BD was undertaken at 0.1 m above the soil surface, adopting a standard measurement employee for trees and shrubs of the Tamaulipan thorn scrub, according to Gómez (2000), Alanís et al. (2008a), Jiménez et al. (2012a). This variable was measured, based on the premise that it supports the generation of relationships for the structuring of allometric

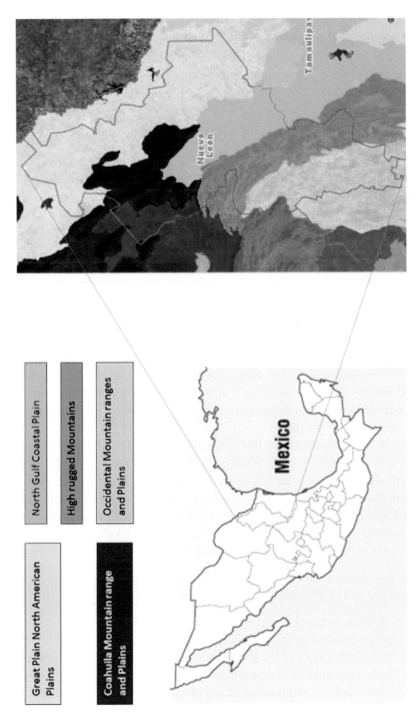

FIGURE 5.3 Physiographical provinces of the Nuevo León state, Mexico.

equations for the estimation of biomass (Méndez, 2001), calculating from this, the basal area. Both BD and DBH were measured by a calibrator.

The total height as a dendrometric variable (*h*) forms part of the main interactions for the construction of allometric equations for biomass estimation (Vanclay, 2009).

5.2.3.2   VOLUME OF WOOD AND CANOPY COVER

The wood volume of each tree was determined according to diameters and total height, applying the formula of Smalian (Moctezuma, 2007) with a morphic coefficient factor of 0.6 (eq. 5.1).

$$V = \left[\left(\left(\frac{D1}{2}\right)^2 \times \pi + \left(\frac{D2}{2}\right)^2 \times \pi \right)\middle/2\right] \times L, \qquad (5.1)$$

where *V* is the volume (m³/ha), D1 and D2 are diameters (cm) of each section (height).

Once the volume was obtained per tree, the mathematical process was carried out to estimate the volume of wood corresponding to each species.

The canopy coverage generally forms part of principal interactions during the construction of allometric equations for the estimation of biomass so that this variable was also considered for the present study. Canfield (1941) defined canopy cover as the vertical downward projection of foliage or the upper part of the plant over the soil or also the proportion of soil occupied by the aerial part of the plants.

According to this definition, this variable was determined by recording the perpendicular projections of the aerial part of each tree over the soil, according the north-south and east-west directions, with the use of metric tape.

From the classical method of calculating the area of a circle, a method adapted to the scrub was developed to calculate the area occupied by each individual (eq. 5.2). From this, the total area occupied by each species and the relative area (in percentage) in each plot and then per hectare was determined.

$$C = \pi\left(\frac{D1}{2}\right)\left(\frac{D2}{2}\right), \qquad (5.2)$$

where *C* is the coverage (m²) of each tree, D1 and D2 are diameters (m) of the canopy projections in the north-south and east-west directions.

The floristic diversity of the woody plant was determined by the evaluation of the ecological attributes proposed by Mueller-Dombois and Ellenberg (1974), when applying the four equations of affinity of Sorensen (1948):

$$FR = \frac{Fi}{F} \times 100, \tag{5.3}$$

where *FR* is the relative frequency, *Fi* the frequency of a species, and *F* the frequency of all the species.

$$DR = \frac{Ni}{N} \times 100, \tag{5.4}$$

where *DR* is the relative density, *Ni* the number of individuals of a species, and *N* the number of individuals of all the species.

$$CR = \frac{Ci}{C} \times 100, \tag{5.5}$$

where *CR* is the relative coverage, *Ci* the coverage of a species, and *C* the coverage of all the species.

$$VI = \frac{FR + DR + CR}{3}, \tag{5.6}$$

where *VI* is the importance value.

5.2.3.3   *STATISTICAL ANALYSIS*

The statistical package used for analysis of scrub productivity data was SPSS version 21, the statistics practiced included an analysis of variance to verify significant differences between growth variables and wood volume, with a 95% confidence interval. The Tukey test was used to determine groups of homogeneity between species and between sites for the aforementioned variables, according to Zar (2010). Since the data resulting from the immediate analysis are percentage values, they were transformed with the sum of square function of the p arcsine, where P = a proportion of the dependent variable (Schefler, 1981).

5.3   RESULTS AND DISCUSSION

5.3.1   *STRUCTURE, DIVERSITY, AND SIMILARITY OF THE STUDIED COMMUNITIES*

In the Nuevo Leon State, the appearance of the mesquite communities (mesquite scrub and woodland) is determined by the occurrence of mesquite trees present in the shrub and arboreal strata, usually of 3–10 m of height, and it is the most outstanding species of these communities which are generally conformed by thorny species that vary in density and size. Humidity plays an important role in the exuberant degree and the species associated in the mesquite scrub and woodland, which affect the density and the insolation degree to the interior of the community. It may be observed that in higher isolation conditions the presence of cactaceous species is common whereas in mostly shady vegetation areas conditions favor the appearance of climbing plants associated to different strata.

5.3.2   FLORISTIC COMPOSITION

A total diversity of 160 taxa pertaining to 59 families was found. The families with greater number of taxa were Poaceae, Asteraceae, and Cactaceae with 47, 36, and 24 taxa, respectively, followed by Fabaceae with 9 taxa and Euphorbiaceae and Acanthaceae with 8 in both cases (Fig. 5.4); the rest of the families mostly presented less than 3 taxa and 23 of them were represented by a single taxon. The number of total species by community varied enormously from 22 taxa in the Great Plain Province of North America (*Puente del Río Salado* site) to 75 in the Coastal Plain Province of the North Gulf (*Los Ebanos* site) and a general average of 46.91 taxa per community. The most common species, considering that they were present in all the sampled communities were *Ruellia nudiflora, Opuntia leptocaulis, Celtis pallida* and *Prosopis glandulosa*. Other species also common in the study sites are *Opuntia engelmannii, Dyschoriste decumbens, Acacia rigidula, Castela texana, Karwinskia humboldtiana, Ziziphus obtusifolia, Acleisanthes obtusa,* and *Tridens muticus*.

It is important to emphasize that during the study, the presence of two endangered species was detected in compliance with the Official Mexican Norm NOM-059-SEMARNAT-2001 (SEMARNAT, 2002). The species were *Echinocereus poselgeri* (Cactaceae) that has the status "subject to special protection" and *Manfreda longiflora* (Agavaceae) with "threatened status." In both cases, deforestation and extensive cattle ranch are the factors that contribute to greater negative impact and inflict loss and deterioration of their habitat (Fig. 5.5). Besides, another relevant factor for the survival is the nodricism required by the species as in the case of *A. poselgeri*. Likewise, the main problem for the establishment of *Manfreda longiflora* is the modification of the habitat and the succulent character of the plant, which makes it attractive to predators (particularly in the early stages of development).

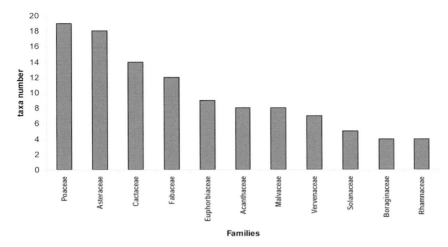

FIGURE 5.4 Families with higher diversity in the mesquite scrub and woodland studied.

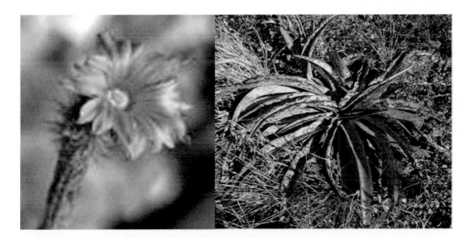

FIGURE 5.5 Species in the NOM (Official Mexican Norm); left, *Echinocereus poselgeri*; right, *Manfreda longiflora.*

5.3.3 DENSITY, CANOPY COVER, AND SIMILARITY BETWEEN COMMUNITIES

The average density of individuals by site was of 14,015 individuals/ha. Maximum values (21,120 individuals/ha) were found in the Great Plain Province of North America (*El Alamo* and *Puente del Rio Salado* sites).

As for the average cover by site it was observed that it was 203.20%, taking in consideration that overlapping between individuals may occur between the accumulated cover from the three strata and even to the interior of each layer. The maximum vegetation cover was reached in the Coastal Plain Province of the North Gulf (*Dulces Nombres* locality) with 314.08%, community with a vegetation very dense and with little uncovered surface. On the other hand, the minimum canopy cover (108.37%) appeared in the Coahuilan Mountain ranges and Plains Province (*Plan del Orégano* site) which has a vegetal community with very few arboreal elements and large open ground areas.

5.3.4 MESQUITE AS A STRUCTURAL ELEMENT OF THE COMMUNITY

In Table 5.2, the participation in relative terms of *Prosopis glandulosa* as a component of herbaceous, shrub, and arboreal strata of the studied communities is shown.

5.3.4.1 VEGETATION COVER

P. glandulosa displayed little cover in the herbaceous layer, going from its absence in some studied sites to a maximum of the 1.02% of the total stratum cover in the Coastal Plain Province of the North Gulf (*Higueras* site). In the shrub layer, its presence is far more noticeable although there are enormous variations between provinces and sampled sites. For example, in the Great Plain Province of North America (*El Alamo* and *El Nogal* sites) vegetal cover is inferior to 1% of the total for the stratum and in other sites. "Puente del Río Salado," "Emiliano Zapata," and "Plan del Orégano" cover values in shrub layer reached 49.73%, 38.46%, and 35.26%, respectively. Finally, in the arboreal layer, *P. glandulosa* showed percentages of cover from 90 to 100% in most of the sites, which is reasonable since in several sites, it constitutes the only species of this layer. In other sites where richness is low and presents greater diversity, the density of other species is low and as a consequence, its cover value is also low (Table 5.2).

5.3.4.2 FREQUENCY

This parameter showed a similar behavior in the vegetation cover, with values less than 1% in most of the cases for the herbaceous layer. Only

TABLE 5.2 Relative Dominance, Frequency, Density, and IVs of Mesquite in the Herbaceous, Shrub, and Tree Layers in Three Physiographic Zones of Northeastern Mexico.

Phisiographic zones		Sampling sites	Vegetation types (canopy)		
			Herb	Shrub	Tree
Relative dominance	Great Plain of North America	2, 4, 5, 6, 7, 9,24,25,26,27	<1	1–50	81–100
	Coastal Plain of the North Gulf	8, 10, 11, 12, 14, 15, 16, 20, 21, 22	1–2	8–30	65–100
	Mountain ranges and plains of Coahuila	1, 3, 13, 17, 18, 19, 23, 27	<1	1–36	94–100
Relative frequency	Great Plain of North America	2, 4, 5, 6, 7, 9,24,25,26,27	0.3–5	2–15	63–100
	Coastal Plain of the North Gulf	8, 10, 11, 12, 14, 15, 16, 20, 21, 22	1–2	4–20	24–86
	Mountain ranges and plains of Coahuila	1, 3, 13, 17, 18, 19, 23, 27	<1	2–11	75–100
Relative density	Great Plain of North America	2, 4, 5, 6, 7, 9, 24, 25, 26, 27	0.1–4.0	0.3–16	42–100
	Coastal Plain of the North Gulf	8, 10, 11, 12, 14, 15, 16, 20, 21, 22	<1	2–36	39–97
	Mountain ranges and plains of Coahuila	1, 3, 13, 17, 18, 19, 23, 27	<1	0.5–14	80–100
Importance value	Great Plain of North America	2, 4, 5, 6, 7, 9, 24, 25, 26, 27	0.2–4.0	0.5–26	53–100
	Coastal Plain of the North Gulf	8, 10, 11, 12, 14, 15, 16, 20, 21, 22	<1	5–29	43–95
	Mountain ranges and plains of Coahuila	1, 3, 13, 17, 18, 19, 23, 27	<1	1–20	83–100

in "Loma Larga" site, the frequency reached 5%. In the shrub stratum its frequency was smaller than 20% in all cases and it was below 5% in most of the sites, which places the frequency with inferior average percentage values than the vegetation cover. The arboreal layer presented very variable frequencies that were ranking from 23.81% in the Coastal Plain Province of the North Gulf ("Dulces Nombres" site) despite it reached one of the highest values of diversity and density, until 100% in the Great Plain Province of North America ("Puente del Río Salado" and "Loma Larga" sites) where mesquite constitutes the only species in the layer (Table 5.3).

5.3.4.3   DENSITY

The relative density of *P. glandulosa* in the herbaceous layer, as well as its cover and frequency, is very low with values going from 0 to 3.91% of the total of individuals/unit of area in of the layer, although in most of them it is smaller than 1%. In the shrub layer, the percentage participation in the density of the layer is increased, although it varies significantly from one site to another since, for example, in the Great Plain Province of North America ("El Alamo" site) reaches scarcely a 0.23% of the total density (this community also presents the smaller density in the herbaceous layer, 0.07%). In contrast, in the Coastal Plain Province of the North Gulf ("Hacienda San Pedro" site) it has a density of the 35.90% of the total of individuals. On the other hand, the arboreal layer has a similar behavior in the cover and frequency, since *P. glandulosa* reaches densities above 70% in most of the cases (Table 5.3).

5.3.4.4   IMPORTANCE VALUE (IV)

As a result of the three previous parameters measured, we can observe that the participation of *P. glandulosa* in the herbaceous layer is very low with IVs inferior to 1% in most of the cases, except by 3.05% in the Great Plain Province of North America ("Loma Larga" site), product of a greater density and frequency in the site. In the shrub layer, *P. glandulosa* showed the most irregular behavior between the studied sites, since its importance goes from sites with a hardly noticeable importance as in the Great Plain of North America (0.52%) and "Level" (0.92%), where species like *Paulothamnus spinescens, Celtis pallida,* and *Porlieria angustifolia* dominated the layer, until 28.12% in the Coastal Plain of the North Gulf, sites where mesquite codominated with species like *Opuntia engelmannii*. There was no site

TABLE 5.3 Higher Importance Values (IV) Average of the Different Strata in the Studied Communities.

Herbaceous	IV (%)	Scrub	IV (%)	Arboreal	IV (%)
Ruellia nudiflora	14.30	*Opuntia leptocaulis*	14.31	*Prosopis glandulosa*	80.31
Opuntia leptocaulis	8.14	*Opuntia engelmannii*	10.41	*Havardia pallens*	20.72
Ruellia sp	7.69	*Prosopis glandulosa*	9.87	*Acacia wrightii*	14.00
Calyptocarpus vialis	7.07	*Celtis pallida*	9.65	*Acacia rigidula*	11.56
Bouteloua trifida	6.41	*Paulothamus spinescens*	8.89	*Pithecellobium flexicaule*	8.51
Oxalis dichondraefolia	6.20	*Acacia rigidula*	7.56	*Celtis pallida*	7.97
Tridens muticus	5.83	*Ziziphus obtusifolia*	7.01	*Condalia hookeri*	7.39
Lantana camara	5.25	*Eupatorium sp.*	5.76	*Bumelia celastrina*	6.92
Dyschoriste decumbens	5.11	*Karwinskia humboldtiana*	5.57	*Acacia farnesiana*	5.88
Setaria sp	4.92	*Castela texana*	5.47	*Cercidium sp.*	3.35

where mesquite had a significantly greater IV than other species in the shrub layer. Finally, the panorama radically changes in the arboreal layer, since in all the cases, *P. gladulosa* had the greater IV of the layer, with greater IV than 80% in the major study sites, some sites with IV between 50% and single 75% and in the Coastal Plain of the North Gulf, its IV was smaller (42.36%), despite this value is superior to the values for the rest of the species of the site (Table 5.3).

5.3.5   FIREWOOD AND WOOD VOLUME DETERMINATION ON PROSOPIS GLANDULOSA

The estimated wood production for each site (Table 5.4) is related to the density of individuals in a representative sample, which includes wood sections of diameter 5 cm or more. The production-density ratio seems to be reversed. When there is a high density of mesquite individuals per hectare, there is a low production volume in cubic meters of wood, for example, in the Province of the Coahuilan Mountain ranges and Plains, for the site 18 "El Puente" of the Salinas Victoria municipality with 1783 individuals/ha, there is a production of 48.95 m^3 and in the site 23 "Ejido Las Presas" of the Lampazos municipality with 2483 individuals/ha, there is a standing production of 9.15 m^3. This tendency was also present in other sites with densities close to 1000 individuals/ha and this productive situation is because in sites with high density, a good number of the trees are of low size and the populations of mesquite are in recovery within community.

On the contrary, some sites such as number 3 "El Llano" in the munici-pality of Los Ramones with a density per hectare of 167, had a production of 84.07 m^3/ha, as well as other sites with densities around 300 trees per hectare presented high productions; in the case of site 11 "Hacienda San Pedro" of the municipality of General Zuazua, located in the Coastal Plain of the North Gulf, there were a low density (750 trees/ha) and high production (116.52 m^3/ha), which could be explained by the fact that the site presented large trees since apparently its use was for livestock purposes because it had characteristics of being an abandoned prairie.

The additions of the extreme results of the densities in relation to their production volumes average a density of 686 mesquite individuals per hectare and yield an average volume production of wood of 43.99 m^3/ha. If we eliminate from the calculations these high densities of 900 or more individuals per hectare, the average production rises to 48.07 m^3/ha; if the most productive sites 9 "El Álamo" and 11 "Hacienda San Pedro" are also

TABLE 5.4 Wood Volume Determination of *Prosopis glandulosa* in Function of Plant Density Per Site and Per Geographic Zones.

Physiographic provinces	Site/municipality	Vol m3/ha	Trees/ha
Great Plain of the North America	2 Ejido Colorados de Arriba, Vallecillo	70.85	250
	4 La Barretosa, Los Herreras	97.44	267
	5 Ejido Emiliano Zapata, Parás	33.40	1060
	6 Puente del Rio Salado, Anáhuac	27.93	540
	7 Loma Larga, General Treviño	24.23	640
	9 Ejido El Álamo, Vallecillo	119.21	500
	24 El Nogal, Anáhuac	10.87	900
	25 Comun. Regantes 26, Anáhuac	56.91	363
	26 Rancho La Ceja, Los Aldama	19.96	467
Average/zone		**46.08**	**539**
Coahuilan mountain ranges and plains	1 Plan del Orégano, Melchor Ocampo	20.40	757
	3 El Llano, Los Ramones	84.07	167
	13 Los Pajaritos, Doctor González	57.21	262
	17 El Resumidero, Salinas Victoria	14.13	1190
	18 El Puente, Salinas Victoria	48.95	1783
	19 Rancho Gomas, Salinas Victoria	41.16	616
	23 Ejido Las Presas, Lampazos	9.15	2483
	27 El cuchillo, China	23.36	767
Average/zone		**37.55**	**1030**
Coastal Plain of the North Gulf	8 Los Ébanos, Los Ramones	33.99	767
	10 Dulces Nombres, Pesquería	36.76	860
	11 Hacienda San Pedro, Gral. Zuazua	116.52	750
	12 Higueras, Higueras	39.61	260
	14 Rancho El Recuerdo, Gral. Terán	39.89	120
	15 Loma La Parada, Marín	23.67	883
	16 El Bajío, Marín	29.71	635

TABLE 5.4 *(Continued)*

Physiographic provinces	Site/municipality	Vol m3/ha	Trees/ha
	20 Kilómetro 80, Los Ramones	11.13	467
	21 Rancho La Bonanza, Gral. Terán	83.39	283
	22 Rancho Nuevo, Gral. Terán	46.13	617
	28 San Pedro de los Escobedo Linares	41.66	367
	29 San Ignacio de Texas, Galeana	11.61	400
	30 Ejido Puentes, Arambarri	49.61	1550
Average/zone		**40.28**	**610**

discarded from the results, the average production volume in relation to the density of individuals would be 41.86 m³/ha with an average density of 480 individuals of mesquite, result that is more conservative in the production of wood, specially of mesquite species or their hybrids in three physiographic zones of the Nuevo Leon State.

Proportionally, the contribution of wood per hectare for each of the sites in relation to the convenient categorization in sizes or diametric classes can be seen in Table 5.5. It is clear that classes between 5 and 25 cm in diameter are present at sites of mesquital, beginning to be scarce, the classes of diameter ranging from 25 to 50 cm, to finally become rare classes, those above 50 cm in diameter.

In general, production averages indicate that in the diametric classes 10–15 and 5–10, with averages of 10.44 and 8.86 m³, the highest production of roundwood was associated with 23.72 and 20.13% of the total average production derived from mesquital sites, and in sum is projected at 43.85%.

Specifically, site 11 Hacienda San Pedro was the one with the highest production values for diameter classes 10–15 and 5–10 with a respective production of 37.20 and 20.49 m³, which is equivalent to 32.76 and 18.04%, which in sum represents about 50% of the production of these classes compared to the remaining ones that were presented at the site.

The analysis of variance (ANOVA) applied to growth variables and firewood volume production, showed high significant differences (P=0.000) between or within groups of the mesquite in each one of the thirty ecosystems. The analysis indicated high significant differences between groups for height (F=20.239; P=0.000), BD (F=12.370; P=0.000), crown projection—density (F=6.550; P=0.000) and firewood volume production (F=3.596; P= 0.000).

The analysis of the frequency distribution demonstrated that most of the sites are constituted by young individuals not very developed. Also, it was stated that the strongest and vigorous trees are located in mesquitals and in the Tamaulipan thorny scrub where some individuals reached heights of 11.1 m, 75 cm of BD and a crown projection of up to 267 m² growing over plain areas with deep soil. Nevertheless, when analyzing the growth variables of mesquite in relation to the structure or type of vegetation, the greater base diameters were found in the Tamaulipan submountain scrub, which can be related to the intraspecific competition as it was indicated by Ainsley et al. (1998) who observed that when the density of mesquite increased, the diameters tend to diminish. We have found that the vigor of the trees in this zone can be related to its benign climate, where the lowest frequency of frost is reported. There are evidences that environmental characteristics such as

TABLE 5.5 Volume Production of Wood Per Site and on Average for the Sizes or Diametric Classes Established.

Sitio <Site>	5–10	10–15	15–20	20–25	25–30	30–35	35–40	40–45	45–50	50–55	55–60	60–65	70–75	75–80	85–90	Total (m3)
							Volume (m³) per Diametric Class (cm)									
1	8.91	3.74	4.21	0.8	1.44	–	1.26	–	–	–	–	–	–	–	–	20.40
2	7.1	14.93	10.67	5.48	5.7	5.7	6.52	3.15	2.97	8.59	–	–	–	–	–	70.85
3	10.17	18.84	16.44	13.9	8.2	0.86	1.66	5.36	–	2.79	–	5.81	–	–	–	84.07
4	11.05	15.41	13.4	10.68	8.45	17.72	–	9.64	11.06	–	–	–	–	–	–	97.44
5	12.88	9.91	2.94	2.42	3.14	–	–	2.09	–	–	–	–	–	–	–	33.40
6	15.87	6.73	2.8	1.45	–	1.045	–	–	–	–	–	–	–	–	–	27.93
7	11.01	9	2.69	1.51	–	–	–	–	–	–	–	–	–	–	–	24.23
8	8.7	8.86	3.34	3.24	5.63	0.58	–	3.61	–	–	–	–	–	–	–	33.99
9	8.29	21.89	12.86	17.3	16.56	2.75	3.38	2.78	6.93	–	6.12	–	13.63	6.7	–	119.21
10	12.57	12.75	6.56	3.42	1.44	–	–	–	–	–	–	–	–	–	–	36.76
11	20.49	37.2	9.92	8.65	6.09	6.02	2.83	4.82	–	–	–	–	17.46	–	–	113.52
12	6.9	10.15	8.16	7.27	3.04	–	1.15	–	–	–	–	2.92	–	–	–	39.61
13	9.29	17.21	12.73	6.28	5.78	0.73	5.15	–	–	–	–	–	–	–	–	57.21
14	3.67	4.05	5.11	11.49	4.73	7.26	3.54	–	–	–	–	–	–	–	–	39.89
15	8.82	9.14	2.51	1.28	1.9	–	–	–	–	–	–	–	–	–	–	23.67
16	9.35	12.16	4.7	1.03	0.91	–	1.52	–	–	–	–	–	–	–	–	29.71
17	5.26	2.94	2.59	3.32	–	–	–	–	–	–	–	–	–	–	–	14.13
18	12.47	8.31	9.72	6.67	7.82	1.4	2.53	–	–	–	–	–	–	–	–	48.95
19	6.42	11.23	7.93	6.24	3.29	1.36	1	–	1.5	–	2.16	–	–	–	–	41.16
20	5.99	3.45	1.51	0.17	–	–	–	–	–	–	–	–	–	–	–	11.13

TABLE 5.5 *(Continued)*

Sitio <Site>	Volume (m³) per Diametric Class (cm)															Total (m3)
	5–10	10–15	15–20	20–25	25–30	30–35	35–40	40–45	45–50	50–55	55–60	60–65	70–75	75–80	85–90	
21	8.89	9.95	8.24	6.88	5.99	5.33	2.08	4.25	6.94	9.5	–	–	–	–	15.35	83.39
22	10.34	14.15	6.45	5.74	3.36	3.96	2.11	–	–	–	–	–	–	–	–	46.13
23	5.48	2.87	0.43	–	0.35	–	–	–	–	–	–	–	–	–	–	9.15
24	1.68	1.47	0.37	1.89	1.02	2.3	–	–	2.11	–	–	–	–	–	–	10.87
25	9.5	13.83	10.17	5.44	3.94	4.33	0.43	4.68	1.52	–	3.03	–	–	–	–	56.91
26	7.03	5.89	3.6	2.05	1.37	–	–	–	–	–	–	–	–	–	–	19.96
27	10.11	7.79	3.46	0.15	1.83	–	–	–	–	–	–	–	–	–	–	23.36
28	6.85	8.99	6.31	3.88	2.45	11.92	1.22	–	–	–	–	–	–	–	–	41.66
29	2.58	1.65	4.32	0.72	–	2.31	–	–	–	–	–	–	–	–	–	11.61
30	8.17	8.74	6.7	10.42	5.54	1.19	1.26	–	2.46	–	–	5.09	–	–	–	49.61
Prom.	8.86	10.44	6.36	4.9923	3.6657	2.5588	1.216	1.3843	1.183	0.70	0.38	0.4607	1.0363	0.2233	0.5117	43.997

minimum average temperatures as well as the frequency and duration of winter frosts limit the establishment and growth of mesquite (Pasiecznik et al., 2001).

5.4   CONCLUSION

In the present study, an ecological characterization of the mesquite scrub and woodland in the north and east of Nuevo Leon State, Mexico was carried out and its wood production potential was evaluated.

The physiognomy of the studied sites was dominated by shrub and arboreal plants where the most outstanding vegetation by its height, density, and cover were mesquite plants. In all the studied sites, the occurring mesquite populations corresponded to the species *Prosopis glandulosa.*

The total floral diversity found was 160 taxa belonging to 59 families, 205 genera, and 302 species, being the most important in number, the families Poaceae (47), Asteraceae (36), Cactaceae (24), Fabaceae (8), and Euphorbiaceae (8). The total number of species by community varied from 22 in "Puente del Río Salado" to 75 in "Los Ebanos" with a general average of 46.91 species per community. The vegetal stratum with highest diversity was the herbaceous layer with 136 taxa and an average of 34.25 per studied site whereas the arboreal stratum displayed the smallest diversity with 13 taxa and a mean value of 3.17 taxa per site.

The species most common in addition to *P. glandulosa* in the arboreal stratum were *Acacia rigidula, Acacia wrightii* and *Celtis pallida, Bumelia celastrina* and *Condalia hookeri.* In the shrub layer the most common species were *Celtis pallida, Opuntia leptocaulis, P. glandulosa, O. engelmannii, Acacia rigidula, Castela texana, Karwinskia humboldtiana,* and *Ziziphus obtusifolia.* In the herbaceous layer the dominant species were *Ruellia nudiflora, Opuntia leptocaulis, Dyschoriste decumbens, Acleisanthes obtusa, Tridens muticus,* and *Mammillaria heyderi.*

The average density of individuals per site considering the three layers was of 274,015 individuals/ha, which 97.99% belong to the herbaceous layer. In the herbaceous stratum the density was 26.84 individuals/m^2 whereas the shrub and arboreal layers presented average densities of 412.74 and 5177.74 individuals/ha, respectively.

The average canopy cover by site, taking in consideration the accumulated cover of the three layers was 203.20%. The cover by stratum was of 30.38, 85.60, and 80.81% for the herbaceous, shrub, and arboreal layers, respectively.

In the herbaceous stratum *Ruellia nudiflora* and *Opuntia leptocaulis* reached the greatest IV with 14.30 and 8.14%, respectively. In the shrub layer *P. glandulosa, O. leptocaulis,* and *O. engelmannii* showed the greatest IV with 11.12, 10.97, and 10.51, respectively. *P. glandulosa* dominates the arboreal layer with an average IV of 80.31%.

The relative frequency of *P. glandulosa* in the herbaceous layer displayed a pattern very similar to the vegetation cover with smaller than 1% values in most of the cases, and only in the Great North American Plains ("Loma Larga" site) it reached a frequency close to 5%. In the shrub layer the percentage value of frequency was smaller than the cover, with lower values than 20% in all the cases, most of them even below 5%. In the arboreal layer the frequencies presented were shown between 23.81% in the Coastal Plains of the North Gulf ("Dulces Nombres" site) to 100% in the Coahuilan Mountain ranges and Plains ("Plan del Orégano" site).

With respect to the relative density of *P. glandulosa* we have that in the herbaceous layer, as for the cover and the frequency, its density is very low with values that go from absence of the species to 3.91% of the total of individuals of the layer. In the shrub stratum, the contribution of this species to the density of the layer increased but it varied significantly from site to site with a minimum density in the Great North American Plains ("El Alamo" site) with 0.23% and a maximum value of the 35.90% in the Coastal Plains of the North Gulf ("Hacienda San Pedro" site). The density in the arboreal stratum displayed values greater than 70 % in most of the cases.

As for the IV of *P. glandulosa* in the community we have that in the herbaceous layer its IV is inferior to 1% in most of the cases, except by the IV of 3.05% in the Great North American Plains ("Loma Larga" site). In the shrub stratum, *P. glandulosa* presented a very irregular pattern with IV hardly noticeable in "the Alamo" (0.52%) and "Llano" (0.92%) and IV as high as 25.50% and 28.12% in "Puente del Río Salado" and "Hacienda San Pedro," respectively. In no place mesquite reached a greater IV than any other species in the shrub layer but in the arboreal layer, *P. glandulosa* showed greater IV than all other species with values higher than 80% in most of the sites.

As for the characteristics pertaining to wood production from *P. glandulosa* we have that in most of the sites the population of mesquite was formed by young individuals with short vegetative development with an average BD of 19.47 cm, a height average of 4.86 m, and an average cover value of 23.03 m^2.

The average density of individuals was 554.87 specimens/ha considering the individuals of all BDs present in the shrub and arboreal layers, whereas the average density considering only those individuals with potential advantage for wood exploitation (BDs greater than 5 cm) was 382.90 individuals/ha.

According to the applied regression models, the volumetric estimation of timber per tree was mainly related to the BD of the individual which could match in a multiplicative mathematical model followed by the relation to the crown projection in an exponential model.

The site "Hacienda San Pedro" situated in the Coastal Plains of the North Gulf presented the greater wood production by plant (0.2299 m^3) and per hectare (126.47 m^3), at least in part, since it displayed individuals with greater height (6.46 m in average), greater crown projection (39.23 m^2), and a density of individuals quite higher than the average (750 individuals/ha).

In contrast, "Plan del Orégano" situated in the Coahuilan Mountain ranges and Plains presented the smallest wood production per plant (0.0204 m^3) and per hectare (9.44 m^3); its individuals displayed the lowest average values in height (3.73 m), average cover (9.83 m^2), BD (14.13 cm), although also showed the second greater density (757.14 individuals/ha).

KEYWORDS

- **ecology**
- **mesquite**
- **biomass**
- **firewood**
- **charcoal**
- **timber**

REFERENCES

Alanís, E.; Jiménez, J.; Aguirre, O. Efecto del uso del suelo en la fitodiversidad del matorral espinoso tamaulipeco. *Ciencia UANL*. **2008,** *11,* 56–62.

Ainsley, R. J.; Treviño, B. A.; Jacoby, P. W. Intraspecific Competition in Honey Mesquite: Leaf and Whole Plant Responses. *J. Range Manag.* **1998,** *51,* 345–352.

Aktuell Meyers Lexikonverlag Mannheim, Leipzig, Wien, Zürich, 2007; p 125.

Archibald, S.; Bond, W. J. Growing Tall vs Growing Wide: Tree Architecture and Allometry of *Acacia karroo* in Forest, Savanna, and Arid Environments. *Oikos* **2003,** *102,* 3–14.

Bainbridge, D. A.; Virginia, R. A.; Jarrell, W. M. *Honey Mesquite. A Multipurpose Tree for Arid Lands;* Network Forest Tree, Winrock International: Morrilton, Arkansas, USA, 1990; p 4.

Beristain, C. I.; Azuara, E.; García, H. S.; Vernon-Carter, E. J. Kinetic Model for Water/Oil Absorption of Mesquite Gum (*Prosopis juliflora*) and Gum Arabic (*Acacia senegal*). *Int. J. Food Sci. Technol.* **1996,** *31,* 379–386.

Bohlman, S.; O'Brien, S. Allometry, Adult Stature and Regeneration Requirement of 65 Tree Species on Barro Colorado Island, Panama. *J. Tropical Ecol.* **2006,** *22,* 123–136.

Canfield, H. R. Application of the Line Interception Method in Sampling Range Vegetation. *J. For.* **1941,** *39,* 333–394.

de la Rosa, A. P. B.; Frias-Hernández, J. T.; Olalde-Portugal, V.; González-Castañeda, J. Processing, Nutritional Evaluation, and Utilization of Whole Mesquite Flour (*Prosopis laevigata*). *J. Food Sci.* **2006,** *71,* 315–320.

Dietze, M. C.; Wolosin, M. S.; Clark, J. S. Capturing Diversity and Interspecific Variability in Allometries: A Hierarchical Approach. *Forest Ecol. Manag.* **2008,** *256,* 1939–1948.

Estrada, C. E.; Yen, M. C.; Delgado, S. A.; Villarreal, Q. J. Legumbres del centro del estado de Nuevo León, México. Anales del Instituto de Biología. Universidad Nacional Autónoma de México. *Serie Botánica.* **2004,** *75,* 73–85.

FAO. Global Forest Resources Assessment 2005, Progress Towards Sustainable Forest Management. Food and Agriculture Organization of the United Nations, Rome, 2006.

Felker, P. Commercializing Mesquite, Leucaena and Cactus in Texas. In *Progress in New Crops*; Janick, J., Ed.; ASHS Press: Alexandria, VA, 1996; pp 133–137.

Franco, L. J.; de la Cruz, A. G.; Cruz, G. A.; Rocha, R. A.; Navarrete, S. N.; Flores, M. G.; Miranda, K. E.; Sánchez, C. S.; Abarca, L. G.; Bedia, S. C. *Manual de ecología.* Ed.; Trillas: Sexta Reimpresión, 2001; pp 266.

Gérardin, P.; Neya, B.; Dumarçay, S.; Pétrissans, M.; Serraj, M.; Huber, F. Contribution of Gums to Natural Durability of *Prosopis africana* Heartwood. *Holzforschung* **2004,** *58,* 39–44.

Gómez A Evaluación de áreas forestales de matorral utilizando un inventario multifásico. Dissertation, Facultad de Ciencias Forestales, Universidad Autónoma de Nuevo León, 2000; p 62.

Hughes, C. Conflict Trees. *Divers. Distrib.* **2001,** *7,* 111–112.

INE. Condiciones generales del ambiente en la frontera norte de México. Resumen ejecutivo, 2005. http://www.ine.gob.mx/ueajei/publicaciones/libros/109/cap2/html

INEGI Estadística del medio ambiente de la zona metropolitana de Monterrey. Aguascalientes, Ags, 2002; pp 311.

Jiménez, J.; Alanís, E.; Ruiz, J. L. Diversidad de la regeneración leñosa del matorral espinoso tamaulipeco con historial agrícola en el NE de México. *Ciencia UANL.* **2012,** *15,* 66–71.

León-Luz, J. L.; Domínguez-Cadena, R.; Díaz-Castro, S. C. Evaluación del peso del leño a partir de variables dimensionales en dos especies de mezquite (*Prosopis articulata* S. Watson y *P. palmeri* S. Watson, en Baja California sur, México. *Acta Botánica Mexicana.* **2005,** *72,* 17–32.

López, B. C.; Rodríguez, R.; Gracia, C. A.; Sabate, S. Climatic Signals in Growth and its Relation to ENSO Events of Two *Prosopis* Species Following a Latitudinal Gradient in South America. *Global Change Biol.* **2006,** *12,* 897–906.

Méndez, E. Ecuaciones de Biomasa para especies de matorral espinoso tamaulipeco del noreste de México. Datos con aplicaciones para inventarios de biomasa. Dissertation, Facultad de Ciencias Forestales. Universidad Autónoma de Nuevo León, 2001.

Meraz, V. S.; Orozco, V. J.; Lechuga, C. J. A.; Cruz, S. F.; Veron, C. J. Mesquite, árbol de gran utilidad. Ciencias 51, 1998.

Moctezuma LG Primer ciclo de seminarios de investigación del CENID-COMEF. México DF. In: *Memorias de Seminario INIFAP-CENID*, 2007; p 38.

Mueller-Dombois, D.; Ellenberg, H. *Aims and Methods of Vegetation Ecology*; Blackburn Press; Caldwell, New Jersey, 1974; pp 45–54 and 93–120.

Návar, J.; Mendez, E.; Graciano, J.; Dale, V.; Parresol, B. Biomass Equations for Shrub Species of Tamaulipan Thornscrub of Northeastern Mexico. *J. Arid Environ.* **2004**, *59*, 657–674.

Pasiecznik, N. M.; Felker, P.; Harris, J. C.; Harsh, L. N.; Cruz, G.; Tewari, J. C.; Cadoret, K.; Maldonado, L. J. The *Prosopis juliflora—Prosopis pallida* Complex: A Monograph. HDRA Coventry UK. Forestry Research Program. Department for International Development, 2001; pp 162.

Pasiecznik, N. *Prosopis* (mesquite, algarrobo): Invasive Weed or Valuable Forest Resource? Forestry Research Programme. HDRA—The Organic Organisation, 2002.

Pasiecznik, N. M.; Harris, P. J. C.; Smith, S. J. Identifying Tropical *Prosopis* Species: A Field Guide, Conventry, UK, 2004.

Richardson, D. M. Forestry Trees as Invasive Aliens. *Conserv. Biol.* **1998**, *12*, 18–26.

Rodríguez, F.C.; Maldonado, A. L. J. Overview of Past, Current and Potential Uses of Mesquite in Mexico. In *Prosopis; Semiarid Fuel Wood and Forage Tree Building Consensus for the Disemfranchised. Center from Semi-arid Forest Resources;* Felker, R., Moss, J., Eds.; Texas A&M University: Washington, DC. EEUU, 1996; pp 6.41–6.52.

Rzedowsky, J. *Vegetación de México*; Limusa, Ed.; México, D. F., 1978; 432 pp.

Rzedowski, J. Análisis de la distribución geográfica del complejo *Prosopis* (Leguminosae, Mimosoideae) en Norteamérica. *Acta Botánica Mexicana.* **1988**, *3*, 7–19.

Salvador, F. J.; Alvarez, S. J. Flora y vegetación. En: Técnicas de muestreo para manejadores de recursos naturales, Bautista, F., Delfín, H., Palacio, J. & Delgado, M. del C. (eds.). Universidad Autónoma de México, Universidad Autónoma de Yucatán, Consejo Nacional de Ciencia y Tecnología, Instituto Nacional de Ecología. 1era. Ed. México. 2004; pp 303–327.

Schefler, W. *Bioestadística*; Fondo Educativo Interamericano, 1981; pp 267.

SEMARNAT. Producción forestal maderable y no maderable. In *Secretaria de Medio Ambiente y Recursos Naturales*, 2007; pp 03–05. http://app1.semarnat.gob.mx/dgeia/indicadores04/07_forestales/ficha_7_2.shtml

Somoza, L.; Vega-Nieva, D.; Ortiz, L. Quality Control of Wood Chips and Wood Pellet from the Biomass Logistic Center of Biopalas. Master's Thesis, University of Vigo, 2014.

Sutton, W. R. J. The Need for Planted Forests and the Example of Radiata Pine. *New For.* **1999**, *17*, 95–110.

USDA. ARS, National Genetic Resources Program. Germplasm Resources Information Network—(GRIN). In *National Germplasm Resources Laboratory*; National Germplasm Resources Laboratory: Beltsville, Maryland, 2007. [Online Database], http://www.ars-grin.gov/cgi-bin/npgs/html/taxgenform.pl?language=en. (accessed January 29, 2007).

Vanclay, J. K. Tree Diameter, Height and Stocking in Evenaged Forests. *Ann. For. Sci.* **2009**, *66*, 702.

Youngquist, J. A.; Hamilton, T. E. Wood Products Utilization. A Call for Reflection and Innovation. *For. Prod. J.* **1999**, *49*, 18–27.

Zamudio, F. J.; Romo Lozano, J. L.; y Cervantes Carrillo, J. O. A. Evaluación financiera y de riesgo de una plantación forestal comercial en Zihuateutla, Puebla. *Rev. Chapingo.* **2010**, *16*, 69–78.

Zar, J. H. *Biostatistical Analysis*, 5th ed.; Prentice-Hall: New Jersey, 2010; p 947.

CHAPTER 6

Research Advances on Native Economic Plants: Trees and Shrubs in Mexico

RATIKANTA MAITI*, HUMBERTO GONZALEZ RODRIGUEZ, and
CH. ARUNA KUMARI

Forest Science Faculty, Universidad de Nuevo Leon, Mexico

Corresponding author. E-mail: ratikanta.maiti@gmail.com

ABSTRACT

The paper narrates a brief review of research advances undertaken by the author and his team on various aspects of native economic plants and also trees and shrubs in Northeast Mexico. Research on native plants includes native crops species, medicinal plants, fiber-yielding plants, cactus spp. The research on medicinal plants in Northeast and highlands of Mexico involved the studies that dealt mainly on ethnobotany, pharmacognosy, phytochemistry, macro- and micronutrients of medicinal plants. Various research methodologies are discussed on different economic plants of Mexico.

The present review makes a synthesis of various aspects of applied biology of more than 30 woody plant species of a Tamaulipan Thorn scrub, Northeastern Mexico on various aspects, such as variability in leaf traits, leaf anatomy, plant characteristics, wood anatomy, wood density, phenology, and few aspects of physiology and biochemistry namely, leaf pigments, leaf epicuticular wax, trees with high nutritional values, carbon fixation, nitrogen and protein contents. The results show a large variability of all the morpho-physiological traits of the woody species related to the coexistence and adaptation of the woody species to the semiarid conditions of Northeast Mexico.

6.1   INTRODUCTION

For more than 30 years as professor and research scientist in two universities, Universidad Autonoma de Nuevo Leeon and Universidad de las Americas in Botany Departments, I have been working on various aspects of economic plants namely, native crop species, medicinal plants, fiber yielding plants, cactus spp., and also on experimental biology of more than 30 woody trees and shrubs at Linares, Northeastern Mexico.

The results have been published as papers in different international journals and books mentioned in the references.

6.2   NATIVE ECONOMIC PLANTS, TREES AND SHRUBS

6.2.1   *NATIVE CROPS IN SEMIARID REGIONS OF NORTHEAST OF MEXICO*

Researches have been undertaken on various aspects of several potential native crop species that are effectively utilized by local inhabitants as food sources. Chile Piquin, wild chili [*capsicum annuum* var aviculare (Dier)]. wild chili, Chile piquin [*Capsicum annuum* var aviculare (Dier)] is of high commercial value for great demand in foreign countries, like USA, domestic culinary values, and medicinal values. This wild chili is grown in its wild habitat on mountains and forests under the shades of trees.

The local inhabitants harvest this wild chili by cutting the branch bearing bunches of round to elongated chili. The seeds of wild chili possess seed dormancy and hard seed coat for which farmers cannot cultivate. The Local inhabitants transplant the plant and grow them in pots that supplies chili for their daily use. An efficient technique was developed to break the dormancy of this wild chili and induce germination.

A small number of seeds are mixed with cow dung extracts in a small flask. The flasks are kept at a low temperature of 4°C for about a week in a refrigerator. The low-temperature induced seeds are then sown superficially in trays that were filled with finely ground soil mixed with organic humus. These trays are given regular slight irrigations so as to keep the soil moist till emergence and growth of the seedlings. When the seedlings are 30 days old, they are transplanted into pots or trays or under the shadow of trees. Wild chili plant requires shade for good growth and productivity.

An efficient technique has been developed by us to break seed dormancy and induce germination. This involves to keep a small number of seeds mixed with extracts of cow dung in a small flask and then keeping it in a refrigerator at 4°C for 7 days and then the treated seeds are sown superficially in trays filled with finely ground soils mixed with organic humus. This needs to be irrigated regularly to keep the soil moist. When the seedlings are about 30 days, we transplant these in pots or trays or under the shadow of trees.

The plant requires shadow for its good growth and productivity. Besides, studies have been undertaken on ecophysiology of this wild chili that included distribution, botany, phenology, pollen viability, biochemistry of chili, macro- and micronutrients, nutritional values, drought resistance related to water potential of the plant (Maiti and Almanza, 1999).

6.2.2   *AMARANTHUS SPP. IN SEMIARID REGIONS OF NORTHEAST MEXICO*

Several species of *Amaranthus* grow in wild conditions in Nuevo Leon, Northeast Mexico.

Studies have been undertaken on botany, anatomy, microsporogenesis, and nutritional values of some species of *Amaranthus*. These studies have shown the presence of large variability in different characteristics among these *Amaranthus* species. A study on nutritional values of vegetable organs of different species of *Amaranthus* showed large variations in nutritional values. Few species, such as *Amaranthus viridis*, *Amaranthus palmeri*, *Amaranthus retroflexus* were found with high-nutritional values, which may be recommended for the nutrition of patients and children but needs to be confirmed.

Therefore, there is a necessity for domestication and cultivation of these selected species as vegetables for human nutrition. A few papers were published that have been mentioned in references.

6.2.3   *PHASEOLUS SPP. PHASELULS VULGARIS*

Beans are very important leguminous crops of high protein content as an important food crop in Mexico, Latin American countries and Asiatic countries. Different aspects of studies have been undertaken on botany and physiology of few wild spp. of *Phaseolus* that grew in Nuevo Leon. Research should be undertaken on the food values of these species.

6.2.4   *BRASSICA SPP.*

Different species of *Brassica* such as *B. campestris, B. oleracea* are important sources of edible oils in the world. We observed that two wild species of *Brassica*, *B. campestris* and *B. oleracea,* grow in wild condition. The studies have been undertaken by us on botany, phenology, and germination of these species (not published). We observed in the case of *B. campestris* that treating its seed in low temperature at 4°C break seed dormancy and induce germination, which needs to be confirmed in future studies. I observed that *B. campestris* was tolerant to cold when most of the plants are killed in one severe winter season.

A study has been made on chemical, nutritional, and functional characterization of *Brassica campestris*. Papers are published on these aspects.

6.2.5   *WILD HELIANTHUS SPP.*

Mexico is considered as the origin of sunflower, *Helianthus*. We observed that this species grows enormously in wild condition. Studies have been undertaken on distribution, botany, and germination of this species. Research needs to be directed on the domestication of this wild species of *Helianthus*.

6.2.6   *MEDICINAL PLANTS*

In Nuevo Leon many native medicinal plants at traditionally used in alleviating various diseases. We analyzed a few macro- and micronutrients of 44 medicinal species used for various diseases. We selected species with high values of macro- and micronutrients.

6.2.6.1   *MACRONUTRIENTS*

A) Species containing high Potassium (K) content on average (mg g^{-1} dw): *Opuntia ficus-indica* (101.47), *Phoradendron villosum* (100.58), *Moringa oleifera* (95.59), *Marrubium vulgare* (91.27), *Melia azadirachta* (90.99), *Hedeoma palmeri* (76.50), *Croton suaveolens* (75.62), *Agave macroculmis* (78.45).

B) Species containing high Magnesium (Mg) content (mg g^{-1} dw): *Opuntia, Ficus indica* (6.39), *Melia azadirachta* (3.41), *Phoradendron villosum* (2.29), *Eriobotrya japonica* (1.78), *Bauhinia forficata* (1.45).

C) Species containing high Phosphorus (P) content (mg g^{-1} dw): *Celtis laevigata* (4.03), *Carya illinoinensis* (2.89), *Phoradendron villosum* (2.40), *Arbutus xalapensis* (1.78), *Hedeoma palmeri* (1.40), *Marrubium vulgare* (1.85).

D) Apart from those mentioned above, there are certain species containing high carbon (C%). These have high carbon dioxide fixation ability. These include the species of *Rhus virens* (50.35), *Arbutus xalapensis* (49.09), *Cinnamomum verum* (49.34), *Tecoma stans* (48.79), *Eriobotrya japonica* (47.98), *Hedeoma palmeri* (46.38), *Moringa oleifera* (45.96), *Buddleja cordata* (45.70), *Carya illinoinensis* (44.27).

E) The species with high Nitrogen (N%) are *Moringa oleifera* (6.25), *Melia azarichta* (5.85), *Marrubium vulgare* (4.56), *Phoradendron villosum* (4.92), *Carya illinoinensis* (3.76), *Buddleja cordata* (3.26), *Celtis laevigata* (3.01).

F) Species containing high C/N ratio: *Agave macroculmis* (30.43), *Arbutus xalapensis* (26.45), *Rhus virens* (22.18), *Cinnamomum verum* (19.78), *Croton suaveolens* (19.37), *Hedeoma palmeri* (16.39), *Eriobotrya japonica* (15.83).

6.2.6.2 MICRONUTRIENTS

A) Species with high Zinc (Zn) content (mg g^{-1} dw) *Tecoma stans* (216.31), *Celtis laevigata* (57.69), *Arbutus xalapensis* (55.20), *Marrubium vulgare* (53.54), *Moringa oleifera* (52.57). B). Species with high Copper (Cu) content (mg g^{-1} dw) *Cinnamomum laevigata* (33.88), *Bauhinia fortificata* (33.40), *Carya illinoiensis* (29.90), *Eryobotria japonica* (26.87).

C) Species with high Iron (Fe) content (mg g^{-1} dw) *Opuntia, Ficus indica* (773.04), *Tecoma stans* (444.82), *Melia azadirachta* (374.78), *Bauhinia forficata* (347.58), *Marrubium vulgare* (334.23).

6.2.6.3 ELITE SPECIES WITH HIGH MACRO- AND MICRONUTRIENTS

A) Potassium, Magnesium, and Phosphorus: *Opuntia, Ficus indica, Phoradendron villosum, Moringa oleifera, Melia azadirachta, Celtis laevigata, Carya illinoinensis.*

B) Nitrogen: *Moringa oleifera, Melia azadirachta, Marrubium vulgare*

C) C/N: *Agave macroculmis, Arbutus xalapensis, Cinnamomum verum, Croton suaveolens, Hedeoma palmeri*

D) Zinc: *Tecoma stans, Celtis laevigata, Arbutus xalapensis*

E) Copper: *Cinnamomum laevigata, Bauhinia forficata, Carya illinoinensis.*

On the basis of macro- and micronutrients we recommend that *Melia azadirachta, Opuntia ficus-indica, Phoradendron villosum, Moringa oleifera, Marrubium vulgare, Celtis laevigata, Carya illinoinensis, Agave macroculmis, Cinnamonum verum, Croton suaveolens,* and *Hedeoma palmeri* could be effectively used for the control of diabetes. Besides, while working in the Biology Department of Universidad de las Americas, I worked in collaboration with Dr. Eugenio Sanchez on ethnobotany and phytochemistry of few medicinal plants used in Puebla for various diseases.

6.2.7   FIBER YIELDING PLANTS

In arid lands of Northeast Mexico, *Agave lecheguilla* and *Yucca carnerosana,* are important sources of fiber, obtained from leaves and also important sources of income of poor arid farmers of this region.

The farmers collected the central young leaf cones, called cogollo, with the help of a hook and then extracted fibers from leaves manually by beating with iron bars or sharp knife or by machine where available. After extraction, they dry the fibers in sun. *Lechuguilla* fibers are strongest fibers used in a polishing machine. Except for few dasonomic studies, no other studies were available on this plant. With the help of students at bachelor, masters, and doctorate levels, we studied various aspects of this fiber plant, such as distribution, ecology, and developmental anatomy of the fibers of this species. Extensive exploitation of this species may lead to extinction.

Overexploitation of many of the native plants may lead to the extinction of these endangered economic plants but no attempts are made for the conservation and propagation of this valuable species of arid lands. On *Yucca carnerosana,* the top of the trunk is cut completely and fibers are extracted manually. This leads to the death of the plants. We made only a few studies on developmental anatomy of the fibers of this plant. In addition, *Henequen, Agave fourcroydes* is cultivated for fiber extraction. A study has been undertaken on developmental anatomy of the fibers of this species.

6.2.8   CACTUS SPP.

Many species of cactus grow in arid lands of Mexico, many of which are endangered. While working in the Universidad las Americas, I undertook a series of studies with the help of my thesis students on various aspects of Cactus spp., botany, morphology, anatomy, phenology, and propagation of species. We developed a simple technique for germination and propagation of more than 60 species. The technique involves sowing the seeds on the soil surface in a tray filled with finely powdered soils mixed with sands and organic matter in a greenhouse.

The trays were covered with polythene sheets with few tube lights fixed above to give light. Cactus needs about 16 h light to induce seed germination. The trays are irrigated regularly with aspersion. Using this novel technique, a greenhouse owner in Puebla could propagate more than 60 species of Cactus with more than 90%.

6.3   RESEARCH ADVANCES ON EXPERIMENTAL BIOLOGY OF WOODY PLANTS OF A TAMAULIPAN THORN SCRUB, NORTHEASTERN MEXICO AND RESEARCH NEEDS

Studies have been undertaken on the biodiversity of leaf traits, leaf anatomy, plant characteristics, wood anatomy, wood density, phenology and few aspects of physiology and biochemistry namely, leaf pigments, leaf epicuticular wax, trees with high nutritional values, carbon fixation, nitrogen, and protein contents. It is suggested that large variations in all these ecophysiological and biochemical components could be related to the coexistence of these species in the semiarid environments of Northeast Mexico.

Some morpho-anatomical traits are considered to be related to adaptation to xeric environments, such as leaf surface, leaf lamina, petiole, venation system, and few wood anatomical and ecophysiological traits, such as pigments, epicuticular wax, leaf nutrients, carbon fixation, etc.

Forests play a great role in offering great service to mankind in reducing carbon dioxide from the atmosphere and converting it to carbon in wood as a source of energy through the process of photosynthesis and supply domestic and industrial products and function as a source of nutrients to grazing animals.

6.3.1   LEAF TRAITS

There exists great diversity in leaf shape, size among woody species for coexistence (Maiti et al., 2015c). Woody plants possess two types of leaves, open canopy (all leaves exposed to sunlight) and close canopy where all leaves are not exposed to sunlight for the capture of solar radiation. It is hypothesized that variability in leaf canopy architecture may be related to photosynthetic efficiency and carbon fixation (which needs to be confirmed in future (Maiti et al., 2014b, 2016d).

6.3.2   LEAF ANATOMY

Leaf anatomical structures, such as leaf surface, leaf lamina, petiole venation pattern, play important roles in the taxonomic delimitation and adaptation of the woody plants to xeric habitats in Northeastern Mexico.

6.3.3   LEAF SURFACE ANATOMY

A study on leaf surface anatomy of 28 species of trees and shrubs showed large variations among species which could be related to drought resistance namely, abundance trichome, sunken stomata on the upper leaf surface, low frequency of stomata. These characteristics could be utilized in the taxonomic delimitation of the species. In the view of the above traits, the species selected for better adaptation to semiarid environments are *Berberis chococo, Celtis laevigata, Condalia hookeri, Diospyros palmeri, Diospyros texana, Ebenopsis ebana, Ehretia anacua, Forestiera angustifolia, Havardia pallens, Helieta parviflora, Karwinskia humboldtiana, Sargantia gregii, Sideroxylon celastriana, Zanthoxylum fagara*. The water relations and drought resistance of the species mentioned should be confirmed in a future study.

6.3.4   ANATOMY OF LEAF LAMINA

A study was undertaken to determine the variability in leaf anatomical traits and its relation to taxonomic delimitation and adaptation of the species to xeric environments. There exists a large variability of anatomical traits with respect to cuticle thickness, presence or absence, the length and compactness of palisade cells of trichomes, etc., which could be related to the taxonomic delimitation and the adaptation of the species to drought conditions. Some species, such as *Karwinskia humoldtiana, Lantana macropoda, Prosopis laevigata, Zanthoxylum fragara, Helieta paviflora, Acacia berlandieri*, possess long and compact palisade cells, which are expected to be efficient in photosynthetic function and adaptation to drought. Future research needs to be directed in this direction (Maiti et al., unpublished).

6.3.5 PETIOLE ANATOMY

A comparative study on petiole anatomy of 36 woody species has revealed a large variability among species in various anatomical traits that can be used in taxonomic delimitation. Species were grouped on the basis of various petiole anatomical traits.

Only five species having large vascular bundle are efficient in the transport of nutrients and water, namely, *Acacia berlandieri, Acacia rigidula, Diospyros palmeri, Fraxinus greggii, Guaiacum angustifolia*, thick petiole (*Acacia berlandieri, Acacia farnesiana, Berberis chococo, Bernardia myricifolia, Eysenhardtia texana*), and mechanical tissues, such as thick cuticle (*Acacia berlandieri, Celtis pallida, Condalia hookeri, Eysenhardtia texana, Gymnosperma glutinosum*), a thick collenchyma *(Acacia farnesiana, Berberis chococo, Bernardia myricifolia, Celtis pallida, Havardia pallens*), and extra sclerenchyma bands that offer mechanical strength (*Acacia berlandieri, Ebenopsis ebano, Eysenhardtia texana, Lantana macropoda, Prosopis laevigata, Xanthoxylum fagara*).

The species having the combination of various desirable traits are expected to be more efficient in the physiological function and mechanical support such as *Acacia berlandieri.*

6.3.6 VENATION PATTERN AND VENATION SYSTEM

Venation gives mechanical strength to the leaf lamina and helps in the conduction of carbohydrates (photosynthates) and nutrients.

Among the species studied *Eysenhardtia texana* had maximum vein islet density, *Ebenopis ebano, Caesalpinia mexicana, Karwinskia humboldtiana*, etc., possessed medium density, whereas *Guaiacum officinale, Amyris madrensis, Sargentia greggii* had low density (Maiti et al., 2015h).

6.3.7   PLANT CHARACTERISTICS AND RELATIONSHIP

Woody plant species show large variations in various plant characteristics, such as type of leaf canopy, tree crown architecture, plant height, canopy cover, basal diameter, branching patterns, and branching density, and there exist relationships among these parameters (Maiti et al., 2015d, Maiti and Rodriguez et al., 2016d).

6.3.7.1   TREE CROWN

Every tree species possesses a typical tree top crown architecture, such as globose, round, irregular architecture, with the association of branches and leaves which help in the capture of solar radiation. Few studies have been undertaken in these aspects.

6.3.7.2   BRANCHING PATTERN AND BRANCHING DENSITY

Branching pattern and crown architecture act as a solar panel in the capture of solar radiation. Three types of branching patterns are found in trees and shrubs, such as monopodial, pseudopodial, and sympodial. The tree crown varies from globose, irregular, to conical patterns (Maiti et al., 2015c).

A study has been undertaken on the perspectives of branching pattern and branching density in 30 woody trees and shrubs. The types of branching observed are monopodial, pseudomonopodial, and sympodial. The branching density observed through animation photography in the field has revealed the presence of three types of branching density, that is, high, medium, and low density. There exist differences in height, biomass, basal trunk, the angle of the primary and secondary branches (Maiti et al., 2015d).

6.3.7.3   WOOD ANATOMY

Wood is an industrial product of great economic importance derived from cambial activity in a tree. Wood is composed of secondary xylem vessels, wood fibers, wood parenchyma, and other products. Significant research inputs have been documented on wood anatomy. Several studies have been undertaken on variability in wood anatomical traits, such as porosity, vessel diameter, their orientations, wood parenchyma, the density of wood sclerenchyma, on the basis of which species may be selected for fabrication of strong furniture or papers, etc.

Most of the species are ring to semiring porous, few diffuse-porous. Fiber cells show large variations in the morphology, length, cell wall thickness, lumen breadth, on the basis of which species may be selected for strong furniture or paper pulp.

Many species possess narrow vessels, which are considered to work against cavitation or occulosis with small narrow vessels, mentioned have a strategy to adapt both to hot and cold climate against cavitation. The species having big vessel diameter may be susceptible to droughts, such as *Celtis pallida*, *Caesalpinia mexicana* or they may have a deep root system for adaptation to semiarid climates in northeast Mexico. Statistically significant differences are observed in all wood anatomical parameters among species studied (Maiti et al., 2016, Maiti et al., 2016d). A study has been undertaken on the variability of wood fiber cell morphology, length, breadth, the cell wall thickness in relation to their potential utility (Maiti et al., 2016; Maiti et al., 2016). Similarly, various studies in different aspects have been published (Maiti et al., 2015, Maiti and Rodriguez, 2015d, Maiti et al., 2016d).

6.3.7.4   REPRODUCTIVE BIOLOGY

In a forest ecosystem trees and shrubs start flowering, fruitification, and finally disperse seeds for maintenance of their life cycles. A study has been undertaken on flowering, fruiting phenology of 12 woody trees at Linares, Northeast Mexico (Maiti and Rodriguez, 2015a). There exists a large variability in the phenological stages among species. The results clearly demonstrate the variation in phenological time schedule among different species.

A study has been made on phenology and pollen viability of four woody species revealing that temperature plays an important role in pollen viability (Maiti and Rodriguez, 2015a).

6.3.8   PHYSIOLOGY AND BIOCHEMISTRY

6.3.8.1   LEAF PIGMENTS

A study has been made on pigment contents (chlorophyll and carotenoid) in 37 species of trees and shrubs in Northeast of Mexico during summer season (Maiti et al., 2016). Large variations were observed in the contents of chlorophyll (a and b and total) and also carotenoids among species. In a study there exists seasonal variation of leaf pigments in trees and shrubs in summer and winter seasons, the species contained lower pigments during winter seasons (Maiti et al., 2016d).

6.3.8.2   EPICUTICULAR WAX

Several woody species in the semiarid regions of Northeastern Mexico possess waxy leaf surface owing to the presence of epicuticular wax. It has been documented that epicuticular wax helps in the reflection of sunlight from the leaf surface, thereby, reducing radiation load and maintaining lower leaf temperature and thereby imparting drought.

A study has been undertaken on the variability of leaf epicuticular wax. Few species were selected with high epicuticular wax namely, *Foresteria angustifolia* (702.04 g/cm^2), *Diospyros texana* (607.65 g/cm^2), *Bernardia myricifolia* (437.53 g/cm^2), *Leucophyllum leucocephala* (388.50 g/cm^2), during summer. These species could be adapted under the semiarid condition for their capacity in the reflectance of radiation load, thereby, reducing gas exchange and probably impart drought resistance, water relations, etc. (Maiti et al., 2015f).

6.3.8.3   MACRO-AND MICRONUTRIENTS

Woody plants possess various leaf nutrients that help in the growth and development of the species and serve as sources of nutrients for grazing animals. A study was undertaken to estimate six nutrients in the leaves, three macronutrients (K, Mg, and P), and three micronutrients (Cu, Fe, and Zn) of 25 woody species (Maiti et al., 2016d).

Macronutrients and micronutrient contents (Cu, Fe, Mn, Zn, Ca, K, Mg, P, C, and N) of 10 native species exhibit large variations among species in the contents of the nutrients. K values ranged from round about 6.80–75.62 mg g^{-1}; Mg content ranges 0.22–5.29 mg g^{-1}, P from 0.09 to 2.43 mg g^{-1}, Cu from 0.09 to 2.8 to 30.71 g gps^{-1}, Fe from 66.32 to 276 g gps^{-1}, Zn from 10.23 to 144.86 g gps^{-1}. *Croton suaveolens* acquired highest level of P (2.43 mg g^{-1}) and K (75.62 mg g^{-1}), whereas *Parkinsonia aculeata* for Mg (5.29 mg g^{-1}), *Cordia boissieri* for both Cu (30.71 g gps^{-1}) and Fe (280.55 g gps^{-1}), on the other hand, *Salix lasiolepis* for Zn (144.86 g gps^{-1}).

These species could serve as excellent sources for ruminants and could adapt and grow well for high nutrient contents. The values of mineral contents were much higher than required by the grazing ruminants. The present study was undertaken to estimate six nutrients in the leaves, five macronutrients (P, Mg, K, C, N), and three micronutrients (Cu, Fe, and Zn).

Among macronutrients, P varied from 0.78 to 243 (mg g^{-1}dw), the species containing high P are *Croton suaveolens*, 2.43; *Eysenhardtia polystachya*, 1.84; *Prosopis laevigata*, 1.65; *Parkinsonia aculeata*, 1.56; *Acacia farnesiana*, 1.54, Mg varied from 0.22 to 9.45 (mg g^{-1}d w). The species containing high Mg (mg g^{-1} dw) are *Ehretia anacua*, 9.45; *Condalia hookeri*, 6.50; *Parkinsonia aculeata*, 5.29.

6.3.8.4   BIODIVERSITY OF LEAF CHEMISTRY (ON PIGMENTS, EPICUTICULAR WAX AND MACRO AND MICRONUTRIENTS)

A study was undertaken on pigments, epicuticular wax, and macro- and micronutrients of 15 woody species (Maiti et al., 2015) showing large variability in leaf chemical components. For example, species with high chlorophyll content were *Ebenopsis ebano* (1.755). Similarly, there were variations in chlorophyll a and chlorophyll b among species.

The species showing high-epicuticular wax load are *Forestiera angustifolia* (702.04 g/cm^2), *Diospyros texana* (607.65 g/cm^2), *Bernardia myricifolia* (437.53 g/cm^2). There is a need to confirm the efficiency of these selected species for productivity and adaptation of the species to the environment (Maiti et al., 2016c, Maiti and Rodriguez, 2015b).

Carbon, nitrogen, and protein content. González Rodrígue et al. (2015c) reported large variation in leaf carbon, nitrogen, and protein content among 44 woody species at Linares, Northeast Mexico. In this study, a few species were selected with high carbon fixation, namely *Eugenia caryophyllata* (61.66%), *Litsea glauscensens* (51.54 %), *Rhus virens* (30.35%), *Gochantia hypoleuca* (49.86%), *Pinus arizonica* (49.32%), *Erybotrya japonica* (4.98%) and *Tecoma stans* (47.79%).

It is recommended that some of these species with high-carbon sequestration capacity may be planted in carbon polluted areas to reduce carbon load from the atmosphere, in addition, these, high-carbon concentration species, could serve as a good source of energy.

In this study, few species were selected with high nitrogen content namely, *Mimosa malacophylla* (8.44%), *Capscicum annum* wild chili (6.84%), *Azadirachta indica* (5.85%), *Eruca sativa* (5.46%), *Rosamarinus officinales* (5.40-%), *Mentha piperata* (5.40-%).

Few species were selected with high C/N ratio namely, *Arbutus xala-pensis* (26.94%), *Eryngium heterophyllum* (24.29%), *Rhus virens* (22.52%), *Croton suveolens* (20.16%), which may be related to high production of secondary metabolites [Maiti et al. (2016))].

6.4   CONCLUSIONS

Maiti et al. (2016e) suggested adaptive morpho-physiological traits of woody plants for coexistence in a forest ecosystem. It is discussed that woody plants being dominant vegetation in a forest ecosystem of semiarid Mexico possess specific morpho-anatomical, ecophysiological, and biochemical traits for adaptation in the semiarid environments with special reference to hot summer and cool winter, similar to the environments prevalent in Mediterranean climates. The paper put forward a few hypothetical concepts for coexistence and adaptation of woody plant species in a Tamaulipan Thorn Scrub, Northeastern Mexico. The hypotheses have been put forwarded on the basis of our results on various morphological, anatomical, and ecophysiological traits of a Tamaulipan Thorn Scrub, Northeastern Mexico. Few future research lines are suggested to confirm the hypotheses.

KEYWORDS

- **economic plants**
- **native crops species**
- **medicinal plants**
- **fiber-yielding plants**
- **cactus spp.**
- **experimental biology**
- **woody plants**

REFERENCES

Alanís G.; Gudalupe, M. Chemical, Nutritional and Functional Characterization of Proteins Extracted from Wild Mustard (*Brassica campestris*, Brassicaceae) Seeds from Nuevo Leon, Mexico. *Econ Bot* **1995,** *49*, 260–268.

Almanza, E. L.; Maiti, R. K. Variation in Nutritional Quality of Wild Chilli "Chile piquín" (*Capsicum annuum* var. *aviculare* Dierb) at Different Stages of Fruit Maturity: A Preliminary Study. *Crop. Res.* **2004**, *27*, 113–115.

Almanza, E. J. G.; Maiti, R. K. El chile piquín (*Capsicum annuum* var. aviculare): Una planta de alto potential alimentcio. *Reforma siglo* **1994**, *27*, 77–86.

Crispin del Rio, Z.; Maiti, R. K. Evaluation of Two Treatments on Germination of *Echinocactus grusonii* (Cactaceae) in Xocoyucan, Tlaxcala, México. *Crop Res.* **2003**, *26*, 175–177.

González, D. I.; García, G. Cuantificación de compuestos antinutricionales de cuatro especies silvestres de *Amaranthus* en Nuevo León. *Turrialba* **1992**, *42*, 487–491.

Gonzalez, R. H.; Maiti, R. K. Phenology (Flowering and fruiting) of Ten Woody Plants in Linares, Mexico. *Int J. Biores. Stress Manag.* **2015**, 6, 438–446.

Gonzalez, R. H.; Maiti, R.; Valencia, N. R. I.; Sarkar, N. C. Carbon and Nitrogen Content in Leaf Tissue of Different Plant Species, Northeastern Mexico. *Int J. Biores. Stress Manag.* **2015**, *6*, 113–116.

Gonzalez, R. H.; Maiti, R. K., Kumari, A., Sarkar, N. C. Variability in Wood Density and Wood Fibre Characterization of Woody Species and Their Possible Utility in Northeastern Mexico. *Am. J. Plant Sci.* **2016**, *7*, 1139–1150.

Gonzalez, R. H.; Maiti, R. K.; Duenas, T. H. A.; Linan, G. M. I.; Gonzalez, J. C. D.; Kumari, A. Variation in Leaf Traits of 34 Trees and Shrubs in Summer Season in Linares, North-Eastern Mexico. *Int J. Biores. Stress Manag.* **2015**, *6*, 707–718.

González, C. O.; Maiti, R. K. Estudio de las plantas alimenticias del Municipio de Matehual, S.L.P., México. *Publicaciones Biológicas* **1991**, *5*, 1–3.

Hernandez, C. B.; Maiti, R. K. Conocimiento sobre la utilización, valor nutricional y composición química del grano de mijo perla (Pennisetum americanum L., Leeke) para alimentación de pollos. *Publicaciones Biológicas* **1992**, *6*, 195–202.

Maiti, R. K.; Almanza, J. Seed Coat Ultrastructure and a Method for Inducing Rapid Germination of the Wild Chili "chile piquín" (Capsicum annuum var. aviculare D. & E., Solanaceae). *Phyton-Intl. J. Exp. Bot.* **1997**, *59*, 73–78.

Maiti, R. K., Luna, O. H. A. Crecimiento y desarrollo de genotipos de frijol (*Phaseolus vulgaris* L.) inoculados con *Rhizobium leguminosarum biovar. phaseoli. Universidad & Ciencia* **1992**, *9*, 83–93.

Maiti, R. K.P; Cuervo P. J A. Morphology and Anatomy of Some Cactus Species Adapted in High Land Valley of Puebla, México. *Crop Res.* **2002**, *24*, 137–144.

Maiti, R. K.; Hernández, P. J. L. Seed Utrastructure and Germination of Some Species Cactaceae. *Phyton Int. J. Exp. Bot.* **1994**, *55*, 97–105.

Maiti. R. K.; Valdez, C. E. El girasol silvestre (Helianthus annus L.) como una alternativa de forraje verde. *Biotam* **1991**, *3*, 27–35.

Maiti, R. K.; Veléz, S. A. Comparative Study of the Germination of Three Species of Cacataceae of Puebla, México. *Crop Res.* **2002**, *24*, 145–148.

Maiti, R. K.; Verde S. J. Evalution of Some Glossy Sorghum Strains for Epicuticular Wax, Chlorophyll and Hydrocyanic Acid Content at the Seedling Stage. *Publicaciones Biológicas* **1991**, *5*, 27–30.

Maiti, R. K.; Wesche, E. P. Especies silvestres de *Amaranthus* en Nuevo León, México. III. Distribución, descripción y morfoanatomía. *Universidad & Ciencia* **1993**, *10*, 17–26.

Maiti, R. K.; Perdomo, V. J. A Novel Technique for the Germination and Propagation of Four Species of *Astrophytum* (Cactaceae). *Crop Res.* **2002**, *24*, 149–153.

Maiti, R. K.; Rodriguez, H. G. Mysetry of Coexistence and Adaptation of Trees in a Forest Ecosystem. *Forest Res.* **2015,** *4,* 4. (DOI:10.4172/2168-9776.1000e120).

Maiti, R. K.; Gómez, B. Germination and propagation of seven species of Cactaceae. *Crop Research.* 2003, *23,* 536–539.

Maiti, R. K.; González De la, C. Estructura floral y microesporogenesis de 5 especies de Amaranthus del Centre de Nuevo León. *Universidad y Ciencia.* **1994,** *11,* 61–76.

Maiti, R. K.; Hernandez, P. J. Variability in Leaf Epicuticular Wax and Surface Characteristics in Glossy Sorghum Genotypes (Sorghum bicolor L. Moench) and its Possible Relation to Shoot Fly (Atherigona soccata Rond.) and Drought Resistance at the Seedling Stage. *Publica'ones Biológicas.* **1992,** *6,* 159–168.

Maiti, R. K.; Hernandez, P. J. L. Seed Ultrastructure and Germination of Some Species of Cactaceae. *Phyton* **1994,** *55,* 97–105.

Maiti, R. K.; Sanchez, A. E. Ethnobotanical Study of 17 Medicinal Plants in Puebla City and Cholula. *Crop Res.* **2003,** *25,* 369–374.

Maiti, R. K.; Almanza, J. G. Some Aspects of the Morphology and Anatomy of the Wild Chili Chile Piquin (*Capsicum annuum* L.) var aviculare, D /E. Solanaceae in Nuevo Leon, Mexico. *BioTAM* **1999,** *11,* 19.

Maiti, R. K.; Baquie L. A. Propagation, conservation, and creation of a germplasm bank of Cactaceae at the Seedling Stage in a Greenhouse Nursery. *Crop Res.* **2002,** *24,* 532–537.

Maiti, R. K.; Baquie, L. A. A Review on *Ferocactus* Species of Cactaceae. *Crop Res.* **2003,** *26,* 208–218.

Maiti, R. K.; Barrillas, G. A. L. Germination and Propagation of Seven Species of Cactaceae. *Crop Res.* **2002,** *23,* 536–539.

Maiti, R. K.; Cuervo, P. J. A. Floral Biology of Three Species of *Mammillaria.* *Crop Res.* **2002,** *24,* 154–160.

Maiti, R. K.; Diaz, D. C. The Methods of Inducing Germination, Seedling Development in the Laboratory and Propagation of Two Species of *Mammillaria* in Green House Culture. *Crop Res.* **2001,** *22,* 241–247.

Maiti, R. K.; Díaz, S. A. Variability in Seed Viability of Seven Species of Cactaceae in Reserve Biosphere of Tehuácan-Cuítlan, Mexico. *Crop Res.* **2002,** *23,* 546–548.

Maiti, R. K.; Perdome H. V. A Novel Technique for the Germination and Propagation of Four Species of *Astrophytum* (Cactacae). *Crop Res.* **2002,** *24,* 149–153.

Maiti, R. K.; Villareal, L. Some Aspects on Pharmacognosy of Ten Species of the Family Solanaceae Utilized in Traditional Medicine. *Caldasia.* **2002,** *24,* 317–321.

Maiti, R. K.; Brrillas, L. A. Management and Intensive Production of Species of Cactaceae in a Greenhouse Nursery: A Model. *Crop Res.* **2002,** *23,* 394–396.

Maiti, R. K.; López, I. M. Evaluación de lineas de sorgo (*Sorghum bicolor* L. Moench.) para su tolerancia a diferentes niveles de temperatura en etapa de plántula. *Publicaciones Biológicas* **1991,** 5, 22–26.

Maiti, R. K.; Martínez, M. A. Quantitative Description of Morphoanatomical Characters and Productivity of Lechuguilla (Agave lecheguilla torr.) (Agavaceae), Villa de García, Nuevo León, México. *Publicaciones biológicas F.C.B.* **1990,** *4,* 29–34.

Maiti R. K.; Velázquez P. H.; Dermal Characteristics of Stems of Five Species of *Astrophytum* (Cactaceae). *Crop Res.* **2003,** *25,* 539–545.

Maiti, R. K.; Olvera, P. R. A. Medicinal Plant Species Selected and Confirmed for Their Efficiency to Cure Different Diseases. *Crop Res.* **2003,** *25,* 550–554.

Maiti R. K.; Prasad R. K. E. Characterisation and Evaluation of Glossy Sorghum Germplasm for Some Agronomic Traits for Their Use in Fodder and Grain Improvement. *Publicaciones Biológicas* **1992**, *6l*, 169–172.

Maiti, R. K.; Ramírez, B. O. Dermal Surface Comparison Between Some Species of Cactaceae and its Possible Relation with Adaptation to Arid Conditions. *Crop Res.* **2002**, *23*, 540–545.

Maiti, R. K.; Sánchez, A. E. Variability in Nutritional Values of Grains of Maize "Criollo" Compared to those of Maize Hybrids. *Crop Res.* **2003**, *25*, 582–584.

Maiti R. K.; Sánchez, A. E. Effects of Different Light-temperature Treatments over Germination Responses and Seedling Development of Some Agave spp. *Res. Crops.* **2005**, *6*, 587–595.

Maiti, R. K.; Sánchez, A. Dermal Surface Characteristics of Leaves in Medicinal Plants as Detective Characters and its Possible Relation with their Medicinal Effects. *Crop Res.* **2002**, *24*, 517–522.

Maiti, R. K.; Valades, M. M. A Study on Floral Morphology and Phenology of Some Species of Cactaceae in the Semi-arid Regions of Nuevo León, Mexico. *Crop Res.* **2001**, *22*, 339–344.

Maiti, R. K.; Marroquin, V. M. A Study on Floral Morphology and Phenology of Some Species of Cactaceae in the Semi-arid regions of Nuevo Leon. *Crop Res.* **2001**, *22*, 57–68.

Maiti, R. K.; Vélez, S. Α. Propagation and Conservation of Cacti (including endangered, rare and vulnerable) in High Land Valleys of Mexico. *Crop Res.* **2002**, *24*, 538–544.

Maiti R. K.; Veléz S. A. Visnaga (*Echinocactus platyacanthus* Link & Otto)- an Endangered Gigantic Cactus: Morphology, Distribution, Germination and Crop Management. *Crop Res.* **2002**, *24*, 545–555.

Maiti, R. K.; Vélez, S. A. Modifying a Technique to Stimulate Natural Conditions for Enhancing seed Germination and Rapid Propagation of Eight Species of Cactaceae. *Crop Res.* **2003**, *25*, 546–549.

Maiti, R. K.; Villarreal, R. Some Aspects on Pharmacognosy of Ten Species of the Family Solanaceae Utilized in Traditional Medicine. *Caldasia* **2002**, *24*, 317–321.

Maiti, R. K.; Wesche E. P. Especies silvestres de Amaranthus de Nuevo León, México. I. Aspectos Ecologicos y Botánicos. *Universidad & Ciencia* **1991**, *8*, 61–67.

Maiti, R. K.; Flores, W. E. A Study on Phenology and Nutritional Values of Wild Species of *Brassica campestris* L. and *Sisumbrium irio* L. (Cruciferae) in the Semiarid Regions of Monterrey, N. L., Mexico. *Crop Res.* **2003**, *26*, 414–419.

Maiti R. K. Seed Grmination Technique For Massive Production of Cactus in Agren House. *Agrobios Newsletter.* **2007**, *4*, 44–45.

Maiti, R. K.; Baquie L. A. Tércnica sencilla de germinación, propagaci'ón and conservación de cactus para campesinos. *Fundación Produce Puebla.* **2002**, 16.

Maiti, R. K.; Carrillo, G. M. J. The Responses of Sorghum with Short and Long Mesocotyl Under Different Stress Conditions. *Publicaciones Biológicas* **1991**, *5*, 18–21.

Maiti, R. K.; De La Riba. General Morphology, Growing Condition and Development of Fiber Filaments in Lechuguilla (*Agave lecheguilla* Torr.). *Turrialba* **1993**, *42*, 45–51.

Maiti, R. K.; Wesche E. P. Especies silvestres de Amaranthus de Nuevo León,México. II. Patrones de crecimiento. *Universidad y Ciencia* **1991**, *8*, 69–76.

Maiti, R. K.; Para, A. C.; Rodriguez, H. G.; Paloma, S. V. Characterization of Wood Fibres of Scrubs and Tree Species of the Tamaulipan Thornscrub, Northeastern Mexico and its Possible Utilization. *Forest Res.* **2015**, *4*, 154.

Maiti, R. K.; Rodriguez, H. G.; Gonzalez E. A.; Kumari, A.; Sarkar, N. C.; Variability in Epicuticular Wax in 35 Woody Plants in Linares, Northeast Mexico. *Forest Res.* **2015,** *5.*

Maiti, R. K.; Rodriguez, H. G.; Kumari A. Nutrient Profile of Native Woody Species and Medicinal Plants in Northeastern Mexico: A Synthesis. *J Bioprocess Biotech* **2016,** *6,* 283.

Maiti, R. K.; Rodriguez, H. G.; Kumari A. Adaptive Morpho-physiological Traits of Woody Plants for Co-existence in a Forest Ecosystem. *Forest Res.* **2016,** *5,* 175.

Maiti, R. K.; Rodriguez, H. G.; Sarkar, N. C.; Kumari, A. Biodiversity in Leaf Chemistry (Pigments, Epicuticular Wax and Leaf Nutrients) in Woody Plant Species in North-eastern Mexico, a Synthesis. *Forest Res.* **2016,** *5,* 170.

Maiti, R. K.; Rodriguez, H. G. M.; Kumari, A.; Díaz, J. C. G. Perspectives of Branching Pattern and Branching Density in 30 Woody Trees and Shrubs in Tamulipan Thornscrub, Northeast of Mexico. *Forest Res.* **2015,** *4,* 4.

Maiti, R. K.; Rodriguez, H. G. Wood Anatomy Could Predict the Adaption of Woody Plants to Environmental Stresses and Quality of Timbers. *Forest Res.* **2015,** *4,* 4.

Maiti, R. K.; Rodriguez, H. G. Eco-physiologically Highly Efficient Woody Plant Species in Northeastern Mexico. *Forest Res.* **2015,** *4,* 4.

Maiti, R. K.; Rodriguez, H. Phenology, Morphology, and Variability in Pollen Viability of Four Woody Trees (*Cordia boissieri, Parkinsonia texana, Parkinsonia aculeate and Leucophyllum frutescens* Exposed to Environmental Temperatures in Linares, Northeastern Mexico. *Forest Res.* **2015,** S1, 002. DOI:10.4172/2168-9776.S1-002.

Maiti, R. K.; Perdomo, V. H.; Singh V. P. Comparative Morphology of Six Species of Mother Plants of *Astrophytum* Grown in a Greenhouse. *Crop Res.* **2003,** *25,* 530–538.

Maiti, R. K.; Rodriguez, H. G.; Sarkar, N. C.; Thakur, A. K. Branching Pattern and Leaf Crown Architecture of Some Tree and Shrubs in Northeast Mexico. *Int J. Biores. Stress Manag.* **2015,** *6,* 41–50.

Maiti, R. K.; Rodriguez H. G.; Ivanova N. S. *Autoecology and Ecophysiology of Woody Shrubs and Trees.* John Wiley and Sons: New Jersey, USA, 2016; pp 331.

Maiti, R. K., Rodriguez, H. G.; Kumari, A. *Applied Biology: A Model*; American Academic Press: 2016; pp 359.

Maiti, R. K.; Rodriguez, H. G.; Karfakis, T. N. S. Variability in Leaf Canopy Architecture may be Related to Photosynthetic Efficiency and Carbon Fixation. IJBSM5 **2014,** *4,* 20–25.

Maiti, R. K.; Rodriguez, H. G.; Kumari A. Wood Density of Ten Native Trees and Shrubs and Its Possible Relation with Few Wood Chemical Composition and Wood Structure. *Am. J. Plant Sci.* **2016.**

Maiti, R. K.; Rodriguez, H. G.; Mermolejo, J.; Gonzalez, M. I. L. Venation Pattern and Venation Density of Few Native Woody Species in Linares, Northeast of Mexico. *J. Biores. Stress Manag.* **2015,** *6,* 719–727.

Maiti, R. K.; Rodriguez, H. G.; Dueñas, T. H. A.; Diaz, J. C., Kumari A. Comparative Petiole Anatomy of 36 Woody Plant Species in Northeastern Mexico and its Significance in Taxonomy and Adaptation. *J. Biores. Stress Manag.* (in press) **2016.**

Maiti, R. K.; Rodriguez, H. G.; Karfakis, T. Variability in Leaf Traits of 14 Native Woody Species in Semiarid Regions of Northeastern Mexico. *IJBSM* **2014,** *5.*

Maiti, R. K.; Perdome, V. H. Comparative Anatomy of Stems of Six Species of *Astrophytum* (Cactaceae): A Preliminary Study. *Crop Res.* **2003,** *25,* 153–158.

Maiti, R. K.; Rodriguez, H.; Kumari, A. Tree and Shrubs with High Carbon Fixation/ concentration. *Forest Res.* **2015,** 94–96.

Moreno, L. S.; Maiti, R. K. Morfología, ultraestructura y contenido de minerales en semilla y desarrollo de las plántula de 5 especies silvestres, una semi-cultivada y una cultivada de frijol (*Phaseolus* spp.) *Phyton* **1994**, *55*, 9–22.

Moreno, L. S.; Maiti R. K. Una revision de los aspectos morfo-anátomicos, fisiológicos y bioquímicos de especies silvestres y cultivadas de frijol. *Universidad Ciencia & Tecnología* **1994**, *2*, 1–13.

Moreno L. S., Maiti R. K. Differential Responses of Two Bean Cultivars (Phaseolus vulgaris L.) Resistant and Suceptible to Water Stress in the Seedling Growth and Mineral Uptake. *Res. Crops* **2000**, *1*, 20–24.

Rodriguez, H. G.; Maiti, R. K.; Kumari, A. Biodiversity of Leaf Traits in Woody Plants in Northeastern Mexico: A Syntheisis. *Forest Res.* **2016**.

Sánchez, A. E., Maiti R. K., Some Aspects on Nutritional Values and Preliminary Phytochemistry of Mexican Wild Chilli "Cihle Piquín" (*Capsicum annuum* var aviculare Dierb.) (D. & E.). *Phyton-Intl. Exp. Bot.* **2003**, *53*, 105–107.

Sanchez, A. E.; Maiti R. K. Contribution to Medicinal Uses and Chemistry of Some Species of Agave: A Review. *Crop Res. J.* **2001**, *23*, 375–381.

Sánchez, A. E.; Maiti, R. K. Ethnomedicine of Cuetzalan, Puebla (Mexico). *Crop Res.* **2003**, *26*, 178–184.

Sanchez, A. E.; Maiti, R. K. Preliminary Study on Pharmacognosy and Phytochemistry of Two Mexican Medicinal Plants, "Gordolobo" (*Bocconia frutescens* L. [Papavaceae]) and "Candelaria" (*Ipomoea bracteata* Cav. [Convolvulaceae]). *Phyton-Int. J. Exp. Bot.* **2002**, 107–111.

Sánchez, A. E.; Maiti R. K. Contributions to Medicinal Uses and Chemistry of Some Species of *Agave*: A Review. *Crop Res.* **2002**, *23*, 375–381.

Sánchez, A. E.; Maiti, R. K. A Preliminary Study on Morpho-anatomical Characters and Secondary Metabolites of Agave "mezcalero" (Agave potatorum). *Phyton-Intl. J. Exp. Bot.* **2003**, *53*, 81–83.

Sánchez, A. E.; Maiti R. K. Contribution to Medicinal Uses and Chemistry of Some Species of *Agave*: A Review. *Crop Res. J.* **2001**, *23*, 156–166.

Sánchez, A. E.; Maiti R. K. A Comparative Preliminary Study on the Phytochemistry of *Ipomoea murucoides* and *Ipomoea arborescence* (Family Convulaceae) of Common use in Cholula, Puebla and other region of Tehuacan, Puebla, México. *Res. Crops.* **2003**, *4*, 254–257.

Sánchez, A. E.; Maiti, R. K. Preliminary Study on Pharmacognosy and Phytochemistry of two Mexican Plants, "Gordolobo" (*Bocconia frutescens* L. (Papavaraceae) and "Candelaria" (*Ipomoea bracteata* Cav. (Convulacae). *Phyton-Intl. Exp. Bot.* **2002**, *107*, 111.

Sánchez, A. E.; Maiti R. K. Therapeutic Properties, Botany and Chemistry of *Origanum majorana*-A Review. *Crop Res.* **2003**, *25*, 385–393.

Sánchez A. E.; Maiti R. K. Therapeutic Properties, Botany and Chemistry of Mexican Arnica (*Heterotheca inuloides*). *Crop Res.* **2002**, *24*, 58–62.

Sánchez, A. E.; Maiti, R. K. Traditional Uses and a Preliminary Study on the Phytochemistry of Nine Medicinal Plant Species of Common Use in High Land of Puebla and Tlaxcala, Mexico. *Crop Res.* **2005**, 30, 113–118.

Torres, C. T. E.; Maiti R. K. Estructura, composición química y valor nutricional del grano de sorgo (Sorghum biocolor (L.) Moench.). *Publicaciones Biológicas.* **1991**, *5*, 97–109.

Villarreal, R. L.; Maiti, R. K. Características morfoanatómicas y productividad de fibra en Agave lecheguilla Torr., en Nuevo León, México. *Turrialba* **1991**, *41*, 423–429.

Villarreal, R. L.; Maiti R. K. Características morfo-anátomicas de la hoja y fibra en Yucca carnerosana (Trel) McKelvey. *Publicaciones Biológicas* **1991,** *5,* 32–35.

Villarreal, R. L.; Maiti R. K. Estudio anatómico de la fibra de henequen (Agave fourcroydes Lemaire). *BioTAM* **1991,** *3,* 9–14.

Villarreal, R. L.; Maiti, R. K. Estudio cuantitativo de las características morfológicas y anatómicas de la hoja en Agave asperrima Jacobi. *Pubicaciones Biológicas* **1991,** *5,* 36–38.

Villarreal, R. L.; Lozano M. E. Productividad de la fibra en hojas de Agave lecheguilla Torrey, en siete localidaddes de Mina, Nuevo Léon, México. *Publicaciones Biológicas* **1991,** *5,* 23–26.

Villarreal, R. L.; Maiti R. K. Crecimiento y desarrollo de la fibra de Yucca carnerosano (Trel.) McKelvey. *Phyton-Int. J. Exp. Botany.* **1994,** *56,* 99–104.

Wesche, E.; Maiti R. K. Contributions to the botany and Nutritional Value of Some Wild *Amaranthus* Species (Amaranthaceae). *Econ Bot.* **1995,** *49,* 423–430.

Wesche, E. P.; Maiti, R. K. Contribuciones al conocimiento de Amaranto silvestre en Nuevo León. Se otorgo el premio anual de investigación en Ciencias Naturales, Universidad Autónoma de Nuevo León, 1990.

Wesche, E. P.; Cuevas H. B.; Maiti R. K. Contenido y tipos de compuestos fenólicos y almidón en granos de 15 variedades de mijo perla (*Pennisetum americanum* L. Leeke). *Publ Biol.* **1991,** *5,* 31–37.

CHAPTER 7

Plant–Water Relations in Native Shrubs and Trees, Northeastern Mexico

HUMBERTO GONZÁLEZ RODRÍGUEZ[*],
HAYDEE ALEJANDRA DUEÑAS TIJERINA, ISRAEL CANTÚ SILVA, and
R. K. MAITI

*Facultad de Ciencias Forestales (School of Forest Sciences),
Universidad Autonoma de Nuevo Leon, Linares, NL 67770, Mexico*

[*]*Corresponding author. E-mail: humberto.gonzalezrd@uanl.edu.mx*

ABSTRACT

Since plant internal water potentials (Ψ) are a consequence of the soil–plant atmospheric continuum, measuring the actual internal plant water potential and soil water status directly in the field gives us reliable information about the water stress plants may suffer. Hence, it is important to measure water potential to identify the plant's capacity and strategy to cope with drought. According to the above mentioned, this chapter deals with the physiological adaptation of native trees and shrubs to drought stress in the semiarid ecosystems of northeastern Mexico. The present study has the objective to relate the soil water content with xylem water potential in native woody species such as *Condalia hookeri* (Rhamnaceae), *Cordia boissieri* (Boraginaceae), *Prosopis laevigata* (Fabaceae), and *Celtis pallida*. Seasonal xylem predawn (06:00 hrs) and midday (12:00 hrs) water potentials were determined at 15 day-intervals. Maximum and minimum seasonal predawn values ranged from −0.67 MPa (*C. pallida*) to −2.92 MPa (*C. hookeri*). At midday, xylem water potential varied from −1.07 MPa (*C. pallida*) to −3.10 MPa (*C. hookeri*). Predawn water potential values were highly and positively correlated with midday ones (*r* values varied from 0.900 in *C. boissieri*, to 0.867 in *C. pallida*) and rainfall (*r* values ranged from 0.894 in *C. hookeri*, to 0.697 in *C. pallida*). Correlation analysis between soil water content at different soil layers with predawn water potential values was weak. During the study, native plant species faced mild to severe drought periods, being the species *P. laevigata* and *C. pallida* the ones that achieved higher predawn and midday water potential values. Thus, these species could be considered as drought-tolerant species while *C. hookeri* and *C. boissieri* showed lower water potentials and could be in a physiological disadvantage under soil water stress. In conclusion, the study shows that the ability of species to control its water status may depend on the response capacity to absorb water and to control the loss of water during the day.

7.1   INTRODUCTION

Water is one of the most important factors influencing the distribution, growth, and development of vegetation and is essential for all vital processes such as photosynthesis and respiration. It forms the essential constituent of cell sap and cell vacuoles. It works as a medium for the absorption of plant nutrients and plant metabolism. Plant cell requires about 90% of water to maintain its vital activity. A substantial decrease in water in the cell causes plasmolysis, thereby, inhibiting all metabolic activities. Water potential plays an important role to maintain a pressure gradient in the plant cells required for the transport of water from one to another. Water absorbed by roots is transported upwards through xylem vessels up to the leaves and other organs to help in metabolic activities and the excess of water is lost through transpiration via the stomatae, thereby, maintaining a water balance in the plant cells. Deficiency of water causes a lowering in plant water potential, excess of water due to flooding affects respiration and plant growth. The sequential process of water absorption, its translocation, and loss by the transpirational flux is discussed in brief below. The deficiency of water called water stress affects the growth and development of the plant. Each species requires an optimum amount of water below which the growth of the species is reduced. The species adapted to drought is called drought resistant. Drought resistant plants have several morphological, anatomical, and biochemical mechanisms of resistance. The density of trichomes, leaf surface with a waxy coating, thick cuticle, compact palisade cells, and few biochemical components, such as proline, sugars, and ABA are related to drought resistance. In the semiarid tropics, several species are tolerant to drought, others not so much. We need to identify them in a forest ecosystem.

7.1.1 PLANT–WATER RELATIONS AND FOREST PRODUCTIVITY

The growth and development of a plant are highly dependent on the availability of soil moisture, soil nutrients and water content in the plant cell. The plant cell requires 85–89% water to maintain the dynamic vital activity and enzymatic processes in a plant cell. A decrease in the water content in the cell below this level reduces the metabolic activity of plant cells and plant growth. Therefore, there is a great necessity to maintain water balance in between plant cells starting from the roots to the leaves. Water content in the cell maintains water potential in the cell and the hydrostatic balance among cells. From the roots up to the leaves, there is a gradual decrease in water content maintaining water potential in the cells which force the movement of water from the root cells up to the leaves leading to the loss of water through transpiration. Plant cells need to maintain this hydrostatic balance for maintaining the plant growth. Water is absorbed by roots and move from the peripheral root cells to the interior of the cells, then reach endodermis and finally to the xylem vessels in the roots owing to the gradients of water potential starting from the peripheral root cells to xylem cells in the roots. Water once entering the xylem vessels is retained in the narrow vessels owing to adhesion force between water molecules. Xylem vessels form capillary tubes connected from the roots upwards to the stems pump water from the roots upwards by root pressures. The loss of water through transpiration creates a vacuum pressure in the leaf mesophyll due to which water in the xylem is under negative pressure and creates cohesive forces in xylem vessels between water molecules to maintain the water columns intact. Thus, roots absorb water from soils owing to the difference of water potential between soil and cells. There is always a gradient of water potential from peripheral cortical cells to the interior cells. Once reaching the xylem vessels water moves up by the suction force called ascent of sap. The adjacent phloem tissue is under positive pressure that is maintained osmotically with assimilated sugars and dissolved minerals. Variability in soil and atmospheric conditions influence the interaction between the pressures and structural properties determine the tissue resistivity against embolism formation under high negative pressures in xylem tissue that threaten the integrity of xylem transport.

7.1.2 PLANT–WATER RELATIONS STUDIES IN NORTHEASTERN MEXICO

The climate in northeastern Mexico is characterized by the alternation between favorable and unfavorable periods of soil water content which affects plant growth and development throughout the year. Plants differ widely in their capacity to cope with drought (Stienen et al., 1989). Adaptations exist to explain these differences and can be conveniently referenced to the capacity to maintain water status (water potential and/or relative water content, RWC). Plants under such conditions regulate their water status using several strategies, namely, osmotic adjustment, stomatal aperture, turgor maintenance, root distribution, and leaf canopy properties (Rhizopoulou et al., 1997). The main type of vegetation in northeastern Mexico, known as the Tamaulipan thorn scrub, is distinguished by a wide range of taxonomic groups exhibiting differences in growth patterns, leaf life spans, textures, growth dynamics, and phenological development (Reid et al., 1990; McMurtry et al., 1996). This semi-arid shrub-land, which covers about 200,000 km^2 including southern Texas and northeastern Mexico, is characterized by an average annual precipitation of 805 mm and a yearly potential evapotranspiration of about 2200 mm. Vegetation is utilized as forage for livestock and wildlife, fuel-wood, timber for construction, traditional medicine, fencing, charcoal, agroforestry, and reforestation practices in disturbed sites (Reid et al., 1990). Since water stress is the most limiting factor in this region, a work was focused to study how seasonal leaf water potentials of native tree species are related to soil water availability and evaporative demand components (González-Rodríguez et al., 2009). The study of native species in this region provides an opportunity to investigate, from an ecophysiological perspective, the response of shrub species to changes in resource availability, in this case, soil moisture content, to gain a better understanding of how such an ecosystem may sustain biomass productivity. Thus, as an approach to understand how seasonal plant xylem water potentials are related to environmental conditions, a study was conducted in four native plant species to describe the adaptive responses.

7.2 MATERIAL AND METHODS

7.2.1 STUDY SITE

This research was carried out at the Experimental Research Station of Universidad Autonoma de Nuevo Leon (24°47' N; 99°32' W; 350 m amsl) in

Linares municipality, Nuevo Leon, Mexico. The climate is subtropical and semi-arid with a warm summer. Mean monthly air temperature ranges from 14.7°C in January to 22.3°C in August. Average annual precipitation is about 800 mm. Soils are predominantly deep, dark-gray, lime clay montmorillonite vertisols (González et al., 2004).

7.2.2 PLANT MATERIAL AND XYLEM WATER POTENTIAL MEASUREMENTS

Four co-existing shrub species, representative of the native plant community and of importance for browsing animals (Domínguez-Gómez et al., 2014) and other multipurpose uses such as wood, charcoal, and timber, have been chosen: *Condalia hookeri* M.C. Johnst. (Rhamnaceae), *Cordia boissieri* A.DC. (Boraginaceae), *Prosopis laevigata* (Humb. & Bonpl. ex Willd) M.C. Johnst. (Fabaceae), and *Celtis pallida* Torr. (Ulmaceae). Five plants of each species were randomly selected within a 20 m×20 m undisturbed thornscrub plot (González et al., 2004) for xylem water potential (MPa) measurements. Xylem water potential measurements were performed on terminal twigs immediately after cutting the sample, at 15-days intervals (between February 21 and June 30, 2017), at 06:00 h (predawn) and 14:00 h (midday), using a Scholander pressure bomb (Model 3005, Soil Moisture Equipment Corp., Santa Barbara, CA) (Ritchie and Hinckley, 1975).

7.2.3 ENVIRONMENTAL DATA

Air temperature (°C) and relative humidity (%) were registered daily using a HOBO Pro Data Logger (HOBO Pro Temp/RH Series, Forestry Suppliers, Inc., Jackson, MS). Daily rainfall (mm) was obtained from a Tipping Bucket Rain Gauge (Forestry Suppliers, Inc.). Gravimetric soil water content (kg kg^{-1} dry soil) on each sampling date was determined in soil cores at layers (four replications) of 0–10, 10–20, 20–30, 30–40, and 40–50 cm.

7.2.4 STATISTICAL ANALYSES

Since xylem water potential and soil water content data were not normally distributed (Kolmogorov-Smirnov test) and variances were not homogeneous for most sampling dates (Levene test), predawn, midday, and soil water content experimental data were subjected to the Kruskal–Wallis nonparametric test (Ott, 1993). The relationships between predawn and midday water potentials and prevailing environmental variables were determined by the Spearman's rank-order correlation analysis since the null hypothesis of normality was rejected at $p = .05$. All applied statistical methods were according to the SPSS® software package (standard released version 13.0 for Windows, SPSS Inc., Chicago, IL).

7.3   RESULTS AND DISCUSSION

The seasonal pattern in gravimetric soil water content at different soil layers as well as the cumulative rainfall registered during the experimental period is shown in Figure 7.1. Cumulative rainfall registered during the experimental period was about 340 mm. Major precipitation peak occurred in June, 2 with 152 mm and minimum rainfall was registered on April, 4 and May, 2 with 0.4 and 2.0 mm, respectively. Seasonal soil water content, at different soil-layer depths, showed a typical response with the onset rainfall events. There were soil water content differences ($p < .05$) among soil layers in two (March, 22 and April, 18) out of the ten sampling dates (Fig. 7.1). During the driest period, April, 4, the soil water content was around 0.10 kg kg^{-1} soil, while during the wettest period, soil water content ranged from 0.218 (depth 0–10 cm) to 0.16 kg kg^{-1} soil (depth 40–50 cm) and coincides with major precipitation peak. The soil moisture content in the soil layer depth 0–10 cm was more responsive to rainfall event than deeper layers.

   The seasonal variation in predawn and midday xylem water potential in the four plant species is shown in Figure 7.2. Predawn xylem water potential values were significantly differed ($p < .05$) among plant species in all sampling dates. At the wettest period (02-Jun), water potential ranged from −0.67 MPa (*C. pallida*) to −0.94 MPa (*C. hookeri* and *C. boissieri*). In contrast, on the driest period (02-May), significantly higher water potential values varied from −1.52 MPa (*P. laevigata*) to −2.92 MPa (*C. hookeri*). With respect to the midday xylem water potential, significant differences ($p < .05$) among native plant were observed in seven sampling dates out of ten. During the wettest sampling date (June, 2), higher midday water potential was recorded in *C. pallida* (−1.07 MPa), while a minimum value was observed in *C. hookeri* (−1.78 MPa). In contrast, during the driest period (May 2), midday water potential values ranged from −1.76 MPa (*C. pallida*) to −3.10 MPa (*C. hookeri*). Predawn water potential values were highly and positively correlated with midday ones (*r* values varied from 0.900, in *C. boissieri*, to 0.867 in *C. pallida*) and rainfall (*r* values ranged from 0.894 in *C. hookeri* to 0.697 in *C. pallida*). Correlation analysis between soil water content at different soil layers with predawn water potential values was weak. During the study and accordingly with water potential data, native plant species faced mild to severe drought periods, being the species *P. laevigata* and *C. pallida* the ones that achieved higher predawn and midday water potential values. Thus, these species could be considered as drought-tolerant species while *C. hookeri* and *C. boissieri* showed lower water potentials and could be in a physiological disadvantage under soil water stress. The study suggests that the first two species may serve as a model to evaluate the strategies of adaptation to drought at high tissue water potential while the latter may serve as an adequate model to study plant adaptation to drought at low tissue water potential. Another explanation for this physiological response is that, perhaps, *P. laevigata* and *C. pallida* seem to tolerate drought using their deeper rooting system, while *C. hookeri* and *C. boissieri* use other physiological or morphological strategies to overcome water stress. Similar findings have been reported by López-Hernández et al. (2010) studying the adaptation of native shrubs to drought stress in northeastern Mexico. The capacity for osmoregulation among native shrubs and trees that grow in the northeastern region of Mexico has suggested a range value between −1.11 and −2.65 MPa (González and Silva, 2001). The results of the present study have indicated that the response of a shrub species to evade drought stress is related to their water and osmotic potentials and to the response of interacting to environmental variables; soil water content, rainfall or evaporative demand components. Also, the ability of native species to cope with drought stress depends on the pattern of water uptake and the extent to control water loss through the transpirational flux. In a humid environment, the rate of transpiration is lower than that in hot summer days which control directly the speed of transpiration and movement of water from the roots upwards to the leaves. This is the driving force for the growth and development of a plant. Optimum moisture is essential for plant growth. Lack of soil moisture causes drought and reduce the growth. In a forest, species susceptible to drought, thereby causing the decrease in growth. Some species are resistant/tolerant to drought due to the presence of morpho-anatomical and physiological mechanisms. Kröber et al. (2015) analyzed leaf morphology of 40 evergreen and deciduous broadleaved subtropical tree species and relationships to functional ecophysiological traits. The authors asked whether the ecophysiological parameters such as stomatal conductance and xylem cavitation vulnerability could be predicted from microscopy leaf.

The implications of this study suggest that the species respond differently to drought through the employment of different strategies and there is scope for forest and range management practices in the selection of drought-tolerant species for planting and reforestation of drought-prone areas.

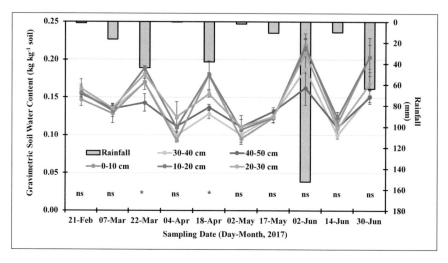

FIGURE 7.1 Seasonal pattern in gravimetric soil water content at five soil depths. Values are means±standard errors ($n = 4$). Cumulative rainfall (mm) for a 15-day period prior to each sampling date is shown. Within the graph, at each sampling date, the asterisk and ns denote significant (*, $p < .05$) or not significant ($p > .05$) differences among soil layers, respectively, in soil water content according to the Kruskal–Wallis test.

Since water availability is the most limiting factor controlling tree growth, survival, and distribution in dry climates (Newton and Goodin, 1989), the great diversity of native shrubs in this region reflects the plasticity among these species to cope with a harsh environment. Therefore, shrub and tree plants have evolved key morphological and physiological traits suited for adaptation to environmental constraints, especially in drought-prone regions. The strategies involve early leaf abscission, limited leaf area, an extensive and deeper root system, epidermal wax accumulation associated with the reduction of water loss by stomatal closure, and accumulation of organic and inorganic solutes (Newton et al., 1991). Shrubs and trees growing in this region under adverse environmental conditions have to seasonally adjust their morpho-physiological traits to cope successfully with changes in soil water availability (Bucci et al., 2008).

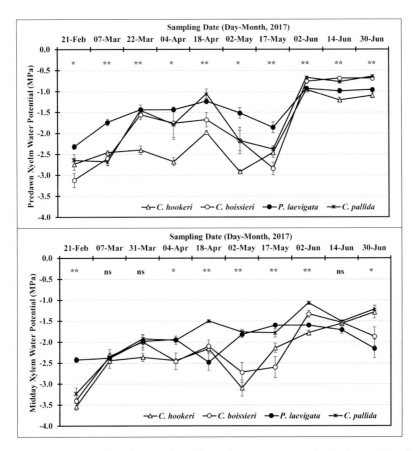

FIGURE 7.2 Seasonal predawn and midday xylem water potential in four native plant species. Values are means ± standard errors ($n = 5$). At each sampling date, the double, and simple asterisks and ns denote significant (**, $p < .01$; *, $p < .05$) or not significant ($p > .05$) differences among plant species, respectively, based on the Kruskal–Wallis test.

KEYWORDS

- **trees**
- **shrubs**
- **water potential**
- **drought resistance**
- **physiological adaptation**

REFERENCES

Bucci, S. J.; Scholz, F. G.; Goldstein, G.; Meinzer, F. C.; Franco, A. C.; Zhang, Y., Hao, G. H. Water Relations and Hydraulic Architecture in Cerrado Trees: Adjustments to Seasonal Changes in Water Availability and Evaporative Demand. *Braz. J. Plant Physiol.* **2008,** *20,* 233–245.

Domínguez, G.; Ramírez, L. T. G.; Rodríguez, H. G.; Cantú, S. I.; Gómez, M. M. V.; Alvarado, M. del S. Mineral Content in Four Browse Species from Northeastern Mexico. *Pak. J. Bot.* **2014,** *46,* 1421–1429.

González, H. G.; Silva, C. I. Adaptación a La Sequía de Plantas Arbustivas del Matorral Espinoso Tamaulipeco. *CiENCiA UANL.* **2001,** *4,* 454–461.

Rodríguez, H. G.; Cantú, S. I.; Gómez, M. M. V.; Ramírez, L. R. G. Plant Water Relations of Thornscrub Shrub Species, Northeastern Mexico. *J. Arid Environ.* **2004,** *58,* 483–503.

Rodríguez, H. G.; Cantú, S. I.; Gómez, M. M. V.; Ramírez, L. R. G.; Pando, M. M.; Molina, C. I. A.; Maiti, R. K. Water Relations in Native Trees, Northeastern Mexico. *Int. J. Agric. Environ. Biotechnol.* **2009,** *2,* 133–141.

Kröber, W.; Heklau, H.; Bruelheide, H.; Leaf Morphology of 40 Evergreen and Deciduous Broadleaved Subtropical Tree Species and Relationships to Functional Ecophysiological Traits. *Plant Biol.* **2015,** *17,* 373–383.

López, H. J. M.; Rodríguez, H. G.; Cantú, S. I.; Ramírez, L. R. G.; Gómez, M. M. V.; Pando, M. M.; Sarquís, R. J. I.; Coria, G. N.; Maiti, R. K.; Sarkar, N. C. Adaptation of Native Shrubs to Drought Stress in North-Eastern Mexico. *Int. J. of Bio-resour. Stress Manag.* **2010,** *1,* 30–37.

Mc, M. C. R.; Barnes, P. W.; Nelson, J. A.; Archer, S. R. Physiological Responses of Woody Vegetation to Irrigation in a Texas Subtropical Savanna. *La Copita Research Area, Consolidated Progress Report.* Texas Agricultural Experiment Station-Corpus Christi, Texas A&M University System, College Station: TX, 1996; 33–37.

Newton, R. J.; Funkhouser, E. A.; Fong, F.; Tauer, C. G. Molecular and Physiological Genetics of Drought Tolerance in Forest Species. *For. Ecol. Manag.* **1991,** *43,* 225–250.

Newton, R. J.; Goodin, J. R. Moisture Stress Adaptation in Shrubs. In *The Biology and Utilization of Shrubs;* McKell, C. M. Ed.; Academic Press: San Diego, CA, 1989; 365–383.

Ott, L. *An Introduction to Statistical Methods and Data Analysis,* 2nd ed.; Duxbury Press: Boston, MA, 1993.

Reid, N.; Marroquín, J.; Beyer, M. P. Utilization of Shrubs and Trees for Browse, Fuelwood and Timber in the Tamaulipan Thornscrub in Northeastern Mexico. *For. Ecol. Manag.* **1990,** *36,* 61–79.

Rhizopoulou, S.; Heberlein, K.; Kassianou, A. Field Water Relations of *Capparis Spinosa* L. *J. Arid Environ.* **1997,** *36,* 237–248.

Ritchie, G. A.; Hinckley, T. M. The Pressure Chamber as an Instrument for Ecological Research. *Adv. Ecol. Res.* **1975,** *9,* 165–254.

Stienen, H.; Smits, M. P.; Reid, N.; Landa, J.; Boerboom, J. H. A. Ecophysiology of 8 Woody Multipurpose Species from Semiarid Northeastern Mexico. *Ann. For. Sci.* **1989,** *46,* 454–458.

CHAPTER 8

Chemical Composition of Woods of 37 Woody Species of Tamaulipan Thorn Scrub, Northeast Mexico: A Case Study

HUMBERTO GONZALEZ RODRIGUEZ[1*], RATIKANTA MAITI[1],
NATALYA S. IVANOVA[2], and CH. ARUNA KUMARI[3]

[1]*Universidad Autónoma de Nuevo León, Facultad de Ciencias Forestales, Carr. Nac. No. 85 Km. 45, Linares, Nuevo León 67700, México*

[2]*Russian Academy of Science, Botanical Garden of Ural Branch, 202a, 8-March street, Yekaterinburg 620144, Russia*

[3]*Crop Physiology, Professor Jaya Shankar Telangana State Agricultural University, Agricultural College, Polasa, Jagtial 505529, India*

Corresponding author. E-mail: humberto.gonzalezrd@uanl.edu.mx

ABSTRACT

The present study was directed to determine the chemical composition of 37 woody trees at Linares, of Tamaulipas Thorn Scrub, Northeast Mexico.

The results show large variability among the species in wood chemical composition, such as neutral detergent fiber (NDF), digestible detergent fiber (ADF), lignin, cellulose, hemicellulose. In these aspects, maximum of amount NDF (94.8%) is observed in *Celtis pallida, Parkinsonia aculeata,* and *Guaiacum angustifolium*. High amount of ADF was found in three species: *Celtis pallida, Parkinsonia aculeata, Lantana macropoda*. With respect to lignin, *Sideroxylon celastrina, Ebenopsis ebano, Ehretia anacua, Amyris texana, Leucophyllum frutescens, Cordia boissieri*, and *Condalia hookeri* have high lignin content (over 24%). On the other hand, maximum of cellulose was observed in *Parkinsonia aculeata, Celtis pallida*, and *Lantana macropoda* have also high levels of cellulose.

Similarly, maximum amount of cellulose was observed in *Bernardia myricifolia*. Close to the maximum content of hemicellulose was revealed in *Celtis laevigata*. With respect to fiber, maximum of fiber is observed in *Celtis pallida*. Close to the maximum content of fiber was found in *Parkinsonia aculeata* and *Guaiacum angustifolium*. The variations in chemical compositions could be related to quality determination and utility of timbers of different woody species.

8.1 INTRODUCTION

Wood is a hard tissue below the bark of a tree. It is of high commercial importance in wood industry. It is used for several domestic uses and also in the manufacture of furniture. Wood quality depends on anatomical structure and chemical composition. Various authors have reported the chemical composition of wood and its relation to wood quality and utilization (Petterson et al., 1984). These studies analyze chemical composition of wood, its methods, structure, hemicellulose components, and the degree of polymerization of carbohydrates. Woods were collected from different countries and analyzed for sugar compositions, such as glucan, galactan, arabinan, and mannan; besides uronic anhydride, aceyle, lignin, were analyzed.

Wood is composed mainly of cellulose, hemicellulose, lignin, and other extractable materials mentioned below. The lignin is present in the cell wall of wood (20–30%). It is cemented in the cell wall of wood, confers rigidity of the same and acts as an obstacle against the degradation of enzymes of the cell wall.

In wood, it is always associated to cellulose but do not occur the same in other cellulosic materials, so that the cellulose may be found practically in a pure condition, for example, in cotton (Ortuno, 1998). Lignin is a tridimensional aromatic polymer in which phenylpropane units are repeated with different types of bonds (ether or C-C) between the monomers. A review was undertaken by Guadalupe Berecenas Pazos and Raymundo Sotelo on the importance of lignin contraction.

On the basis of literature, it is confirmed that the shrinkage of wood can be partially attributed to the content of lignin in the wood. It was assessed that temperate hard wood obtained both from Mexico and the United States had a higher shrinkage capacity than tropical woods.

Specific gravity is found to be the most important variable; however, the influence of lignin is also significant. They remarkedly suggested that it is necessary to carry out experimental studies on the effect of these variables on dimensional changes, along with other important traits such as extractives and ray volume. All the plants and especially woody species are constituted by majority the components like C, H, O, and N and also contain small quantities of Ca, K, and Mg. The elements C, H, and O are combined to form organic components of wood, such as cellulose, hemicellulose, and lignin, as well as pectins (Ortuno, 1998). The components of the cell wall are lignin and the polysaccharides constituted by cellulose and hemicellulose. Cellulose is the main constituent of the cell wall of all higher plants with the majority of wood fibers (40–45%).

This is constituted by D-glucose in form of pyranose linked together by 1-4 glycosidic bonds with the formation of cellobiose residues. The hemicellulose is associated with cellulose in the cell wall. This is formed by pentose and hexose distinct from glucose (mannose, xylose, glucose, galactose, and arabinose), linked together with a polymerization grade from 100 to 200. The chemical structure and composition vary according to species.

Similarly, all the hemicelluloses are insoluble in H_2O but can be dissolved in strong alkalis and easily hydrolyzed by acids. Its amorphic structure and low molecular weight confer greater solubility and susceptibility to hydrolysis than cellulose (Ortuno, 1998). The cellulosic fraction—cellulose and hemicellulose—of wood may be separated in its components, depending on its solubility in NaOH at 17.5%, according to their grade of polymerization (Ortuno, 1998). The pectins or pectic substances are also the hydrates of carbon, form cell wall of young cells.

It is difficult to separate lignin of wood; besides it alters with the method of extraction. The molecular weight of the separated product may vary between 1000 and 20,000 g/mol (Lu and John, 2010). Owing to the high content of this aromatic and phenolic compounds, the lignins shows dark color and are easily oxidized, are relatively stable in aqueous acidic minerals, but are soluble in aqueous bases and hot bisulfite.

The wood also contains a series of extractable compounds of varied chemical compositions, such as gums, resins, fats, alkaloids, and also tannins. Tannins can be extracted from woods, which can be extracted from wood by cold or hot water or with organic solvents, including alcohol, benzene, acetone, or ether. The proportion of these substances is from 1% to 10%, whereas some tropical species may contain up to 20% of the same. The inorganic compounds are not soluble in the mentioned solvents but sometimes are included among the extracts (Ortuno, 1998).

Berland and Holmbom (2004) investigated the pattern of distribution of wood components along a radial cross-section of the stem using microscale analytical technique. The results reveal that heartwood had more lignin but less cellulose than sapwood. The total content of hemicellulose was similar along the radial direction.

There were significant differences in the distribution of sugars units in hemicellulose. Latewood contained galactoglucomannan in earlywood but less pectin. Jones et al. (2006) used diffuse reflectance near infrared spectroscopy for nondestructive estimation of wood's chemical composition from wood strips. Besides, they estimated cellulose, hemicellulose, lignin, arabinan, galactan, mannan, and xylan by using standard analytical chemistry methods.

Sriraam et al. (2012) reported the average chemical contents of wood mentioned below. Elements share, % of dry matter weight, carbon 45–50%, hydrogen 6.0–6.5% oxygen 38–42%, nitrogen 0.1–0.5%. Sulfur max 0.05. They observed large variations of cellulose, hemicellulose, lignin, and total extractives among scot pine, spruce, eucalyptus, silver birch.

A study has been undertaken by Memet Baharloglu et al. (2013) to determine the effects of the anatomical and chemical composition of wood on the quality of particleboard containing woods of different species. They concluded that anatomical and chemical composition of wood species determine physical properties of particleboard that are related to the length and number of cells and fibers. Panels containing more of pinewood gave higher mechanical strength and lowest thickness values and there were significant differences in physical and mechanical properties among particle boards that were related to length, thickness, and the number of cells and fibers.

Similarly, a study was undertaken by Agata Pawlika et al. (2013) on chemical composition of wood species of Africa. They estimated holocellulose, pentosans, and substances soluble in organic solvents, such as 1% NaOH, in cold and hot water, and also determined mineral substances.

Their results are shown below. Constituents: Koto Sip Mahogany, cellulose: 43.03, 41.59, 43.14; holocellulose 71.76, 64.28, 59.91; lignin 22.43, 30.36, 30.20. Very recently Scharnweber et al. (2016) studied variations of wood's chemistry among trees using X-ray fluorescence. They observed the variation of chemical composition between one coniferous and one broadleaf (*Castanea sativa*) grown in different conditions. Pine showed greater values.

The common signal was stronger for pine than for chestnut.

Maiti et al. (2015) studied variability of wood-density of ten woody species and its possible relation with wood's chemical composition at Linares, Northeast Mexico. They observed large variations in the wood's density and wood's chemical composition. In general, though there was no clear relationship between wood density and other chemical composition of wood, it is observed that the species having wood of moderate and high-wood density contained >30% sulfur, >40% cellulose, and more or less 20% (Maiti et al., 2016) lignin.

The present study was undertaken on the chemical composition of 37 woody shrubs and trees in Northeast Mexico.

8.2 MATERIALS AND METHODS

In the present study, 37 woody trees and shrubs are taken for the chemical composition of wood (species are shown in the graphs in results).

The woody species included in the study are mentioned below.

Family	Growth type	Scientific name
Rutaceae	Shrub	*Helietta parvifolia* (A. Gray) Benth.
Zygophyllaceae	Shrub	*Guaiacum angustifolium* (Engelm.) A. Gray.
Scrophulariaceae	Shrub	*Leucophyllum frutescens* (Berland) I. M. Johnst.
Euphrobiaceae	Shrub	*Bernardia myricifolia* (Scheele) S. Watson.
Fabaceae	Shrub	*Eysenhardtia polystachya* (Ortega) Sarg.
Fabaceae	Shrub	*Leucaena leucocephala* (Lam.) de Wit
Fabaceae	Tree	*Ebenopsis ebano* (Berland.) Barneby & J. W. Grimes
Rutaceae	Tree	*Sargentia greggii* S. Watson
Ebenaceae	Shrub	*Diospyros palmeri* Eastw.
Leguminoseae	Shrub	*Acacia rigidula* Benth.
Rutaceae	Shrub	*Amyris texana* (Buckley) P. Wilson.
Boraginaceae	Shrub	*Cordia boissieri* A.DC.
Ulmaceae	Shrub	*Celtis pallida* Torr.
Rutaceae	Shrub	*Zanthoxylum fagara* (L.) Sarg.
Asteraceae	Shrub	*Gymnosperma glutinosum* (Spreng.) Less.
Leguminoseae	Shrub	*Acacia farnesiana* (L) Willd
Leguminoseae	Shrub	*Acacia farnesiana*
Verbenaceae	Shrub	*Lantana macropoda* Torr.
Oleaceae	Shrub	*Forestiera angustifolia* Torr.
Euphrobiaceae	Shrub	*Croton suaveolens* Torr.
Berberidaceae	Shrub	*Berberis trifoliata* Torr.
Boraginaceae	Shrub	*Ehretia anacua* I. M. Johnst.
Rhamnaceae	Shrub	*Condalia hookeri* M. C. Johnst.
Ebenaceae'	Shrub	*Diospyros texana* Scheele
Sapotacee	Tree	*Sideroxylon celastrina* (Kunth) T. D. Penn.

TABLE *(Continued)*

Family	Growth type	Scientific name
Leguminoseae	Tree	*Caesalpinia mexicana* A. Gray
Rhamnaceae	Shrub	*Karwinskia humboldtiana* (Willd. ex Roem. & Schult.) Zucc.
Mimosaceae	Tree	*Acacia schaffneri* (S.Watson) F. J. Herm.
Fabaceae	Tree	*Prosopis laevigata* (Humb. & Bonpl. ex Willd.) M. C. Johnst.
Fabaceae	Tree	*Acacia berlandieri* Benth.
Leguminosae	Tree	*Cercidium macrum* I. M. Johnst.
Fagáceae	Tree	*Quercus polymorpha* Schltdl. & Cham.
Caesalpiniaceae	Tree	*Parkinsonia aculeata* L
Salicaceae	Tree	*Salix lasiolepis* Benth.
Fabaceae	Tree	*Acacia wrightii* Benth.
Oleaceae	Tree	*Fraxinus greggii* A. Gray
Ulmaceae	Tree	*Celtis laevigata* Willd.
Fabaceae	Tree	*Harvadia pallens* (Benth.) Britton & Rose.

Triplicate samples of wood are collected from each of 37 species and then were subjected to chemical analysis for neutral detergent fiber (NDF), and detergent fiber lignin (ADL) contents following Anken procedure. Hemicellulose (NDF-ADF) and cellulose (ADF-lignin) were obtained by difference by cambium but its contents decrease in old trees (Technique of Ankon).

Estimation of each component was done in five replications. The procedures are mentioned below:

Estimation of each component was done in five replications.
The procedures mentioned below:

A—scientific name
B—common name
C— dry matter
D—dry weight
E—P. sample
F—FDN
G— (F2−[D2*1.00507611])
H—% NDF = (G2/[E2*C2])*100
I—% NDF corr = (H2−S2)
J—ADF

K—(J2/D2)
L—% ADF = ([J2−{D2*1.001191319}]/[E2*C2]*100)
M—% ADF corr = (L2−S2),
N—lignina,
O—lignin corr = ([N2−{D2*1.00045152}]/[E2×C2])*100)
P—% lignin = (O2−S2) ………Q = peso del crisol, R = cenizas,
S—% ashes = ([{R2−Q2}−0]/[E2*C2])*100
T—hemicel = (H2−L2)
U—cellulose = (L2−P2)
V—% cellulose = ([E2−{N2−D2}/E2]*100)*(L2/100)
W—% lignina = ([N2-D2]−[R2−Q2]/E2)*100*(L2/100)
X—% acid insoluble detergent fiber = (R2−Q2)/E2*100*(L2/100)

8.2.1 DATA ANALYSIS

Comparison of average values is a way of comparing relationships between species. Statistical analysis of the variables are undertaken, such as analysis of variance (ANOVA), among and between groups.

A statistically significant result, when a probability (p value) is less than a threshold (significance level), justifies the rejection of the null hypothesis (Box.1953). ANOVA tests the null hypothesis about equality of the means of all the groups that are compared; however, this statistic only demonstrates the presence or absence of difference between species and groups, it answers the question, whether we should accept or reject the null hypothesis. We also analyzed Tukey's HSD test to evaluate the differences between species.

If the null hypothesis is rejected (differences are statistically significant), then we should search the answer to a question which of the species and groups is actually different from others. Parametric variants of ANOVA calculate for this purpose so-called post hoc (after the event) tests, which are aimed to point the group being different from others. Multiple comparison procedures and statistical tests were carried out (Morrison et al., 2013)

8.3 RESULTS AND DISCUSSION

We analyzed the characteristics for 37 species. Statistically significant differences between species was observed for all studied characteristics NDF ($F_{(36, 148)} = 21{,}642$, $p = 0$) (Fig. 8.1), ADF ($F_{(36,148)} = 18{,}783$, $p = 0$) (Fig. 8.3), lignin ($F_{(36,148)} = 39{,}030$, $p = 0$) (Fig. 8.5), cellulose ($F_{(36,148)} = 25{,}237$,

$p = 0$) (Fig. 8.7), hemicellulose (F(36,148) = 9,4778, $p = 0$) (Fig. 8.9), fiber (F(36,148) = 21,660, $p = 0$) (Fig. 8.11). Means are given in Table 8.1.

8.3.1   NEUTRAL DETERGENT FIBER

Maximum of NDF (94.8%) is observed in *Celtis pallida* (Fig. 8.1, Table 8.1). *Parkinsonia aculeata* and *Guaiacum angustifolium* have also high values of NDF. These species do not have statistically significant differences from each other but they are different from other species (Figs. 8.1 and 8.2). Acacia farnesiana has a minimum of NDF (74.86%). This species has a maximum number of statistically significant differences from other species (Fig. 8.2). Minimum of statistically significant differences from other species is observed in *Harvadia pallens* (Fig. 8.2).

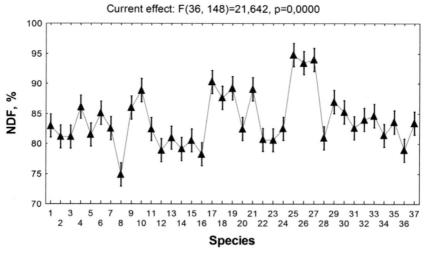

FIGURE 8.1   NDF content (%) of woody tree species in 1: *Acacia schaffneri*, 2: *Fraxinus greggii*, 3: *Helietta parvifolia*, 4: *Forestiera angustifolia*, 5: *Cordia boissieri*, 6: *Salix lasiolepis*, 7: *Karwinskia humboldtiana*, 8: *Acacia farnesiana*, 9: *Diospyros texana*, 10: *Croton suaveolens*, 11: *Acacia berlandieri*, 12: *Sargentia greggii*, 13: *Acacia rigidula*, 14: *Ebenopsis ebano*, 15: *Amyris texana*, 16: *Ehretia anacua*, 17: *Celtis laevigata*, 18: *Quercus polymorpha*, 19: *Bernardia myricifolia*, 20: *Prosopis laevigata*, 21: *Lantana macropoda*, 22: *Eysenhardtia polystachya*, 23: *Cercidium macrum*, 24: *Zanthoxylum fagara*, 25: *Celtis pallida*, 26: *Guaiacum angustifolium*, 27: *Parkinsonia aculeata*, 28: *Leucaena leucocephala*, 29: *Leucophyllum frutescens*, 30: *Condalia hookeri*, 31: *Acacia wrightii*, 32: *Harvadia pallens*, 33: *Gymnosperma glutinosum*, 34: *Berberis trifoliata*, 35: *Caesalpinia mexicana*, 36: *Sideroxylon celastrina*, 37: *Diospyros palmeri*.

TABLE 8.1 The Chemical Composition and Fiber Content of the Tree Species.

A: mean, B: standard deviation

№	Species	NDF, %		ADF, %		Lignin, %		Cellulose, %		Hemicellulose, %		Fiber, %	
		A	B	A	B	A	B	A	B	A	B	A	B
1	*Acacia schaffneri*	83.01	1,43	60.16	0,83	19.05	0,35	41.21	0,51	22.85	0,79	83.10	1,41
2	*Fraxinus greggii*	81.17	1,07	55.43	0,40	15.28	0,25	40.29	0,49	25.74	0,70	81.31	1,05
3	*Helietta parvifolia*	81.15	0,94	60.73	0,72	20.40	1,32	40.53	1,17	20.42	0,58	81.34	0,82
4	*Forestiera angustifolia*	86.12	2,50	63.88	2,59	20.72	0,74	43.28	1,85	22.25	0,35	86.24	2,44
5	*Cordia boissieri*	81.50	2,81	61.56	1,84	24.36	1,33	37.34	1,66	19.94	1,03	81.64	2,81
6	*Salix lasiolepis*	85.14	1,94	63.56	1,57	17.85	0,94	45.92	1,85	21.58	0,58	85.36	1,96
7	*Karwinskia humboldtiana*	82.57	0,74	60.02	0,58	21.93	0,40	38.27	0,66	22.55	0,42	82.76	0,79
8	*Acacia farnesiana*	74.86	0,63	50.89	1,02	17.31	0,48	33.70	1,25	23.97	0,43	74.98	0,61
9	*Diospyros texana*	86.01	2,30	62.15	1,07	18.71	1,18	43.59	0,54	23.86	1,25	86.15	2,29
10	*Croton suaveolens*	88.89	2,96	61.52	1,12	19.51	1,20	42.18	0,64	27.37	2,06	89.06	2,89
11	*Acacia berlandieri*	82.43	0,55	61.48	0,70	16.93	0,85	44.98	1,49	20.95	0,43	82.86	0,50
12	*Sargentia greggii*	78.92	0,78	59.61	0,61	18.67	1,47	41.05	1,41	19.32	0,74	79.05	0,78
13	*Acacia rigidula*	81.01	1,25	60.55	0,87	19.30	3,03	41.36	2,60	20.47	0,41	81.13	1,29
14	*Ebenopsis ebano*	79.13	0,65	60.14	0,26	27.80	4,50	32.55	4,69	18.99	0,56	79.34	0,61
15	*Amyris texana*	80.56	2,32	60.33	1,46	24.85	3,59	35.62	4,63	20.23	1,38	80.71	2,35
16	*Ehretia anacua*	78.27	0,72	62.38	4,54	24.93	2,75	37.68	3,59	15.89	4,41	78.49	0,77
17	*Celtis laevigata*	90.27	3,80	60.09	0,93	14.60	0,33	45.57	0,90	30.18	3,10	90.35	3,80
18	*Quercus polymorpha*	87.63	1,95	59.72	0,52	19.57	0,32	40.29	0,39	27.91	1,50	87.77	2,00
19	*Bernardia myricifolia*	89.23	2,88	58.84	0,81	20.12	0,31	38.85	0,81	30.39	3,09	89.36	2,84

TABLE 8.1　(Continued)

№	Species	NDF, %		ADF, %		Lignin, %		Cellulose, %		Hemicellulose, %		Fiber, %	
		A	B	A	B	A	B	A	B	A	B	A	B
20	Prosopis laevigata	82.48	5,06	60.72	4,67	16.76	0,55	44.16	4,23	21.76	8,80	82.68	5,00
21	Lantana macropoda	89.06	0,43	71.37	0,42	19.08	0,16	52.56	0,40	17.69	0,39	89.32	0,42
22	Eysenhardtia polystachya	80.67	0,38	62.22	0,60	17.66	0,17	44.85	0,71	18.44	0,62	80.96	0,32
23	Cercidium macrum	80.61	0,63	63.05	0,80	15.63	0,23	47.61	0,69	17.55	0,30	80.79	0,63
24	Zanthoxylum fagara	82.52	2,12	65.46	4,52	18.45	0,81	47.10	4,14	17.06	3,34	82.61	2,12
25	Celtis pallida	94.80	1,61	77.58	11,43	17.18	0,67	60.51	11,65	17.22	9,99	94.91	1,60
26	Guaiacum angustifolium	93.45	2,32	65.13	2,58	21.23	0,44	44.06	3,05	28.33	3,35	93.62	2,34
27	Parkinsonia aculeata	93.99	2,87	77.14	2,91	15.43	0,40	61.85	2,87	16.85	5,65	94.14	2,91
28	Leucaena leucocephala	80.96	0,96	64.42	0,81	18.97	0,35	45.60	1,08	16.54	0,84	81.11	0,95
29	Leucophyllum frutescens	86.97	0,91	67.25	0,53	24.67	1,62	42.88	1,33	19.72	0,59	87.27	0,91
30	Condalia hookeri	85.28	7,18	64.65	4,70	24.14	1,49	40.67	3,31	20.64	2,96	85.44	7,23
31	Acacia wrightii	82.63	0,39	58.55	0,79	15.43	0,23	43.29	0,63	24.08	0,79	82.80	0,34
32	Harvadia pallens	84.03	0,57	60.13	0,48	16.49	0,26	43.65	0,26	23.90	0,49	84.04	0,53
33	Gymnosperma glutinosum	84.67	1,59	59.04	1,25	11.94	0,49	47.23	0,88	25.63	1,37	84.80	1,60
34	Berberis trifoliata	81.40	0,15	54.88	0,38	15.06	0,51	39.95	0,37	26.52	0,44	81.53	0,14
35	Caesalpinia mexicana	83.63	0,36	58.67	0,37	17.16	0,20	41.53	0,41	24.96	0,30	83.65	0,33
36	Sideroxylon celastrina	78.94	0,46	58.25	0,83	28.57	0,83	29.80	0,49	20.69	0,62	79.07	0,37
37	Diospyros palmeri	83.45	0,46	58.77	0,49	14.26	0,65	44.63	0,37	24.67	0,67	83.56	0,47
	Total	83.98	4,90	61.90	5,61	19.19	4,00	42.87	6,69	22.08	4,63	84.14	4,89

Another nine species also did not have much difference from other species: *Acacia schaffneri, Acacia berlandieri, Acacia wrightii, Salix lasiolepis, Karwinskia humboldtiana, Prosopis laevigata, Condalia hookeri, Caesalpinia mexicana, Diospyros palmeri.*

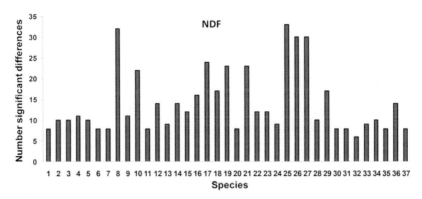

FIGURE 8.2 Results of Tukey's HSD ($p < 0.05$) for NDF in woody tree species.

8.3.2 DIGESTIBLE DETERGENT FIBER

ADF of most species is close to the average and statistically significant differences were not detected (Fig. 8.3). Much more ADF was found in three species *Celtis pallida, Parkinsonia aculeata*, and *Lantana macropoda*. Significantly smaller ADF was detected in *Acacia farnesiana*.

These species are different from other species significantly (Fig. 8.4). In addition, many significant differences were detected in *Leucophyllum frutescens, Berberis trifoliata*, and *Fraxinus greggii*. This parameter of other species is very similar.

8.3.3 LIGNIN

Different plant species have different lignin content (Fig. 8.5). The lignin content of the investigated plants varies from 11.94 to 28.57%.

Sideroxylon celastrina, Ebenopsis ebano, Ehretia anacua, Amyris texana, Leucophyllum frutescens, Cordia boissieri, and *Condalia hookeri* have high lignin content (over 24%) (Table 8.1). Extremely low lignin content was found in *Gymnosperma glutinosum, Diospyros palmeri*, and *Celtis laevigata* (<14.6%). We have found a significant difference in many cases. The greatest difference of *Cordia boissieri, Ebenopsis ebano, Amyris texana,*

Ehretia anacua, Leucophyllum frutescens, Condalia hookeri, Gymnosperma glutinosum, and *Sideroxylon celastrina* from other plant species is lignin content (Fig. 8.6).

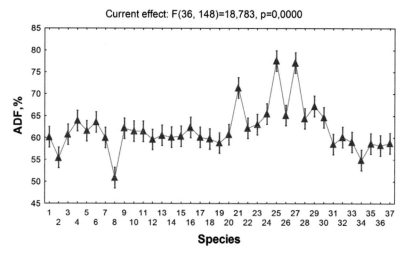

FIGURE 8.3   ADF content (%) in woody tree species. 1: *Acacia schaffneri*, 2: *Fraxinus greggii*, 3: *Helietta parvifolia*, 4: *Forestiera angustifolia*, 5: *Cordia boissieri*, 6: *Salix lasiolepis*, 7: *Karwinskia humboldtiana*, 8: *Acacia farnesiana*, 9: *Diospyros texana*, 10: *Croton suaveolens*, 11: *Acacia berlandieri*, 12: *Sargentia greggii*, 13: *Acacia rigidula*, 14: *Ebenopsis ebano*, 15: *Amyris texana*, 16: *Ehretia anacua*, 17: *Celtis laevigata*, 18: *Quercus polymorpha*, 19: *Bernardia myricifolia*, 20: *Prosopis laevigata*, 21: *Lantana macropoda*, 22: *Eysenhardtia polystachya*, 23: *Cercidium macrum*, 24: *Zanthoxylum fagara*, 25: *Celtis pallida*, 26: *Guaiacum angustifolium*, 27: *Parkinsonia aculeata*, 28: *Leucaena leucocephala*, 29: *Leucophyllum frutescens*, 30: *Condalia hookeri*, 31: *Acacia wrightii*, 32: *Harvadia pallens*, 33: *Gymnosperma glutinosum*, 34: *Berberis trifoliata*, 35: *Caesalpinia mexicana*, 36; *Sideroxylon celastrina*, 37; *Diospyros palmeri*.

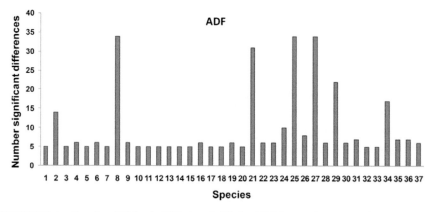

FIGURE 8.4   Results of Tukey's HSD ($p < 0.05$) for ADF in woody tree species.

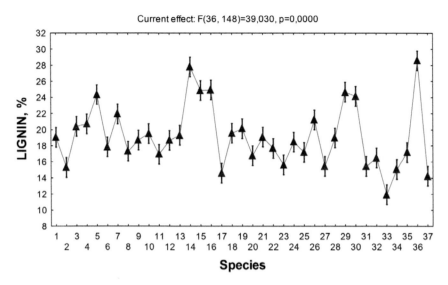

FIGURE 8.5 Lignin content (%) in woody tree species. 1: *Acacia schaffneri*, 2: *Fraxinus greggii*, 3: *Helietta parvifolia*, 4: *Forestiera angustifolia*, 5: *Cordia boissieri*, 6: *Salix lasiolepis*, 7: *Karwinskia humboldtiana*, 8: *Acacia farnesiana*, 9: *Diospyros texana*, 10: *Croton suaveolens*, 11: *Acacia berlandieri*, 12: *Sargentia greggii*, 13: *Acacia rigidula*, 14: *Ebenopsis ebano*, 15: *Amyris texana*, 16: *Ehretia anacua*, 17: *Celtis laevigata*, 18: *Quercus polymorpha*, 19: *Bernardia myricifolia*, 20: *Prosopis laevigata*, 21: *Lantana macropoda*, 22: *Eysenhardtia polystachya*, 23: *Cercidium macrum*, 24: *Zanthoxylum fagara*, 25: *Celtis pallida*, 26: *Guaiacum angustifolium*, 27: *Parkinsonia aculeata*, 28: *Leucaena leucocephala*, 29: *Leucophyllum frutescens*, 30: *Condalia hookeri*, 31: *Acacia wrightii*, 32: *Harvadia pallens*, 33: *Gymnosperma glutinosum*, 34: *Berberis trifoliata*, 35: *Caesalpinia mexicana*, 36: *Sideroxylon celastrina*, 37: *Diospyros palmeri*.

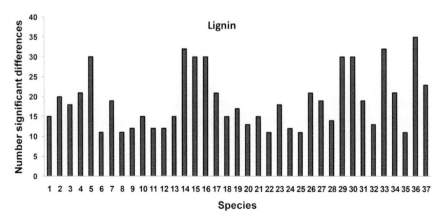

FIGURE 8.6 Results of Tukey's HSD ($p < 0.05$) for lignin content in woody tree species.

8.3.4 CELLULOSE

The cellulose content of the investigated plants varies from 29.80% to 61.85% (Fig. 8.7). Maximum of cellulose content is observed in *Parkinsonia aculeata*. *Celtis pallida* and *Lantana macropoda* have also high levels of cellulose.

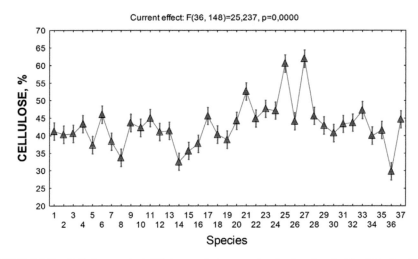

FIGURE 8.7 Cellulose content (%) in woody tree species. 1: *Acacia schaffneri*, 2: *Fraxinus greggii*, 3: *Helietta parvifolia*, 4: *Forestiera angustifolia*, 5: *Cordia boissieri*, 6: *Salix lasiolepis*, 7: *Karwinskia humboldtiana*, 8: *Acacia farnesiana*, 9: *Diospyros texana*, 10: *Croton suaveolens*, 11: *Acacia berlandieri*, 12: *Sargentia greggii*, 13: *Acacia rigidula*, 14: *Ebenopsis ebano*, 15: *Amyris texana*, 16: *Ehretia anacua*, 17: *Celtis laevigata*, 18: *Quercus polymorpha*, 19: *Bernardia myricifolia*, 20: *Prosopis laevigata*, 21: *Lantana macropoda*, 22: *Eysenhardtia polystachya*, 23: *Cercidium macrum*, 24: *Zanthoxylum fagara*, 25: *Celtis pallida*, 26: *Guaiacum angustifolium*, 27: *Parkinsonia aculeata*, 28: *Leucaena leucocephala*, 29: *Leucophyllum frutescens*, 30: *Condalia hookeri*, 31: *Acacia wrightii*, 32: *Harvadia pallens*, 33: *Gymnosperma glutinosum*, 34: *Berberis trifoliata*, 35: *Caesalpinia mexicana*, 36: *Sideroxylon celastrina*, 37: *Diospyros palmeri*.

Minimum of cellulose is observed in *Sideroxylon celastrina*. *Acacia farnesiana* and *Ebenopsis ebano* have also low levels of cellulose. These species have the greatest number of significant differences from other plant species (Fig. 8.8).

8.3.5 HEMICELLULOSE

Hemicellulose content among these investigated plants varied from 19.89% to 30.39% (Fig. 8.9). Maximum of cellulose is observed in *Bernardia myricifolia*. Close to the maximum content of hemicellulose was revealed in *Celtis laevigata*.

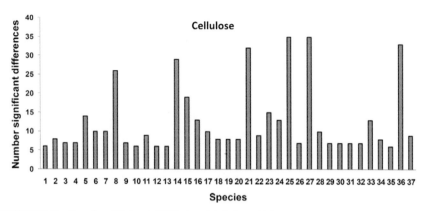

FIGURE 8.8 Results of Tukey's HSD ($p < 0.05$) for cellulose content in woody tree species.

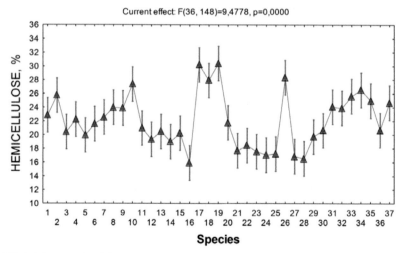

FIGURE 8.9 Hemicellulose content (%) in woody tree species. 1: *Acacia schaffneri*, 2: *Fraxinus greggii*, 3: *Helietta parvifolia*, 4: *Forestiera angustifolia*, 5: *Cordia boissieri*, 6: *Salix lasiolepis*, 7: *Karwinskia humboldtiana*, 8: *Acacia farnesiana*, 9: *Diospyros texana*, 10: *Croton suaveolens*, 11: *Acacia berlandieri*, 12: *Sargentia greggii*, 13: *Acacia rigidula*, 14: *Ebenopsis ebano*, 15: *Amyris texana*, 16: *Ehretia anacua*, 17: *Celtis laevigata*, 18: *Quercus polymorpha*, 19: *Bernardia myricifolia*, 20: *Prosopis laevigata*, 21: *Lantana macropoda*, 22: *Eysenhardtia polystachya*, 23: *Cercidium macrum*, 24: *Zanthoxylum fagara*, 25: *Celtis pallida*, 26: *Guaiacum angustifolium*, 27: *Parkinsonia aculeata*, 28: *Leucaena leucocephala*, 29: *Leucophyllum frutescens*, 30: *Condalia hookeri*, 31: *Acacia wrightii*, 32: *Harvadia pallens*, 33: *Gymnosperma glutinosum*, 34: *Berberis trifoliata*, 35: *Caesalpinia mexicana*, 36: *Sideroxylon celastrina*, 37: *Diospyros palmeri*.

Quercus polymorpha, Croton suaveolens, and *Berberis trifoliata* (chococo) have also low levels of hemicellulose. Significant differences were found among the species (Fig. 8.10).

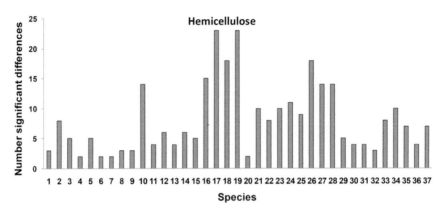

FIGURE 8.10   Results of Tukey's HSD ($p < 0.05$) for hemicellulose content in woody tree species.

8.3.6   FIBER

It is observed that not only there were statistically significant differences in the chemical composition of wood samples of the investigated plants; they also exhibited variability in the fiber content. The fiber content among these plant species varied from 74.98% to 94.91% (Fig. 8.11).

Maximum of fiber is observed in *Celtis pallida.* Close to the maximum content of fiber was revealed in *Parkinsonia aculeata* and *Guaiacum angustifolium.* Minimum of fiber content is observed in *Acacia farnesiana.* This species shows máximum number of statistically significant differences from other species (Fig. 8.12*). Croton suaveolens, Celtis laevigata, Bernardia myricifolia,* and *Lantana macropoda* have also many significant differences from other plant species.

8.3.7   RESULTS OF TUKEY'S HSD TEST FOR EACH PLANT SPECIES (P < 0.05)

The investigated plant species differ in lignin contents to the greatest degree (Fig. 8.13). The greatest similarity of the studied species is traced on the content of hemicellulose and ADF (Fig. 8.1). However, some plant species have the features. *Croton suaveolens, Guaiacum angustifolium,* and *Sargentia greggii* have the highest number of statistically significant differences in the content of fiber and NDF. *Acacia farnesiana* has the highest number of statistically significant differences in the content of fiber, ADF, and NDF. *Celtis laevigata, Bernardia myricifolia,* and *Quercus polymorpha* have the highest number of statistically significant differences in the content of hemicelluloses, fiber, and NDF. *Lantana macropoda* has the highest number of statistically significant differences in the content of NDF and cellulose. *Celtis pallida* and *Parkinsonia aculeata* have the highest number of statistically significant differences in the content of celluloses, fiber, ADF, and NDF.

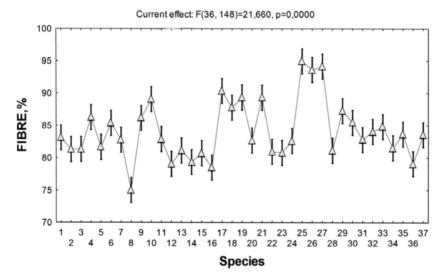

FIGURE 8.11   Fiber content (%) in woody tree species. 1: *Acacia schaffneri,* 2: *Fraxinus greggii,* 3: *Helietta parvifolia,* 4: *Forestiera angustifolia,* 5: *Cordia boissieri,* 6: *Salix lasiolepis,* 7: *Karwinskia humboldtiana,* 8: *Acacia farnesiana,* 9: *Diospyros texana,* 10: *Croton suaveolens,* 11: *Acacia berlandieri,* 12: *Sargentia greggii,* 13: *Acacia rigidula,* 14: *Ebenopsis ebano,* 15: *Amyris texana,* 16: *Ehretia anacua,* 17: *Celtis laevigata,* 18: *Quercus polymorpha,* 19: *Bernardia myricifolia,* 20: *Prosopis laevigata,* 21: *Lantana macropoda,* 22: *Eysenhardtia polystachya,* 23: *Cercidium macrum,* 24: *Zanthoxylum fagara,* 25: *Celtis pallida,* 26: *Guaiacum angustifolium,* 27: *Parkinsonia aculeata,* 28: *Leucaena leucocephala,* 29: *Leucophyllum frutescens,* 30: *Condalia hookeri,* 31: *Acacia wrightii,* 32: *Harvadia pallens,* 33: *Gymnosperma glutinosum,* 34: *Berberis trifoliata,* 35: *Caesalpinia mexicana,* 36: *Sideroxylon celastrina,* 37: *Diospyros palmeri.*

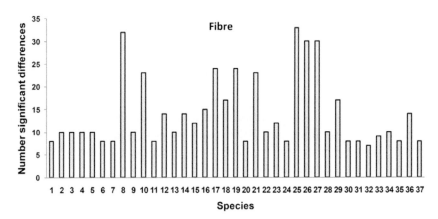

FIGURE 8.12   Results of Tukey's HSD ($p < 0.05$) for fiber content in woody species.

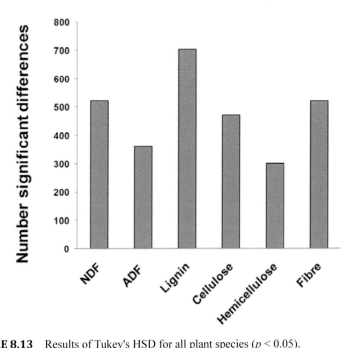

FIGURE 8.13   Results of Tukey's HSD for all plant species ($p < 0.05$).

8.3.8   CONCLUSIONS

In conclusion, it may be noted that the investigated plant species, to the greatest degree, differ in lignin contents. This information may be helpful in the selection of species for a particular purpose. The greatest similarity of the studied species is traced on the content of hemicelluloses and ADF.

Table 8.1 depicts the chemical composition of woods of 37 woody species (percentage of NDF, ADF, lignin, cellulose, hemicellulose, and fiber) at Linares, Northeast Mexico. Table 8.1 reveals that there exist large variations among woody species in the percentage of NDF, ADF, lignin, hemicellulose, cellulose, and fiber) among species. For example, percentage of NDF on an average ranged from 75 to 94; ADF, 51–77; lignin, 11–28; hemicellulose, 16–36; cellulose, 29–62; and fiber, 74–05. The variability in these chemical components are represented in Figures 8.2–8.4 and Tukey's HSD for each element at the last.

In this respect, few studies are documented on the wood chemical composition of woods of few woody plants, but studies on the percentage of NDF, ADF, and fiber observed in the present study on a large number of woody species are rare in the literature. We mention herein few of these results on different woody species in other countries, some of which coincide with our results.

In this respect, Petterson (1984) reported the chemical composition of woods of few species mentioning the variation of lignin from 18% to 35%. Ortuno (1998) reported the chemistry of cellulose, hemicellulose, and pectins. On the other hand, Gudalupe Barcenas Pozas and Raymondo Deavalas Sotelo (1999) made a comprehensive review on importance of lignin stating that lignin offers resistance to shrinkage and movement of moisture and specific gravity also plays a great role. This reflects the quality of a particular wood. In other studies, Guadalupe Berland and Bjarme Holman (1999) reported that distribution of lignin in a particular wood varied radially from heartwood, softwood, and transition zone wood, lignin is maximum in heartwood and medium in softwood. But our study was concentrated on groundwood of different species. There is a necessity to study the variation of lignin and other composition in different zones similar to that as done by Gudalupe Barcenas Pozas and Raymondo Deavalas Sotelo (1999). On the other hand, Agata Pawlika et al. (2013) reported variation in chemical composition, such as lignin, holocellulose, pentosans of exotic wood species obtained from countries, including the United States. They reported that cellulose varied from 41.59 to 43.14; lignin from 22.43 to 30.36. The results more or less coincide with our findings.

Maiti et al. (2016) working on wood's chemical composition of ten woody species at Linares reported that lignin varied from 15.28% to 24.35%; hemicellulose, 19.94% to 27.36%; cellulose, 33.69% to 45.92%. They mentioned the role of chemical compositions, such as lignin and cellulose, on the wood density of the species. On the other hand, Scharnweber et al. (2016) reported that the chemical composition varied in two species, pine and chestnut, cellulose from 41% to 43% and lignin from 22% to 30%, which coincides with the results of few species studied particleboard.

With respect to the role of chemical composition on wood quality Sriraam et al. (2012) working on wood chips and pellets of scot pine, spruce, eucalyptus, and silver birch reported that cellulose ranged from 39.5% to 45.00%. Eucalyptus showing the maximum Hemicellulose ranged from 19.20% to 32.40% and lignin from 22% to 31.30%. Eucalyptus had a maximum lignin percentage. Similarly, Mehmet Baharlogu et al. (2013) reported the effects of anatomical composition on the quality of particleboard. They concluded that pine wood produced strong particleboard.

We selected woody species for containing high-percentage of different chemical contents:

- High % NDF: *Celtis pallida* (94.80); *Parkinsonia aculeata* (93.99); *Guaicum angustifolium* (93.46); *Celtis laevigata* (90.27); *Quercus polymorpha* (87.63); *Croton suaveolens* (88.89).
- High % ADF: *Celtis pallida* (77.58); *Parkinsonia aculeata* (77.14); *Lantana macropoda* (71.37); *Leucophyllum frutescens* (67.27); *Guiacum angustifolium* 65.10).
- High % lignin: *Siderxylon celastrina* (28.67); *Ebenopsis ebano* (27.80); *Amyris texana* (24.85); *Ehretia anacua* (24.93); *Leucophyllum frutescens* (24.67), *Guiacum angustifolium* (21.23); *Condalia hookeri* (24.14); *Cordia boissieri* (24.36).
- High % hemicellulose: *Bernardia myricifolia* (30.39); *Celtis laevigata* (30.18); *Guiacum angustifolium* (28.33); *Quercus polymorpha* (27.91); *Croton suaveolens* (27.37).
- High % cellulose: *Parkinsonia aculeate* (61.85); *Celtis pallida* (60.51); *Lantana macropoda* (52.56); *Prosopis laevigata* (44.16); *Cercidium macrum* (47.61); *Salix lasiolepis* (45.92); *Leucaena leucocephala* (45.60), *Celtis laevigata* (45.57), *Eysenhardtia polystachya* (44.85).
- High % fiber: *Celtis pallida* (94.91); *Parkinsonia aculeate* (94.14); *Guiacum angustifolium* (93.62); *Celtis laevigata* (90.35); *Bernardia myricifolia* (89.36); *Lantana macropoda* (89.32); *Croton suaveolens* (89.06); *Quercus polymorpha* (87.77); *Leucophyllum frutescens* (87.27); *Forestiera angustifolia* (86.24); *Diospyros texana* (86.15).

It is expected that high percentages of NDF, ADF, lignin, and fiber contribute to strength of wood for making of strong furniture and offer resistance to strong winds and storms. We selected few species with high lignin percentage such as *Siderxylon celastrina* (28.67); *Ebenopsis ebano* (27.80); *Amyris texana* (24.85); *Ehretia anacua* (24.93); *Leucophyllum frutescens* (24.67), *Guiacum angustifolium* (21.23); *Condalia hookeri* (24.14); *Cordia boissieri* (24.36), for high NDF namely, *Celtis pallida* (94.80); *Parkinsonia aculeata* (93.99); *Guaicum angustifolium* (93.46); *Celtis laevigata* (90.27); *Quercus polymorpha* (87.63); *Croton suaveolens* (88.89); for high ADF namely, *Celtis pallida* (77.58); *Parkinsonia aculeata* (77.14); *Lantana macropoda* (71.37); *Leucophyllum frutescens* (67.27); *Guiacum angustifolium* (65.10); and high fiber percentage namely, *Celtis pallida* (94.91); *Parkinsonia aculeate* (94.14); *Guiacum angustifolium* (93.62); *Celtis laevigata* (90.35); *Bernardia myricifolia* (89.36); *Lantana macropoda* (89.32); *Croton suaveolens* (89.06); *Quercus polymorpha* (87.77); *Leucophyllum frutescens* (87.27); *Forestiera angustifolia* (86.24); *Diospyros texana* (86.15).

The timber of these species could produce strong furniture as well as function against shrinkage and strong winds/storm stress. Besides, high wood density could impart strength in wood. Rodriguez et al. (2016) reported that there exists a large variability in wood density among woody species.

It is expected that high cellulose and high hemicellulose may contribute to good paper quality; hemicellulose has a good adhesive capacity in the paper. In this study, we selected few species for containing high values of these components. For high cellulose percentage, we selected *Parkinsonia aculeata* (60.85); *Celtis pallida* (60.61); *Lantana macropoda* (52.56); *Prosopis laevigata* (44.16); *Cercidium macrum* (47.61). On the other hand, we selected a few species for high hemicellulose percentage such as *Bernardia myricifolia* (30.39), *Celtis laevigata* (30.18). These hypotheses need to be confirmed in future study.

8.4 CONCLUSIONS

A study on analysis of few chemical components of woods of 37 woody species of Tamaulipan Thorn Scrub at Linares, Northeast Mexico reveals significant differences in percentages of NDF, ADF, lignin, cellulose, hemicellulose, and fiber contents. The species have been selected on the basis of high values of each component. The species with a high percentage of NDF, ADF, and fiber are recommended for the fabrication of strong furniture, doors, and instruments for domestic uses. The timber of these species may act against shrinkage and strong winds. The species selected for high cellulose and hemicellulose are recommended for the manufacture of paper. All these hypotheses need to be confirmed in future studies.

ACKNOWLEDGMENTS

Valuable technical assistance provided by Elsa González Serna is gratefully acknowledged. We thank two anonymous reviewers for critically reading the manuscript and for their constructive comments that helped to improve the manuscript. This research was funded, in part, by Universidad Autónoma de Nuevo León (Proyecto PAICYT Grant CT259-15) and Consejo Nacional de Ciencia y Tecnología (Grant 250732).

KEYWORDS

- **chemical composition**
- **woods**
- **ADF**
- **NDF**
- **lignin**
- **cellulose**
- **hemicellulose**
- **variability**
- **Tamaulipan thorn scrub**

REFERENCES

Baharoloğlu a M.; Nemli, G.; Sarı, B.; Birtürk T.; Bardak S. Effects of Anatomical and Chemical Properties of Wood on the Quality of Particleboard. *Composites* **2013,** *52*, 282–285.

Berland, F.; Holmbom, B. Chemical Components of Early and Heartwood in Norway spruce Heartwood and Sapwood and Transition Zone. *Wood Sci. Technol.* **2004,** *38*, 245–256.

Chandrasekaran, S. R.; Hopke, P. K.; Rector, L.; Allen, G.; Lin, L. Chemical Composition of Wood Chips and Wood Pellets. *Energ. Fuels* **2012,** *26*, 4932–4937.

Box, G. E. P. Non-normality and Tests on Variances. *Biometrika* **1953,** *40*, 318–335.

Fisher, R. A. Studies in Crop Variation. I. An Examination of the Yield of Dressed Grain from Broadbalk. *J. Agri. Sci.* **1921,** *11*, 107–135.

Gelman, A. Analysis of Variance? Why it is More Important Than Ever. *Annal. Stat.* **2005,** *33,* 1–53.

Jones, P. D.; Laurence, R.; Gary F. S.; Richard, F. P., Clark, D. A. Nondestructive Estimation of Wood Chemical Composition of Sections of Radial Wood Strips by Diffuse Reflectance Near Infrared Spectroscopy. *Wood Sci. Technol.* **2006,** *40,* 709–720.

Maiti, R. K.; Rodriguez H. G.; Kumari A. Wood Density of Ten Native Trees and Shrubs and Its Possible Relation with Few Wood Chemical Composition and Wood Structure. *Am. J. Plant Sci.* **2016,** 7.

Morrison, S.; Sosnoff, J. J.; Heffernan, K. S.; Jae, S. Y.; Fernhall, B. Aging, Hypertension and Physiological Tremor: The Contribution of the Cardioballistic Impulse to Tremorgenesis in Older Adults. *J. Neurol. Sci.* **2013,** *326,* 68–74.

Ortuño, A. V. Introducción a la química industrial. Editorial Reverté. *Alhambra Universidad.* **1998,** p 636.

Pawlicka A.; Waliszewska B. Chemical Composition of Selected Species of Exotic Wood Derived from the Region of Africa. *Acta Sci. Pol. Silv. Colendar. Rat. Ind. Lignar.* **2013,** *10,* 37–41.

Petterson, R. The Chemical Composition of Wood. Chaper 2. The Chemistry of Soft Wood. *Adv. Chem.* **1984,** *207,* 57–126.

Pazos, G. B.; Sotelo, R. D. Importancia de la lignina en las contracciones de la madera: revisión bibliográfica. *Madera y Bosques.* **1999,** *5,* 13–26.

Ray, R. N.; Chowdhury, M. C.; Jan, T. K. Wood Chemistry and Density: An Analog for Response to the Change of Carbon Sequestration in Mangroves. *Carbohy. Polym.* **2012,** *90,* 102–108.

Rodriguez, H. G.; Maiti, R.; Sarkar, N. C.; Kumari, A. Variability in Wood Density and Wood Fibre Characterization of Woody Species and Their Possible Utilityin Northeastern Mexico. *Am. J. Plant Sci.* **2016,** *7,* 1139–1150.

Scharnweber, T.; Hevia, A.; Buras, A.; van der Maaten E.; Wilmking M. Common Trends in Elements? Within- and Between-tree Variations of Wood-chemistry Measured by X-ray Fluorescence—A Dendrochemical Study. *Sci.Total Environ* **2016,** *566–567,* 1245–1253.

Tukey, J. W. Comparing Individual Means in the Analysis of Variance. *Biometrics* **1949,** *5,* 99–114.

CHAPTER 9

Carbon Sequestration by Woody Trees and Shrubs in Northeastern Mexico: A Synthesis

RATIKANTA MAITI,[1] HUMBERTO GONZALEZ RODRIGUEZ,[1*] CH. ARUNA KUMARI,[2] and NARAYAN CHANDRA SARKAR[3]

[1]Universidad Autónoma de Nuevo León, Facultad de Ciencias Forestales, Carr. Nac. No. 85 Km. 45, Linares, Nuevo Leon 67700, México

[2]Professor Jaya Shankar Telangana State Agricultural University, Agricultural College, Jagtial, India

[3]Department of ASEPAN, Institute of Agriculture, Visva-Bharati, PO Sriniketan, Birbhum, West Bengal 731236, India

*Corresponding author. E-mail: humberto.gonzalezrd@uanl.edu.mx

ABSTRACT

Carbon sequestration reveals the capacity of plants in fixation of carbon dioxide through leaves and stores them in plant biomass and wood, thereby reducing carbon load from atmosphere.

The present chapter makes a brief review of research undertaken globally with special reference to woody trees and shrubs in Northeastern Mexico. In this study, a few species with high carbon fixation/carbon content in leaves such as *Leucophyllum frutescens*, 49.97%; *Forestiera angustifolia*, 49.47%; *Acacia berlandieri*, 49.18%; *Bumelia celastrina*, 49.25%; and the species with moderately high carbon—*Acacia rigidula*, 48.23%; *Acacia farnesiana*, 46.17%; *Gymnospermum glutinosum*, 46.13%; *Croton suaveolens*, 45.17%; *Sargenia greggii*, 44.07%, and so on were selected. Few other species contained carbon ranging from 31% to 43%. It is recommended that these native plants could be transplanted in areas contaminated with high carbon load. The species with high carbon concentration are good sources of energy and growth of these species, besides sources of charcoal for the forest dwellers.

9.1   INTRODUCTION

Trees and shrubs are our life savers for reducing carbon dioxide emitted by greenhouse gases (GHGs) and supplying oxygen for our respiration. These trees and shrubs in the semiarid regions of Tamaulipan thorn scrub serve as important sources of timbers for furniture and sources of forage and nutrients for wild grazing animals for possessing various micro and macronutrients required for wild animals in Northeast of Mexico (Ramirez, 1998; Ramirez-Lozano, 2015). The availability of nutrients in leaves is essential for efficient plant function (Chaplin, 1982).

Trees also have the ability to fix atmospheric Carbon dioxide in the biomass and besides their ability to contribute to plant growth and productivity they supply nutrients also. We narrate here a brief review of research undertaken in carbon fixation and its impact in climate change. Many research activities have been directed on nutrient content and metabolism in leaves (Chapman et al., 1990). Plants have capacity to capture carbon dioxide from the atmosphere during the process of photosynthesis and finally store carbon in biomass and wood as sources of bioenergy. Variation in carbon fixation by photosynthesis is related to variation of carbon deposition in plant species.

Carbon is the source of energy for plants. During photosynthesis, plants take in CO_2 and give off the oxygen (O_2) to the atmosphere. The oxygen released is available for respiration. The plants retain and use the stored carbon for growth to guide all metabolic functions. Finally, carbon is stored in plant organs and timber serving as an important source of energy. On the other hand, as a consequence of global climatic change generated, there is an eventual increase in the aerial temperature and an increase of GHGs, particularly CO_2.

There are two methods of sequestration of carbon dioxide from atmosphere, land management practice for maximizing the storage of carbon in soil and another by plant for long term as mentioned above. Geologic sequestration involves a process in carbon sequestration process (CCS/0 Process). In this process, carbon is stored through agricultural and forestry practices. This involves also injection of carbon dioxide captured from the atmosphere is injected deep underground where carbon dioxide oxide is stored permanently. Carbon fixation in trees is a micro optimization process leading to the accumulation of carbon in plant organs. Two alternative economic-analog models of carbon fixation are developed by John Holt (1990). The second model takes into consideration of carbon revenue as the minimum of two functions involving carbon gain to leaf and root biomass, respectively. In both of these models, leaves and roots are the limiting factors. Coleman et al. (1995) undertook a study on the photosynthetic productivity of aspen clones varying in sensitivity to tropospheric ozone revealing the influence of environments on this activity. Increasing global warming associated with incessant logging, illegal anthropogenic activities and conversion of forest to agriculture have enhanced the accumulation of GHGs mainly carbon dioxide in the atmosphere, thereby increasing pollution and climate change (Alig et al., 2002). The constant emission of carbon dioxide by burning of fossil fuels is a menace to enhance atmospheric pollution and is endangering the security of mankind and animals. This has direct impact on climate changes, thereby, reducing crop productivity and aggravating poverty. Different technologies are adopted to mitigate it in different developed countries in relation to carbon dioxide capture and sequestration but these high-cost technologies are beyond the reach of developing countries to adopt this technology. This urges a great necessity to reduce CO_2 load from the atmosphere.

In this respect, plants have capacity to capture carbon dioxide load from the atmosphere during the process of photosynthesis, synthesis of carbohydrate which is stored as carbon. Variation in carbon fixation by photosynthesis is related to variation of carbon deposition in plant species. Carbon is the source of energy for plants. Carbon fixation through the process of photosynthesis leads to the production of biomass and dry matter production in the forest plants.

The accumulation of forest biomass determines the amount of carbon store in forest plants (Brown, 1999). During the process of photosynthesis, plants take in CO_2 and give off the oxygen (O_2) to the atmosphere. This oxygen that is released is made available for our respiration. The plants retain and use the stored carbon for growth to guide all metabolic functions (Lincoln Taiz and Edwardo Zeger, 1998). In order to mitigate carbon pollution, forest plantation is done to capture and retain carbon. Forests play an important role in the global C cycle (Brown, 1999).

There exists a great diversity among plat species in growth habit, leaf size, lea shape, canopy and capacity of carbon fixation needed for photosynthesis and respiration (Wright et al., 2001). The fixation of CO_2 into living matter maintains all life on Earth and the biosphere with geochemistry. Braaakman and Smith (2012) developed a model for early evolution of biological carbon fixation process. This finally leads to all modern pathways to a single ancestral form. From this has arisen most early divergence of tree life. This in turn integrates fully their metabolic and phylogenetic constraints.

In the United States storage of carbon is forests is encouraged not for paying carbon tax. In Eastern United States and South Et Colorado, Keller et al. (2003) adopted a strategy for sequestration of carbon dioxide for managing future climate change and optimum economic growth framework. They developed first, a simple analytical model, and second, by using a numerical optimization model with an objective to explore the problem in a more realistic manner.

The incessant increase of GHGs caused by logging, illegal human activities is a menace to our life security. This particular greenhouse gas levels were increased several folds leading to pollution and climate change (Alig Adoms and Mc Cor, 2002).

It is well known that the increased global warming is attributed to the increased concentration of various GHGs as carbon dioxide, methane, nitrous oxide, sulfur dioxide, chlorofluorocarbon, ozone and water vapor (Garduno, 2004). On the other hand, the excess atmospheric carbon being released in the atmosphere can be absorbed by photosynthesis by trees and ecosystems (Rodriguez et al., 2008) Carbon sequestration has significant role in reducing global warming (Pimients et al., 2007). It is suggested by Adam Martin and Sean Thomas that an accurate knowledge of carbon content in live wood is a great necessity for quantification of tropical forest carbon stocks. They reported that wood carbon content differed significantly among species from 41.9% to 51%.

In Mexico, various studies have been undertaken on the variability of carbon content in the above-ground biomass (Gyosco and Guarine, 2005; Yemena et al., 2012a). Jimenez et al. (2013) estimated Wood carbon contents of some representative species of the pine-ok forest of Sirra Madre Oriental. The species included are *Pinus pseuditrobus, Juniperus fláccida, Quercus laceyi, Quercus rysophyla, Quercus canby* and *Arbutus xalapens*. The highest wood carbon was obtained from *Junipeus fláccida* (51.18%) while *Quercus crysophylla* contained the lowest (47.98%); the component with the highest carbon concentration was the leaves of *Arbutusxala pensis* (55.05%), while the bark of Quercus laceyi had the lowest (43.65%) Highly significant differences were observed for the average carbon concentration by group of species. Coniferous species contained an average of 50.76% while that of broad leaf was 48.85%.

In the context of the above literatures we undertook two studies on carbon fixation of a number of trees and shrubs at Linares, Northeastern Mexico. In the context of the above literature survey, we undertook two studies on carbon fixation/carbon sequestration in two sets of plants.

9.2   STUDY 1

Gonzále Rodriguez et al. (2015a) estimated carbon fixation (sequestration) of 37 mostly trees in Linares, northeast of Mexico with the main objective to select species with carbon fixation for recommendation of plantation in carbon dioxide polluted areas.

9.2.1   MATERIALS AND METHOD

The study was located in the experiment station of Forest Science Faculty of Universidad Autonoma de Nuev Leon, at Linare (24°47′N, 99°32′W), at elevation of 350 m. The climate is subtropical or semiarid with warm summer, monthly mean air temperature varies from 14.7°C in January to 23°C in August, but during summer may rise to 45°C. The annual precipitation is 805 mm. The vegetation Tamaulipan thorn scrub soil is deep, dark gray, lime-gray, and vertisol.

9.2.2   CHEMICAL ANALYSIS

The leaves of woody and shrubs were collected during autumn, and placed to dry on newspaper for a week. The leaves are collected, separated from plants, dried in an oven at 65° for 3 days in an oven (precision model, 16eg) and passed two times through a mesh of 1×1 mm in diameter using a mill (Thomas Willey) and then stored in desiccator. A 2 mg of the sample weighed in an AD 600 Perkin balance Elmer was kept in Chon's analyzer Perkin Elmer Model 2400 for estimation of carbon, hydrogen and nitrogen. For estimation of mineral contents, the samples were incinerated in a muffle oven for 5 h. Then shed sample is digested in a solution of HCL and HNO3 using wet digestion (Cherney, 2000).

The carbon content (% dry weight basis) was estimated in 0.020 g of milled and dried leaf tissue using CHN analyzer (Perkin Elmer, model 2400). Carbon contents (% dry weight basis Protein content is determined by a factor Nitrogen content ×6.25.

9.2.3   RESULTS AND DISCUSSION

In this study, we selected few species with high carbon fixation/carbon content in leaves such as *Leucophyllum frutescens*, 49.97%; *Forestiera angustifolia*,

TABLE 9.1 Leaf Nutrients Content in Different Plant Species MET). Data are Means and Standard Deviation ($n = 5$).

Name scientific	Family	Type	% C	% N	C/N	% Protein
Helietta parvifolia	Rutaceae	Shrub	31.13 ± 1.03	2.43 ± 0.25	12.84 ± 4.16	15.19
Amyris texana	Rutaceae	Shrub	38.06 ± 1.89	3.72 ± 0.33	12.79 ± 5.65	23.25
Leucophyllum frutescens	Scrophulariaceae	Shrub	49.97 ± 0.94	2.25 ± 0.27	22.17 ± 3.51	14.06
Acacia rigidula	Fabaceae	Shrub	48.23 ± 1.56	2.60 ± 0.22	18.58 ± 6.96	16.25
Zanthoxylum fagara	Rutaceae	Shrub	40.35 ± 3.15	2.98 ± 0.90	13.56 ± 3.50	18.63
Karwinskia humboldtiana	Rhamnaceae	Shrub	31.35 ± 0.70	2.84 ± 0.10	11.03 ± 6.91	17.75
Celtis pallida	Ulmaceae	Shrub	38.66 ± 0.88	4.12 ± 0.67	9.38 ± 1.32	25.75
Guaiacum angustifolium	Zygophyllaceae	Shrub	41.89 ± 3.56	2.90 ± 0.42	14.44 ± 8.48	18.13
Acacia farnesiana	Fabaceae	Shrub	46.17 ± 2.63	3.41 ± 0.18	13.54 ± 14.61	21.31
Lantana macropoda	Verbenaceae	Shrub	42.91 ± 3.74	4.43 ± 0.39	9.68 ± 9.53	27.69
Bernardia myricifolia	Euphrobiaceae	Shrub	42.69 ± 1.13	4.21 ± 0.49	10.13 ± 2.30	26.31
Forestiera angustifolia	Oleaceae	Shrub	49.47 ± 0.43	3.00 ± 0.41	16.47 ± 1.04	18.75
Croton suaveolens	Euphrobiaceae	Shrub	45.17 ± 0.35	2.33 ± 0.53	20.16 ± 0.67	14.56
Gymnosperma glutinosum	Asteraceae	Shrub	46.19 ± 1.04	5.89 ± 0.29	7.85 ± 3.54	36.81
Eysenhardtia polystachya	Fabaceae	Shrub	36.26 ± 0.58	4.06 ± 0.27	8.94 ± 2.15	25.38
Berberis trifolilata	Berberidaceae	Shrub	36.91 ± 1.25	2.43 ± 0.19	15.17 ± 6.71	15.19
Cordia boissieri	Boraginaceae	Tree	43.43 ± 1.20	3.28 ± 0.09	13.23 ± 13.38	20.50
Ehretia anacua	Boraginaceae	Tree	34.09 ± 2.51	2.44 ± 0.10	13.97 ± 25.10	15.25
Caesalpinia mexicana	Fabaceae	Tree	41.12 ± 1.96	2.91 ± 0.38	14.13 ± 5.16	18.19
Condalia hoockeri	Rhamnaceae	Tree	30.07 ± 2.81	3.06 ± 0.41	9.83 ± 6.85	19.13
Sargentia gregii	Rutaceae	Tree	44.07 ± 1.22	1.91 ± 0.45	23.13 ± 2.71	11.94

TABLE 9.1 *(Continued)*

Name scientific	Family	Type	% C	% N	C/N	% Protein
Diospyros palmeri	Ebenaceae	Tree	37.59 ± 1.72	2.17 ± 0.12	17.36 ± 14.33	13.56
Diospyros texana	Ebenaceae	Tree	40.79 ± 1.46	1.89 ± 0.06	21.58 ± 24.33	11.81
Bumelia celastrina	Sapotacee	Tree	49.25 ± 1.56	2.42 ± 0.36	20.35 ± 4.38	15.13
Ebenopsis ébano	Fabaceae	Tree	37.57 ± 1.21	3.86 ± 0.20	9.73 ± 6.05	24.13
Quercus polymorpha	Fabaceae	Tree	43.02 ± 2.38	1.96 ± 0.18	21.95 ± 13.22	12.25
Acacia berlandieri	Fabaceae	Tree	49.18 ± 1.25	3.82 ± 0.14	12.88 ± 8.89	23.88
Acacia shaffneri	Fabaceae	Tree	39.52 ± 0.99	4.32 ± 0.16	9.15 ± 6.19	27.00
Leucaena leucocephala	Fabaceae	Tree	43.16 ± 1.98	3.78 ± 0.50	11.42 ± 3.96	23.63
Prosopis laevigata	Fabaceae	Tree	41.64 ± 0.71	3.85 ± 0.21	10.83 ± 3.38	24.06
Celtis laevigata	Ulmaceae	Tree	39.45 ± 0.51	3.01 ± 0.18	13.13 ± 2.78	18.81
Cercidium macrum	Fabaceae	Tree	43.41 ± 3.44	4.01 ± 0.30	10.83 ± 11.47	25.06
Parkinsonia aculeata	Caesalpiniaceae	Tree	36.63 ± 3.25	3.04 ± 0.41	12.05 ± 7.93	19.00
Salix lasiolepis	Salicaceae	Tree	33.37 ± 4.58	2.06 ± 0.50	16.24 ± 9.16	12.88
Harvadia pallens		Tree	43.49 ± 1.24	2.97 ± 0.15	14.64 ± 8.27	18.56
Acacia wrightti	Mimosaceae	Tree	36.59 ± 1.11	3.96 ± 0.18	9.25 ± 6.22	24.75
Fraxinus greggii	Oleaceae	Tree	38.06 ± 1.89	2.15 ± 0.14	17.69 ± 13.85	13.44

49.47%; *Acacia berlandieri*, 49.18%; *Bumelia celastrina*, 49.25%, while the species with moderately high carbon were Acacia rigidula, 48.23 %; *Acacia farnesiana*, 46.17%; *Gymnospermum glutinosum*, 46.13%; *Croton suaveolens*, 45.17%; *Sargenia greggii*, 44.07%. Other species contained carbon ranging from 31% to 43%.

The species with high carbon concentration are good sources of energy and growth of these species, besides sources of charcoal for the forest dwellers. The species also showed large variability in nitrogen (2–5%), C/N (7–36%) and protein contents (11–37%) representing the nutritional value for forage for animals.

9.3   STUDY 2

Carbon fixation in relation to leaf characteristics and wood density Though wood is an important source of carbon of high commercial value, the information with respect to the role of plant characteristics and carbon fixation capacity on wood quality such as density and wood structural characteristics is rare.

The present study was undertaken to determine carbon fixation, leaf canopy, leaf nutrients (% C, N, protein, C/N) with their possible relation with wood density of 18 native woody species at Linares, Mexico.

9.3.1   *MATERIALS AND METHODS*

We selected the following 18 species of economic importance in the region for analyzing their nutrient content and carbon fixation ability. We investigated the following aspects: Leaf nutrients (N, C/N, protein). Carbon fixation.

Leaf canopy architecture—open, semi close, close depending on the mode of exposure to solar radiation (Maiti et al., 2014). Density: We collected 10 pieces of wood of 5 cm long from the branches of the tree of each species and then dried in an oven at 80°C for 3 days, then cooled and kept in a desiccator to prevent absorption of water from the atmosphere. Then each wood species was dipped in water in a measuring cylinder for measuring the volume of the wood. The density of wood was calculated as follows:

$$\text{Density} = \frac{\text{Weight of wood } (g)}{\text{Volume } (cm^3)}$$

9.3.2 RESULTS AND DISCUSSION

Table 9.2 depicts leaf canopy, C %, N %, C/N, protein, and wood density of 18 species. It is observed from Table 9.1, that the leaf canopy of the species studied varies from open, semi-closed, and close. Most of the species have semi-close and open canopy leaves.

The tree canopies are classified depending on the mode of exposure to solar radiation and probable efficiency in photosynthesis. The species with open leaf canopy is expected to be more efficient in the capture of solar radiation and greater photosynthesis compared to those having semi-close and close canopy ones. In this context, the species showed variability in carbon fixation ranging from 30% to approximately 50%.

The species with high carbon fixation are *Leucophyllum frutescens* (49.97%), *Forestiera angustifolia* (49.47%), *Bumelia celastrina* (49.25%), *Acacia berlandieri* (49.18%), and *Acacia farnesiana* (46.17%). Interestingly all these have open leaf canopy, except *Forestiera angustifolia* (semi-close, shrub), which indirectly support the hypothesis by Maiti et al. (2014).

This needs to be verified with further study. Nitrogen and protein content serve in nitrogen metabolism and enzyme function thereby contributing to forage value for animal health. Nitrogen content varied approximately from 2% to 4%, while C/N varied from 8% to 22%. On the other hand, protein content varied from 11 to 26%, reasonably high value from the stand point of animal nutrition. Several species have more than 20% protein.

The species showing high value of protein content are *Bernardia myricifolia* (26.31%), *Celtis pallida* (25.75%), *Eysenhardtia polystachya* (25.38%), *Cercidium macrum* (25.06%), *Ebenopsis ebano* (24.13%), *Acacia berlandieri* (23.38%), which are excellent sources of protein for animal health. It is expected that high carbon fixation could contribute to high accumulation of carbon in wood, thereby possibly increase of wood density. In this respect wood density varied from 0.62 to 0.95. The species showing higher values of wood density are *Bernardia myricifolia* (0.97), *Prosopis laevigata* (0.95), *Ebanopsis ebano* (0.91), *Eysenhardtia polystachya* (0.91), *Cercidium mexicana* (0.90), *Karwinskia humboldtiana* (0.88), *Cordia boissieri* (0.87), *Acacia berlandieri* (0.87), Condalia hoockeri (0.85), and *Celtis pallida* (0.77).

It is interesting to note that all these species possess open to semi open leaf canopy, thereby indicating that the species with open canopy have high carbon fixation as well as high wood density.

TABLE 9.2　Leaf Nutrients Content in Different Plant Species.

S. No	Scientific name	Family	Type/leaf canopy	% C	% N	C/N	% Protein	Density g/cm^3
1	Diospyros texana	Ebenaceae	Tree (semi-close)	40.79 ± 1.46	1.89 ± 0.06	21.58 ± 24.33	11.81	0.642 ± 0.055
2	Bumelia celastrina	Sapotacee	Tree (open)	49.25 ± 1.56	2.42 ± 0.36	20.35 ± 4.38	15.13	0.785 ± 0.078
3	Cercidium macrum	Fabaceae	Tree (open)	43.41 ± 3.44	4.01 ± 0.30	10.83 ± 11.47	25.06	0.901 ± 0.104
4	Prosopis laevigata	Fabaceae	Tree (open)	41.64 ± 0.71	3.85 ± 0.21	10.83 ± 3.38	24.06	0.954 ± 0.077
5	Condalia hoockeri	Rhamnaceae	Tree (semi-open)	30.07 ± 2.81	3.06 ± 0.41	9.83 ± 6.85	19.13	0.851 ± 0.143
6	Celtis laevigata	Ulmaceae	Tree (close)	39.45 ± 0.51	3.01 ± 0.18	13.13 ± 2.78	18.81	0.717 ± 0.035
7	Harvadia pallens	Fabaceae	Tree (open)	43.49 ± 1.24	2.97 ± 0.15	14.64 ± 8.27	18.56	0.707 ± 0.061
8	Ebenopsis ebano	Fabaceae	Tree (semi-close)	37.57 ± 1.21	3.86 ± 0.20	9.73 ± 6.05	24.13	0.910 ± 0.065
9	Cordia boissieri	Boraginaceae	Tree (semi-close)	43.43 ± 1.20	3.28 ± 0.09	13.23 ± 13.38	20.50	0.620 ± 0.048
10	Acacia berlandieri	Fabaceae	Tree (open)	49.18 ± 1.25	3.82 ± 0.14	12.88 ± 8.89	23.88	0.876 ± 0.063
11	Forestiera angustifolia	Oleaceae	Shrub (semi-close)	49.47 ± 0.43	3.00 ± 0.41	16.47 ± 1.04	18.75	0.634 ± 0.033
12	Karwinskia hum boldhiana	Rhamnaceae	Shrub (open)	31.35 ± 0.70	2.84 ± 0.10	11.03 ± 6.91	17.75	0.885 ± 0.080
13	Acacia farnesiana	Fabaceae	Shrub (open)	46.17 ± 2.63	3.41 ± 0.18	13.54 ± 14.61	21.31	0.808 ± 0.090
14	Leucophyllum frutescens	Scrophulariaceae	Shrub (open)	49.97 ± 0.94	2.25 ± 0.27	22.17 ± 3.51	14.06	0.787 ± 0.183
15	Eysenhardtia polystachya	Fabaceae	Shrub (open)	36.26 ± 0.58	4.06 ± 0.27	8.94 ± 2.15	25.38	0.911 ± 0.084
16	Bernardia myricifolia	Euphorbiaceae	Shrub (open)	42.69 ± 1.13	4.21 ± 0.49	10.13 ± 2.30	26.31	0.975 ± 0.092
17	Celtis pallia	Ulmaceae	Shrub (open)	38.66 ± 0.88	4.12 ± 0.67	9.38 ± 1.32	25.75	0.777 ± 0.065
18	Zanthoxylum fagara	Rutaceae	Shrub (open)	40.35 ± 3.15	2.98 ± 0.90	13.56 ± 3.50	18.63	0.661 ± 0.043

9.4 CONCLUSIONS

The study showed large variability in carbon fixation (carbon concentration), nitrogen among 37 species during Autumn, in northeast Mexico thereby giving good opportunity in the selection of species with high carbon concentration. The species with high carbon fixation with arboreal habit could be planted in polluted areas and town planning to reduce carbon dioxide load. It is desirable to select species with landscape architecture and high capacity of carbon fixation to fulfill our objectives. Further study is needed to estimate carbon fixation of these species during summer season to determine the influence of environment on carbon fixation. There is also necessity to select species with high carbon fixation and good landscape architecture. The study also demonstrates a large variability in nitrogen, C/N, and protein content among the species studied which may be used in the selection of species for high nutritive values of forage for animals.

KEYWORDS

- **carbon sequestration**
- **variability in carbon sequestration**
- **species with high carbon sequestration**
- **contamination**

REFERENCES

Adam, R.; Sean, M.; Thomas, C. A Reassessment of Carbon Content in Tropical Trees. *PLoS One* **2011,** *6* (8), e23533. (https://doi.org/10.1371/journal.pone.0023533).

Adoms, A. R. J. R.; McCorL, B. Projecting impacts on Global Climate Change on the US Forest and Agriculture Sectors and Carbon Budgets. *Forest Ecol. Manag.* **2002,** *169,* 21–23.

Braakman, R.; Smith, E. The Emergence and Early Evolution of Biological Carbon-Fixation. *PLoS Comput. Biol.* **2012,** *8* (4), e1002455. (doi:10.1371/journal.pcbi.1002455).

Brown, S. *Guidelines for Inventorying and Monitoring Carbon Effects in Forest-Base Projects Winrock International for the World Bank*; Arlington: Virginia, U.S.A., 1999; p11.

Chaplin, F. S. The Mineral Nutrition of Wild Plants. *Ann. Rev. Ecol. Syst.* **1982,** *19,* 233–260.

Chapman, F. S. The Ecology and Economics of Storage in Plants. *Ann. Rev. Ecol. Syst.* **1990,** *21,* 423–447.

Cherney, D. J. R. Characterization of Forages by Chemical Analysis. In *Forage Evaluation in Ruminant Nutrition*; Givens, D. I., Owen, O., Axford, R. F. E., Omed, H. M., Eds.; CAB International: Wallingford, 2000; pp 281–300.

Coleman, M. D.; Isebrands, J. G.; Dickson, R. E.; Karnosky, D. F. Photosynthetic Productivity of Aspen Clones Varying in Sensitivity to Tropospheric Ozone. *Tree Physiol.* **1995**, *15*, 585–592.

Garduno, R. Que es el efecto invernadero. In *Cambioclimatico: Una vision desde Mexico*; Martinez, J. Y., Fernandez, A., Eds.; INE-SEMARNAT, Mexico. D.F., 2004; pp 29–39.

Gayoso, J.; Guerra, J. Contenido de carbono en lo biomoso aéreo de bosques nativos en Chile. *Bosque* **2005**, 33–38.

Rodriguez, H. G.; Maiti, R. K.; Valencia, N. R. I.; Sarkar, N. C. Carbon and Nitrogen Content in Leaf Tissue of Different Plant Species, Northeastern Mexico. *Int. J. Bio-resour. Stress Manag.* **2015**, *6*, 113–11.

Jiménez, P. J.; Treviño, G. E. J.; Yamallel, J. I. Carbon Concentration in Pine-Oak Forest Species of the Sierra Madre Oriental. *Revista mexicana de ciencias forestales* **2013**, *4* (17), 50–61.

Hof, J. J. Carbon Fixation in Trees as a Micro Optimization Process: An Example of Combining Ecology and Economics. *Ecol. Econ.* **1990**, *2*, 243–256.

Keller, K.; Yang, Z.; Hall, M., Bradford, D. F. *Carbondioxide Sequestration: When and How Much*; Center for Economic Policy Studies (CEPS), Princeton University September; 2003, p 4.

Lincoln, T.; Zeger, E. Plant Physiology Second Edition. Sinauer Associates, Inc. Publishers. Massachusets. Lindroth, R. L., Osien, T. L., Burnhill, H. R. H., Wood, S. A. (2002). Effects of Genotype and Nutrient Availability on Photosensitivity of Trembling Aspen (Populus tremoides Mich) During Leaf Senescence. *Biochem. Sys. Ecol.* **1998**, *30*, 297–307.

Pimienta. *Estimacion de biomasay contenido de carbono de Pinus cooperi Banco e Pueblo Nuevo*; Madera y Bosque: Durango, 2007; Vol. 13, pp 35–36.

Ramirez, R. G. Food Habits and Nutrient Techniques of Small Ruminants, Extensive, Management Systems. *Small Ruminants Res.* **1998**, *34*, 215–220.

Ramirez, L. R. G. Native Shrubs: Edible Foliage for Small Ruminants. In: *Applied Botany*; Maiti, R. K. et al., Eds.; Puspa Publishing House: Kolkata, India, 2015; p 222.

Rodriguez, R. Carbono contenido en un bosque troicalsubcadicifolio en la reserva de la Biosfera E Cielo, Tamaulipas, Mexico. *Reseta Latinoamericano de Recursos Naturales* **2008**, *4*, 215–222.

Wright, L. J. P. B. Strategy Shifts in Leaf Physiology, Structure and Nutrient Content Between Species of High- and Low-Rainfall and High- and Low-Nutrient Habitats. *Funct. Ecol.* **2001**, *15*, 423–434.

Yemena, Y.; Jimnez, J.; Trevino, G.; Alanis, R. Caracterizacion de carbono en el fueste de 21 especies de conifers de noreste de Mexico. *Revista Mexican de Ciancias forestal* **2012**, *3*, 490–506.

Yemana, Y.; Jimnez, J.; Aguiree, P. A.; Trevino, G. *Contenido de carbono total de especies arboreoud y arbustos de diferentes usos en el matoral de matoral Tamaupan*; Bosque, Mexico, 2012; Vol. 33, pp 145–152.

CHAPTER 10

Mangrove Forest and Plantation

PRADEEP KHANNA*

Former Chief Conservator of Forest, Gujarat, India.

Corresponding author. E-mail: pradeep.khanna@gmail.com

ABSTRACT

Mangroves, which were once considered wastelands, are being increasingly recognized for their ecological services that they perform as inshore stabilization, protection from cyclones/storms/tsunami, home to marine biodiversity, etc. Mangroves prosper in warm tropical regions. More than 40% of world mangroves are found in Asia. Mangrove forests in India extend over 4921 km^2 in 12 states and union territories. The Sundarbans, recognized as a heritage site, extending to over 6000 km^2 in India and Bangladesh support a contiguous patch of mangrove forests that are the largest mangrove forests of the world. Gujarat coasts support the second largest area of mangrove with 1140 km^2 of mangrove forests. Mangroves received attention, and efforts for its rejuvenation started, after the declaration of Marine National Park in 1980. The mangrove cover increased from an estimated 427 km^2 in 1987 to 1140 km^2 in 2017, over two-and-a-half-fold increase. Gujarat is the only state of India that has reported such significant increase in mangrove forests. Though the diversity of species of mangrove species in Gujarat is restricted to fourteen species, the education awareness has played a significant role in making a success of mangrove conservation program in Gujarat. The GEER Foundation has made a significant contribution in providing research inputs with support of Mangrove for Future and IUCN. Detailed mapping of mangroves and potential areas for mangrove has been done.

10.1   INTRODUCTION

Mangroves now recognized for their high productivity and variety of economic and ecological services were considered as wastelands holding little intrinsic value till first half of the twentieth century and attracted little attention. Large mangrove areas were reclaimed for a variety of economic activities. It was in later part of the 20th century that importance and value of mangroves were recognized.

Mangroves are highly productive ecosystems. They are a special type of vegetation occupying the mudflats at the boundary of marine and terrestrial environment. They stand with their roots in tidal region in salty marine water. Thus, one of the special characteristics of this group of vegetation is its salt tolerance. They are predominantly found in tropics. They thrive in the environment near mouths of large rivers, where river deltas provide lot of sediment. The mangrove cover in the world is estimated at 18 million ha with about 40% in Asia (Spalding, 1997). Countries with large tracts of mangrove forests are Indonesia (45,421 km^2; Spalding, 1997), Brazil (13,800 km^2; Spalding, 1997), Bangladesh (5767 km^2, Spalding, 1997), and India (4921 km^2, Anonymous SFR, 2017).

Last 50 years we observed increasing appreciation of ecological importance of mangrove forests for a variety of ecological services they provide. These include:

a) Shoreline stabilization: Mangroves function as a stabilizer of sediment that is deposited by the geomorphological process.

b) Protection from cyclones and storms: Mangroves are susceptible to damage from storms and cyclones. Yet they provide protection from the severity of devastation caused by storms, cyclone, and even tsunami.

c) Maintenance of channel depth: Stabilization of coastal sands helps to maintain channel depth for uninterrupted navigation.

d) Marine life conservation: Mangrove provides an environment for the conservation of a variety of marine life that includes fishery and wild marine life. It includes marine life that thrives in the mangrove region as also marine life beyond the mangroves.

e) Coral conservation: Mangroves contribute to coral conservation by retaining silt from moving over corals and restricting algal growth due to eutrophication.

f) Wildlife conservation: Mangroves are safe home to a large variety of birds, resting and feeding areas for migratory birds and are known to support large heronries.

g) Timber and fodder for the local community

h) Offer ecotourism opportunities that provide employment opportunities to the local community.

i) Carbon sequestration: Mangrove forests are efficient for carbon sequestration. The primary productivity of mangroves is amongst the highest of natural ecosystems (Ong, 2013).

Mangroves prefer warm tropical regions. However, there are variations in the latitude range for mangrove occurrence in different geographic regions. In Pacific Asia where over 40% of the mangrove forests occur the northern limit of mangrove is defined at 31°22′ N latitude. In the Western and Eastern Australia, the southern limit of the mangrove is defined at 33°16′ S and 38°45′ S, respectively. The region for mangroves is identified as 32°20′ N and 28°56′ S in Atlantic America and 30°15′ N and 5°32′ in Pacific America. The latitude range for mangroves in the Atlantic Africa is 19°50′ N to 12°20′ S. However, in Eastern Africa/Red Sea the latitude range for mangrove is reported as 27°40′ N to 32°16′ S. The cause of variation in ranges of latitude in which mangroves are found in various geographic regions seems to relate to variation in temperature range (World Mangrove Atlas, 1997, Spalding et al., 1997).

10.2 MANGROVES OF INDIA

Mangrove forests in India extend over 4921 km^2 in 12 States and union territories (Anonymous SFR, 2017). Significant mangrove forests are in the states Andhra Pradesh 404 km^2, Gujarat 1140 km^2, Maharashtra 304 km^2, Odisha 243 km^2, West Bengal 2114 km^2, and Andaman & Nicobar Islands 617 km^2 (Anonymous SFR, 2107). Sundarbans' mangroves estimated as over 6000 km^2 (Bangladesh, 4050 km^2; India, 2050 km^2) form a continuum across India and Bangladesh is the largest tract of mangroves in the world (Spalding, 1997). The Sundarbans' mangroves of India constitute the largest Mangrove area of India. Sundarbans mangrove forests occupy the deltaic region of Ganga, Brahmaputra, and Meghna rivers. There are numerous islands in the region. In some literature, Sundarbans is recognized as a wonder of the world for its occurrence in a densely populated region. The Sundarbans are declared a heritage site of UNESCO with Indian Sundarbans listed as Sundarbans National Park while Bangladesh Sundarbans as Sundarbans heritage site. Sundarbans support large biodiversity that includes a diversity of mangrove species, wildlife, including the Royal Bengal Tiger, estimated at about 500, and host of other terrestrial, amphibians, and aquatic wildlife.

10.3   MANGROVES OF GUJARAT

Gujarat has a 1600-km long coastline that accounts for about 30% of India's coastline. The coastal region along this long coast varies significantly in topography, climate, and edaphic factors. Mangroves are largely concentrated in the Saurashtra and Kutch regions. Singh reported in 1999 that the notified mangrove forest's area in Kutch, Jamnagar, (now divided into Jamnagar and Devbhumi Dwarka), and Rajkot (now Morvi) districts is 1324.40 km².

Gujarat coasts support the second largest area of mangrove with 1140 km² of mangrove forests (Anonymous SFR, 2017). Story of mangrove conservation in Gujarat is unique for the major gains in conservation. In early 1980s, there was an emergence of interest in the conservation of marine flora and fauna. The first marine protected area of India Marine National Park (MNP) and Sanctuary constituted along the southern coast of Gulf of Kutch in 1980. The new administrative unit constituted to develop and manage the newly constituted marine-protected area initiating a variety of efforts that included mapping of mangrove areas, identification of coral-rich sites, biodiversity survey for marine life in the region and also included mangrove plantation experiments.

Although over 1325 km² of the area is notified as mangrove forests, the actual mangrove cover was much less. There are large blanks including hypersaline mudflats included in notified mangrove forests. It also includes 103.25 km² area leased out to 21 salt industries in Jamnagar district. There are few patches of mangrove near Kandla port, Surajbari, Mundra port, and in Kori creek that are not notified as forests (Singh, 1999).

The Imperial Gazetteer of India, Vol. XVIII (1908), mentions that in Navanagar (now Jamnagar) state, mangrove swamps line the shore of Gulf, affording large supplies of firewood and pasture. The Saurashtra and Kutch are semiarid and arid and have high evapotranspiration. There is no major river system or perennial river in the region. The conditions thus are not conducive to rich and luxuriant mangrove forests. However, Chavan (1985) recorded dense high forests with a height of up to 14 m albeit supporting little diversity of tree species in mangroves of Jamnagar.

The mangrove areas in other parts of Gujarat received little attention and recognition. The meager mangroves in Gulf of Cambay are mainly restricted to Surat and Valsad districts with virtual absence at Khambhat and its adjoining areas and little documentation reflect at little attention they received.

10.4 THE REJUVENATION

Increased interest and thrust in the conservation of marine biodiversity and mangrove conservation was observed, In early 1980s, Southern coastal region in the Gulf of Kutch with the islands that supported corals and significant biodiversity of marine fauna were notified as a sanctuary and the high diversity core area as MNP. The 457.92 km^2 area of the intertidal zone and the islands, locally called Bets, were notified as a marine sanctuary under the Wildlife Protection Act, 1972. The high biodiversity critical areas, 162.89 km^2, were at the same time notified as MNP under the same act. A special unit headed by a conservator of forest was constituted to manage the wildlife and mangrove areas in the southern region of Gulf of Kutch. Until 1982, Digvijay Cement Company had lease to dredge coral areas including that of Pirotan, Kalvan, Jindra, Dhani, Dera, and Goose for calcium carbonate for cement manufacture. The advent of MNP changed the situation to favor conservation. The dredging of corals stopped as the state government canceled the lease and the MNP authorities started conservation efforts for corals and mangroves.

10.5 MANGROVE AFFORESTATION

Although there is mention of mangrove plantations being carried out in Kutch in the first 5-year plan period (1951–1956), the concerted efforts at mangrove afforestation may be considered to have started in 1983 by the management of the MNP with plantation of 7 ha mangrove area. The foresters at MNP experimented and evolved technology for mangrove plantation. The success enthused the field foresters. The effort increased in geometrical progression and spread to other potential mangrove areas.

The mangrove forest area reported by the Forest Survey of India (FSI) for various years beginning in 1987 depicts this resurgence. The mangrove cover increased from an estimated 427 km^2 in 1987 to 1140 km^2 in 2017, over two-and-a-half-fold increase. It may also be observed that significant and consistent increase, over time is recorded in Gujarat state only. The mangrove-cover increase in India was reported at about 700 km^2 is almost wholly accounted for by Gujarat state.

Early mangrove plantations were largely carried out using poly pot raised *Avicennia* spp. Foresters experimented and innovated to develop methods of planting with seed sowing and added *Rhizophora mucaronta* and *Ceriops tagal* in their afforestation program. The program of mangrove afforestation was extended to Kutch. It needed the effort to standardize seed collection time for these species and method and time for sowing in the field and for raising seedlings. Changing soil erosion/deposition pattern, algae deposition to the extent of strangulating the new recruits and inaccessibility and deep mud presented difficulties in raising plantations. Soil erosion and algae occasionally resulted in complete failure too.

Raised bed with the sowing of about 20 propagules to afford protection to central recruits in the raised bed from soil erosion and algae strangulation was innovated with success. Difficulties due to hostile site conditions and evolving methods, the program did not deter the efforts. The afforestation program continued vigorously with afforestation targets multiplying manifold reaching to as high as 10,000–12,000 ha. It extended to the Gulf of Cambay regions. The success in Khambhat region has been remarkable. Though young and low in height, the plantation grew with remarkable success in the region where the pioneering workers of the region state that they could hardly see any mangrove. One of the sarpanch, head of the democratic village body stated during one of the visits of the author that he could see only one tree of Cher (local name for *Avicennia* spp.). The coastal mudflats of Ahmedabad in areas nearing Bhavnagar though were not designated forest areas were afforested on the initiative of local authorities. The learning and adaptation were quick in making available the seeds in time. Cooperation with pioneers in MNP was intensive both for learning and seed sourcing. There was greater reliance on learning, adaptation, and cooperation to make seeds available timely. Innovative approaches, like cluster planting of seeds on raised beds, were used to stabilize moving in the early period of plantation establishment and protect young seedling from algae deposition using peripheral seedling as a protective cover.

All these efforts resulted in increasing mangrove area in estimated by the Forest Survey of India as stated in Table 10.1.

It may be interesting to see the mangrove areas at various points of time by regions rather than districts. The mangrove area in the Gulf of Cambay region more than doubled in the period 2001–2015 (Table 10.2). In the Gulf of Cambay, there are regions in Anand and Kheda districts where there was hardly any existence of mangrove that now support significant young mangrove trees.

10.6   EDUCATION AND AWARENESS

The afforestation efforts of potential mangrove areas, the coastal mudflats, were accompanied with program to raise awareness for mangroves and marine biodiversity. The Nature education program was widely used in mangrove and MNP areas to educate and raise awareness towards the mangroves and faunal marine diversity. It helped masses especially the young population to be aware of natural heritage, its role on the ecology of the region. This helped with increased support and commitment for conservation amongst local as well as civil communities. It also raised curiosity that leads to increased participation in research work on mangroves leading to synergy. The Nature Education program of the Gujarat Forest Department played a pivotal role in raising awareness and spreading scientific knowledge. The nature education camps conducted by the MNP organization, with youth being primary target, included various sections of the society with specially designed camps for target groups need special mention in spreading message and information that lead to concern and support of civil society and local communities for conservation of mangrove and corals that were unknown to common people. Gujarat Ecology Commission, GEER Foundation, and forest department officials of coastal regions of Gujarat and Gujarat Ecology Society too contributed significantly in making the message reach all the sections of society. The results bear evidence to the conservation technique created by these efforts.

TABLE 10.1 Mangrove Cover in States of India (Area in km^2).

Year	Andhra Pradesh	Gujarat	Maha-rashtra	Odisha	Tamil Nadu	West Bengal	A&N Islands	Others	Total
1987	495	427	140	199	23	2076	686	0	4046
1989	405	412	114	192	47	2109	973	3	4255
1991	399	397	113	195	47	2119	971	3	4244
1993	378	419	155	195	21	2119	966	3	4256
1995	383	689	155	195	21	2119	966	5	4533
1997	383	901	124	211	21	2123	966	8	4737
1999	397	1031	108	215	21	2125	966	8	4871
2001	333	911	118	219	23	2081	789	8	4482
2003	329	916	158	203	35	2120	658	29	4448
2005	354	991	186	217	36	2136	635	26	4581
2009	353	1046	186	221	39	2152	615	27	4639
2011	352	1058	186	222	39	2155	617	34	4663
2013	352	1103	186	213	39	2097	604	34	4628
2015	367	1107	222	231	47	2106	617	43	4740
2017	404	1140	304	243	49	2114	617	50	4921

Source: State of Forest Report series 2001, 2003, 2005, 2009, 2011, 2013, 2015, 2017.

TABLE 10.2   Mangrove Forest Area in Various Regions of Gujarat (area in km^2).

Year	Gulf of Kutch	Gulf of Cambay	Other areas	Total
2001	849	61	1	911
2003	892	67	1	916
2005	859	76	1	991
2009	934	112	0	1046
2011	939	117	2	1058
2013	960	139	4	1103
2015	963	140	4	1107
2017	986	148	6	1140

Source: State of Forest Report series 2001, 2003, 2005, 2009, 2011, 2013, 2015, 2017.

10.7   RESEARCH AND SURVEY

Lack of information, data, and increased concern raised through an awareness program triggered research and survey of mangroves. Early efforts were aimed at assessment of resource and potential areas for mangrove afforestation. It included:

1. assessment and mapping of mangrove cover in various regions of the state;
2. mangrove biodiversity in different areas, the history, and the factors having impact on diversity and growth;
3. growth pattern and rate;
4. physiology of mangrove species occurring in Gujarat;
5. assessment and mapping of potential mangrove areas;
6. carbon sequestration by mangrove species;
7. community dependence and role of community in making success of mangrove afforestation.

On each of these aspects, detailed studies were conducted with the state-supported Gujarat Ecological Research Foundation playing the pivotal role and Gujarat Ecology Society contributing significantly.

10.8   MANGROVE SURVEY

GEER Foundation, using LISS-III data of November 1998, mapped mangrove forests of Gujarat on a scale of 1:50,000. This was a significant improvement over the Forest Survey of India assessment at that time that was at the scale of 1:250,000 till then. The study simultaneously identified mudflats that hold promise as potential mangrove area. It reported dense mangrove over 455.6 km^2 sparse mangrove 482.8 km^2 totaling to 938.4 km^2 of mangrove cover in Gujarat. This was lower than reported by FSI in FSR 1999 as 1031 km^2 FSI too, in its SFR 2001 report based on changes in scale and technology, found the mangrove cover in Gujarat as 911km^2 that is close to the estimates of GEER. It simultaneously estimated potential mangrove area as 637.2 km^2 with other mud flats estimated at 2094.4 km^2.

These reports generated interest in mangroves of Gujarat at various fora. It stimulated policy inputs, investment for research, survey, and regeneration. Protective role of mangroves got further highlighted by the observation that mangroves played a significant role in mitigating damage due to the 2004 Tsunami that impacted Andaman Nicobar Islands and eastern coast of South India. It also gave recognition to the concept bio-shield at the highest policy level.

10.8.1   THE IUCN-SPONSORED PROJECT UNDER MANGROVE FOR FUTURE PROGRAM

In 2009, the mangrove areas of south Gujarat were surveyed for their floristic diversity and natural regeneration under a project funded by Mangrove for Future (MFF) program sponsored by International Union for Conservation of Nature (IUCN) at Gujarat Ecological Education and Research (GEER) Foundation.

Detailed mapping of the mudflats was performed in south Gujarat and Gulf of Cambay to identify and locate potential mangrove afforestation areas. The study identified areas that are larger than 100 ha. It identified 70 such potential areas totaling 79155.17 ha. This study categorized these potential areas into A, B, and C zones. The zone A included intertidal areas adjacent to creeks/water sources, which have either clay or clay dominated mixed soils receiving tidal inundation for 7–15 days in the tidal cycle of 15 days. Zone A areas are ideal for mangrove afforestation. The area of Zone A was reported to be 20129.68 ha. The zone B included areas that are generally behind zone A areas and receive tidal inundation for 4–6 days in the tidal cycle of 15 days. This is inadequate inundation for mangroves. These areas required intervention to facilitate frequent marine water movement for raising mangrove species. Zone B area was estimated to be 37483.41 ha. The zone C areas are further inland with inundation limited to 1–3 days are suited for mangrove associates. Zone C area was estimated to be 21542.08 ha. Each area with its zone was mapped and maps have been made available to field units to plan afforestation/regeneration program.

The detailed study of the floristic diversity of the mangrove forests of Gulf of Cambay included mangrove areas of Valsad, Navsari, Surat, Bharuch, Vadodara, Anand, Kheda, Ahmedabad, and Bhavnagar districts. The study surveyed the diversity of mangroves, mangrove associates, species richness, and natural recruitment in various zones of the study region. It also studied preferred substrata for various mangrove species occurring in the region. The study revealed interesting community usage and dependency on mangrove and vegetation in intertidal regions.

The study identified occurrence of 14 mangrove species that included 12 of earlier reported species and two species that were not reported earlier. It identified 122 mangrove associates that included 21 monocots.

Mangrove species of Gulf of Cambay:

1. *Avicennia marina* (Forsk.) Vierh
2. *Avicennia officinalis* L.
3. *Avicennia alba* Bl.
4. *Ceriops tagal* (Perr.) Robinson
5. *Cerops decandra*
6. *Aegiceras corniculata* (L.) Blanco
7. *Exoecaria agallocah* L.
8. *Sonneratia apetala* Buch.- Ham.
9. *Rhizophora mucoronata* Lamk.
10. *Bruguiera cylinderica (L.) Bl.*
11. *Acanthus ilicifolius* L.
12. *Bruguiera gymnorhiza* (L.) Savingny.
13. *Kandelia candel* (L.) Druce
14. *Lumnitzera racemosa* Willd.

Common mangrove associates of Gulf of Cambay:

1. *Aeluropus lagopoides* (L.) Trin. Ex Thw.
2. *Cressa cretica* L.
3. *Porteresia coarctata* (Roxb.) Tateoka
4. *Sesuvium potulacastrum* (L) L
5. *Salvadora persica* L
6. *Saclicornia brachiate* Roxb
7. *Salicornia nudiflora* Roxb
8. *Clerodendrum inerme* (L.) Gaertn. F.

The study reported some of the lesser known mangrove areas in the estuaries of Purna River.

Direct dependence of local community on mangroves was observed for fodder and fuel. Village women were seen going for fodder collection to smaller islands near the village on a shared boat. Villagers also reaped benefits of fish collection and at least in one of the villages, there is a tradition of protecting mangroves; for their protection, they offer to the village from natural calamities. It may be inferred that there were local traditions in the region for protection of mangrove but have fallen in disuse with time.

10.8.2 RESEARCH ON REPRODUCTIVE ECOLOGY OF MANGROVE OF GUJARAT

The GEER Foundation undertook research on pollination biology and reproductive ecology of three major mangrove species with the funding from Ministry of Environment and Forest, Government of India, (2005–2008), viz.,

1. *Aegiceras corniculatum* (L.) Blanco,
2. *Ceriops tagal* (Perr.) C.B. Robinson
3. *Rhizophora mucronata* Lamk

The study was conducted in the Gulf of Kutch. It studied flower production, flowering synchrony, pollinators, and their visitation and developmental biology. The study explored relationship of different environmental parameters with breeding success and integrated data on these aspects to arrive at logical conclusions that are useful to develop conservation plans for the selected species of mangroves.

The study of floral biology detailed the periods and processes of transformation from matured bud to seed setting stage. Pollen production and viability with identification and visitation pattern of pollinators for the three species have been detailed in the report. The detailed sequence extent of anther dehiscence, pollen dispersal, stigma receptivity, nectar secretion, and pollinator visits when placed on a time axis that divided the total life of flower from anthesis to completion of fertilization into 10 sequential floral stages revealed interesting observations regarding the reproductive strategy of these species.

10.8.2.1 AEGICERAS CORNICULATUM

The study inferred that for *A. corniculatum* anther dehiscence and stigma receptivity are broadly out of phase except during a small period of overlap during stage-4 and stage-5 when the level of receptivity for stigma is very low. Further, the period of high-stigma receptivity is during the later stages when anther dehiscence has already completed and pollen grains are not available. This implies that the species favors cross-breeding through protandry. However, during stage-4 and stage-5, weak presence of anther dehiscence and stigma receptivity was observed that indicates a the small possibility of self-breeding also, usually found in mangrove species to help propagate in isolated populations. It is also indicated that there is a possibility of pollination by pollen of other flowers of the same inflorescence or the same tree (geitonogamy), which helps the propagation of species as an isolated population.

10.8.2.2   *CERIOPS TAGAL*

Anther dehiscence and stigma receptivity are found to be broadly out of phase for *C. tagal* except during a small period during stage-4 when the level of stigma receptivity is very low. Further, the period of high stigma receptivity is during later stages when anther dehiscence has already been completed and pollen grains are not available. This implies that the species favors cross-breeding through protandry. However, during stage-4, weak presence of anther dehiscence and stigma receptivity is observed indicating that the species holds a small possibility of self-breeding also. Like *A. corniculatum* in the case of *C. tagal* to there are conditions wherein there is possibility of pollination by pollen of other flowers of the same inflorescence or the same tree (geitonogmay) that helps propagation of species as an isolated population.

10.8.2.3   *RHIZOPHORA MUCRONATA*

Anther dehiscence and stigma receptivity are widely out of phase for *R. mucronata*. The anther dehiscence is completed during stage-2, whereas the significant stigma receptivity is observed during stage-6 onwards. Hence, anther dehiscence and stigma receptivity are widely separated overtime without any overlap unlike in the case of *A. corniculatum* and *Ceriops tagal*. However, this time gap is bridged by the function of petal corona that effectively increases the pollen presentation time and makes some pollen available up to stage-7 when the stigma receptivity is considerably high. Therefore, petal performs an extra reproductive function keeping alive some possibility of self-breeding in a flower, which otherwise strongly favors cross-breeding, through very pronounced protandry. The presence of corona on lateral margins of petals regulates the pollen dispersal and effectively increases the pollen presentation period. Thus, corona plays the role of holding some pollen grains, though a very small proportion of the total, until the period of stigma receptivity just starts. Therefore, there are very small chances that some pollen grains held by corona may remain viable until stigma receptivity just starts. It is inferred that the possibility of self-breeding is extremely low for *R. mucronata* though not ruled out. This small possibility of self-breeding helps *R. mucronata* to propagate even as isolated populations.

It is also interesting to note that the pollinator's visits are in two distinct phases, that is, stage-3 to stage-5 and stage-7 to stage-9. The visit during the first phase is prompted by pollen as a reward (bees, ants, and beetles). The reward of pollen during the first phase facilitates cross-breeding because the stigma is not receptive and the pollinators may carry the pollen grains outside the flower. The reward during the second phase also favors cross-breeding because, during this phase, pollen grains from the same flower are not available and the pollinators seeking the reward may bring in the pollen grains from other flowers.

The study of breeding mechanism of indicated occurrence of autogamy, geitonogamy, and xenogamy in all the three species, that is, *Aegiceras corniculatum*, *Ceriops tagal*, and *Rhizophora mucronata*. None of these species are purely self-breeding or purely cross-breeding.

10.9   REGENERATION

The research work also documented the species' preference for site conditions (such as the type of substratum and the inundation) in natural regeneration of major mangrove species and their associates. It was species increases as the clay component in soil increases. As the sand increases in soil mangrove associates appear to have greater success.

The overall status of natural recruitment of different mangrove species and mangrove associates was found as follows:

Aviccennia marina	68%
Aegiceras corniculatum	04%
Ceriops tagal	17%
Rhizophora mucronata	01%
Mangrove associates	10%

The research work on the three species indicated reproductive success as *A. corniculatum (42%) C. tagal* (3%), and *R. mucronata* (1%) (Pandey and Pandey, 2009). In case of *A. corniculatum,* despite a better breeding success, the natural recruitment has been found to be low indicating that the availability of matured propagule may be there but the chances of establishment are relatively less. This may be due to preference of crabs for the propagules of *A. corniculatum* as it has less fiber and tannin content. Though *Ceriops tagal* has lower reproductive success there is better recruitment as its propagules are not preferred by herbivores as it has relatively high-fiber and tannin content.

10.10 SUBSTRATUM REQUIREMENT

The substratum preference by different species for natural recruitment was studied. The study reported that the substrata with sand being its predominant content supported non-mangrove species and *Avicennia marina.* The area with substrata having some clay and more sand was found to be occupied by *A. marina* and *R. mucronata.* The substrata with higher clay content than sand in the region is occupied by *A. marina, R. mucronate,* and *C. tagal.* Substrata having clay as its predominant content is occupied by *Ceriops tagal* and *A. corniculatum.* The hard clay was found to be the place for *A. marina, Ceriops tagal*, and non-mangroves.

10.11 CARBON SEQUESTRATION IN MANGROVES FORESTS OF GUJARAT

The detailed biometric exercise was conducted to study carbon sequestration in the mangrove forests of Gujarat. The tree numbers were estimated for nine major mangrove species in girth classes. Biometric exercise was conducted to estimate biomass for each species in various girth classes for below ground and above-ground biomass and soil carbon was also estimated. The coast of Gujarat was divided into four regions, viz., Kutch, Gulf of Kutch, Saurashtra, and South Gujarat. In each region, the mangrove areas were categorized to dense, moderately dense, and sparse mangrove areas. Thus, the mangrove area of Gujarat was divided into 12 categories. In Kutch region, the carbon sequestration ranged between 41.65 ton per ha and 91.47 ton per ha averaging to 67.73 ton per ha. In Gulf of Kutch, the carbon sequestration is higher ranging from 19.66 to 118.83 ton per ha averaging to 82.90 Ton per ha.

Mangroves of South Gujarat region have the highest carbon sequestration per unit area with an average of 180.24 ton per ha. The total carbon sequestration in mangrove forests of Gujarat is estimated to be 5.874 million ton in soils and 2.242 million ton in plants totaling to 8.116 million ton.

10.12   CONCLUSION AND RESEARCH NEEDS

Research interest in mangroves has been only a few decades old. Most of the research reports are empirical observations that need to be pursued and confirmed. Some of the research areas are detailed below that may be considered priority concerns.

1.   Growth pattern: Initial research on growth pattern has thrown many interesting observations. Pandey et al. (2012) observed two growth seasons for Avecinia spp. in the Gulf of Kutch. It may be explored if there are two growth periods in other regions and for other species. How the growth periods relate to local climate with the variation in growth rate. It may also have a relation with underground growth of the root system and so the establishment of the new recruits. This may help optimize the planting season.

2.   Mangrove ecosystem functioning: The variations in coastal environment call for long-term research to have adequate understanding of cause-effect phenomena in mangrove ecosystems. The nutrient cycling in mangroves needs to be better understood. It will help appreciate their role in regulating water quality, thereby, learning how mangroves maintain nutritional homeostasis while being subjected to high rates of water turn over (ocean and freshwater) that certainly must leach large amounts of nutrients.

3.   Reproductive biology: The research on reproductive biology of few species have enlightened on the misconceptions about mangrove reproduction. The details of role of local biodiversity in the reproduction of mangroves and symbiotic relationship between large diversity of fauna with mangrove vegetation have been observed. The research on reproductive biology is fundamental to understanding the mangrove species need to be pursued with greater inputs.

4.   The ecological role of mangroves: Almost all the reports on mangroves have highlighted the ecological role of mangrove in the marine ecosystem. The contribution of mangrove in sustaining the diversity of marine life, enhancing fish catches, stabilizing coasts,

arresting silt is reported. Some authors have reported on contribution of mangroves to sustaining corals by reducing silt load and eutrophication in the region. The mangrove ecosystems have been observed to be highly productive; however, they need scientific investigation to establish cause–effect relationship.

5. Role of mangroves in recycling heavy metal: There are studies indicating the ability of mangroves to address ecotoxic waste containing heavy metal. A valid question that may be researched - Can mangroves recycle heavy metals in an environmentally safe and scientifically sound manner?

6. Economic valuation of the ecological services by mangroves: In modern world discussions often continue on the importance, need and future hidden in the rich biodiversity, ecological stability, and environmental conservation. But hard economic considerations with often narrow national and even regional biases guide the decisions. It is, therefore, of immense importance that the economic contribution of mangroves is evaluated and quantified as in local, regional, and global categories.

KEYWORDS

- **mangrove forests**
- **ecological services**
- **mangrove mapping**
- **potential areas**
- **carbon sequestration**

REFERENCES

Anon. *The State of Forest Report*, Forest Survey of India, Dehradun, 1987, p 84.
Anon. *The State of Forest Report*, Forest Survey of India, Dehradun, 1989, p 50.
Anon. *India's Wetlands, Mangroves and Coral Reefs.* World Wide Fund for Nature India for Ministry of Environment & Forests Governement of India, New Delhi, 1992, p 61.
Anon. *India State of Forest Report*, Forest Survey of India, Dehradun, 1997, p 72.
Anon. *India State of Forest Report*, Forest Survey of India, Dehradun, 2001, p 130.
Anon. *India State of Forest Report*, Forest Survey of India, Dehradun, 2013, p 252.
Anon. *India State of Forest Report*, Forest Survey of India, Dehradun, 2015, p 300.

Anon. *India State of Forest Report*, Forest Survey of India, Dehradun, 2017, p 363.

Biswas, N. *The Gulf of Kutch Marine National Park and Sanctuary: A Case Study.* International Collective in Support of Fishworkers, Chennai, 2006, p 46.

Ong, J. E.; Gong, W. K. *Structure, Function and Management of Mangrove Ecosystems.* ISME Mangrove Educational Book Series No. 2. International Society for Mangrove Ecosystems (ISME): Okinawa, Japan, and International Tropical Timber Organization (ITTO): Yokohama, Japan, 2013; p 81.

Pandey, C. N.; Pandey R. *Study of Floristic Diversity and Natural Recruitment of Mangrove Species in Selected Mangrove Habitats of South Gujarat.* GEER Foundation, Gandhinagar, 2009, p 92.

Pandey C. N.; Pandey R. *Pollination Biology and Reproductive Ecology of Major Mangrove species of Gujarat.* GEER Foundation: Gandhinagar, 2009; p 918.

Pandey, C. N.; Pandey, R.; Mali M. *Carbon Sequestration by Mangroves of Gujarat.* GEER Foundation: Gandhinagar, 2012; p 159.

Pandey, C. N.; Pandey, R., Khokhariya, B. *Potential Area Mapping for Mangrove Restoration in South Gujarat.* GEER Foundation: Gandhinagar, 2012; p 248.

Singh, H. S. *Mangroves in Gujarat (Current status and strategy for conservation).* GEER Foundation: Gandhinagar, 1999; p 127.

Sigh, H. S.; Yennawar, P.; Asari, R. J.; Tatu, K.; Raval, B. R. *An Ecological and Socio-Economic Study in Marine National Park and Sanctuary in the Gulf of Kutch* (A Comprehensive Study on Biodiversity and Management Issues). GEER Foundation: Gandhinagar, 2006.

Spalding, M. D.; Blasco, F.; Field, C. D., Eds.; *World Mangrove Atlas.* The International Society for Mangrove Ecosystems: Okinawa, Japan, 1997; p 178.

PART III
Crop Resources Management

CHAPTER 11

Management of Seed Crops

ASHOK K. THAKUR* and SUJATA KUMARI

Department of Seed Science and Technology, University of Horticulture and Forestry, Nauni 173230, Solan, Himachal Pradesh, India

Corresponding author. E-mail: ashok.horticulture@gmail.com

ABSTRACT

Seed is a vital input in agriculture. The quality and genetic production capacity of seed determines the quantity as well as quality of produce, and also determines economics of production. In a crop production system, seed quality is the basic input to which other inputs are added to have desired output. It ensures other agroproduction and protection inputs to be productive and cost-effective. The management of mother crop plays pivotal role in quality of produced seed. Seed production requires specialized skills and knowhow, unlike general crop production. It involves crop and region-specific genetic as well as agronomic principles that have to be precisely practiced to achieve desired quality of seed. Seed having good quality is the basic input for enhancement of crop as well as other inputs productivity. Well planned evaluation and release of cultivars, systematic production, and supply of seed, seed testing, certification and enforcement of seed legislation, in toto, is essential to exploit the technological breakthroughs in crop production system. This chapter describes seed quality, its components, and factors governing seed quality. The genetic, agronomic, legislative mechanisms for controlling seed quality are described to have better understanding of seed production. However, the main emphasis remains on management of seed quality at preharvest as well as postharvest level.

11.1 CONCEPT OF SEED QUALITY

Seed as input is crucial, critical, vital, and basic in crop production. Seed quality is directly and positively correlated to crop productivity and quality.

Hence, seed quality plays a pivotal role in improving agricultural economy is one of the most essential and effective inputs. Seed quality, according to Thompson (1979) is a complex of several components and their relative importance in different sets of production systems. These components have been categorized as (1) analytical quality, (2) species purity, (3) freedom from weeds, (4) cultivar purity, (5) germination capacity, (6) vigor, (7) size, (8) uniformity, (9) health, and (10) moisture content. These components were categorized in more systematic manner by Nema (1985) into four major components: (1) Genetic quality, (2) physical quality, (3) physiological quality, and (4) health quality.

The importance of quality seed is well understood around the globe. In India, seed quality attained the central stage after introduction of high yielding cultivars of field crops like Bajra, sorghum, and wheat during 6th decade of 20th century. History of grain production in developing countries clearly reveals that quality seed was one of the keys to the Green Revolution. The introduction of dwarf and high yielding varieties of wheat resulted in 3–4 times increase in wheat productivity. The quick and intense enhancement of wheat productivity founded the Green Revolution. Production and availability of quality seeds of these novel cultivars played an equally important role in the Green Revolution.

In crop production, seed quality is basic input to which other inputs are applied to have desired output. The productivity and cost-effectiveness of other production inputs are also dependent on the quality of seed sown. It is the combination of seed quality and other agroinputs that results in productivity enhancement (Fieistrizer, 1975). Well-planned evaluation and release of improved varieties, systematic seed production, and supply, seed testing, certification and enforcement of seed legislation, in toto, are essential to exploit the technological breakthroughs in crop production.

11.2 COMPONENTS OF SEED QUALITY

The seed quality components can be categorized into four major groups:

  i)   genetic quality,
 ii)   physical quality,
iii)   physiological quality, and
 iv)   seed health.

These components, independently and their interaction at all levels, sum up to constitute the overall seed quality.

11.2.1 GENETIC QUALITY

Genetic quality or purity of a cultivar means all the seeds of a sample (variety) are genetically pure, that is, uniformly possess the essential characteristics of the cultivar in question, without any contamination from seeds of other variety of the same crop. The genuineness of variety attains the prime position among the most important characteristics of seed quality. In scientific seed production, every care is taken at every stage to maintain the genuineness of variety. In spite of this, varieties may become impure. To verify the genuineness of variety before selling seed is, therefore, an insurance against the supply of impure seed. Genetic purity is an important requirement to maximize the potential of improved varieties.

11.2.2 PHYSICAL QUALITY

Physical seed quality is the proportion of pure seed in the seed lot. It also explains the other constituents of seed lot, namely, inter matter, broken seeds, other crop(s) seeds, seeds of other distinguishable varieties of the same crop, weed seeds, and inert matter, etc. Inert matter includes soil, dust, chaffs, broken seeds, having less than half size, and any material other than seeds. Proportion or percentage of pure seed forms the basis of quality. Higher proportion of pure seed is desired. Other parameters, such as germination and vigor, are determined on the pure seeds after removing all other physical impurities.

11.2.3 PHYSIOLOGICAL QUALITY

The degree of excellence of seeds with respect to all physiological processes that enable a seed to germinated and develops into seedling or plant is collectively is the physiological quality. The main components of physiological quality are viability, germination, and vigor. The speed of germination or germination index is also measured to have a detailed description of germination and vigor. A pure live seed is another parameter that evaluates the physical as well as the physiological quality of seed lot. It is a function of seed purity and germination of seeds. It explains the real worth of seed to have proper crop stand. It is also termed as planting value of seed lot. Planting value is the product of pure seed and germination and expressed in percentage.

11.2.4   SEED HEALTH

Seed is prone to many diseases and pests and many of these are carried by seed from one generation of the crop to others. The freedom from seed-borne biotic stress-causing agents is often termed as seed health. Seed health plays an important role not just in seed quality but other issues related to seed trade like quarantine, etc.

The quality of seed means that seed is superior and pure in terms of its genetic constitution, physiologically strong enough to produce a plant of the desired kind in a wide range of environmental conditions, free from physical impurities and biotic stress-causing agents.

The seed quality is, therefore, the degree of excellence of seed or seed lot in terms of these parameters. There are minimum limits of different seed quality parameters that are imposed legally are Indian Minimum Seed Certification Standards (IMSCS, 2013). Hence, the seed lot possessing the values of parameters more than minimum limits is the quality seed.

11.3   FACTORS AFFECTING SEED QUALITY

There are major three groups of the factor affecting seed quality as listed below. The constituents of the individual group are detailed below.

11.3.1   ENVIRONMENTAL FACTORS

The environmental factors include adaptability, light, temperature, sun, rain, wind, soil, and pollinators, etc.

11.3.2   PREHARVEST TECHNOLOGY

The preharvest factors affecting seed quality are cropping history, seed source, isolation, rouging, weeding, plant protection, irrigation, nutrition, and other intercultural operations.

11.3.3   HARVEST AND POSTHARVEST TECHNOLOGY

The harvest and post-harvest operations affecting seed quality are harvesting, curing, drying, grading, seed treatment, bagging, packing, labeling, sealing, storage and transit.

11.4 MECHANISM OF SEED QUALITY CONTROL

Both quality assurance (QA) and quality control (QC) mechanisms are deployed to manage quality seed production and distribution as well. There are minimum standards for seed quality to regulate seed quality. In India, IMSCS (2013) are in place. The standards are mandatory to produce certified seeds. Seed certification system involving inspections of fields, processing units and issuing of certificate by designated authority provides a mechanism of QA in production chains. This mechanism is applicable only to the foundation and certified classes of seeds of notified varieties of crops. However, certification is not compulsory. Thus, certification is having limited applicability restricted to certified seeds of notified varieties only. Hence, truthfully labeled seeds do not fall in the regulation of certification.

To overcome this limitation of seed certification, another mechanism of compulsory truthfully labeling has been devised. The labeling is compulsory irrespective of seed class and notification status of variety. There are different labels, also called as tags, are listed below:

- Golden yellow tag (breeder seed)
- White tag (foundation seed)
- Azure blue tag (certified seed)
- Opel green tag (truthfully labeled seed)

These tags are inscribed with the information about the seed in the packs to which these tags are attached or sealed with. Seed quality information on tag includes:

- germination,
- genetic purity, and
- physical purity.

The truthful labeling is essential for QC of seeds. The seed quality information must have compliance to IMSCS and must be true to seed lot when seed samples are tested for various seed quality parameters. Seed sampling and testing is QC mechanism applicable to all seeds produced and sold. It includes seed testing for physical and physiological parameters and grow-out test and laboratory techniques to assess genetic purity.

In addition, there are laws and legislations for international trade of seeds that take care of the quality of seed produced outside the country and are not covered under the above mechanisms.

11.5   BASIC PRINCIPLES OF SEED PRODUCTION

Quality-seed production is specialized production system. It involves high scientific and technical skills and involves high investments. Strict compliance of genetic and agronomic principles and legislative standards is needed to fulfill the minimum prescribed quality of particular crop and class of seed.

11.5.1   GENETIC PRINCIPLES

Seed production, unlike food production, needs to follow certain genetic principles as the genetic purity is of utmost importance among components of seed quality. These principles are described below.

11.5.1.1   DETERIORATION OF VARIETIES

Genetic purity of a variety is determined by many factors during seed production cycles. These are enumerated by Kadam (1942) as listed below:

11.5.1.2   DEVELOPMENTAL VARIATION

The unfavorable environment causing stress to the plants leads to developmental variation. These are the result of differential growth response. The seed crops should, therefore, be cultivated in area and season of adoption to avoid or minimize such variations in varietal characters.

11.5.1.3   MECHANICAL MIXTURES

Mixing of other variety's seeds at various stages of production and processing leads to varietal deterioration. The deterioration is further aggravated if such plants are not rogued out in cross-pollinated crops.

11.5.1.4   MUTATIONS

Mutations are spontaneous and have minor often nondetectable changes that having no remarkable deterioration on varietal characters. However, the detectable mutations need to be rogued out in seed-production fields.

11.5.1.5 NATURAL CROSSING

Natural cross pollination with rogues and off-types deteriorates the varietal purity in seed production cycles. Bateman (1947) suggested factors that determine natural crossing are the breeding system of species, isolation, varietal mass, and pollinating agent.

11.5.1.6 MINOR GENETIC VARIATIONS

Minor genetic variations are often not phenotypically visible. They may even exist in variety at the time of their release. These variations may get eliminated or may appear with larger magnitude in production cycles. Yield trials of lines propagated from nucleus or breeder seeds have been suggested to eliminate or minimize these variations (Hann, 1953).

11.5.1.7 SELECTIVE INFLUENCE OF DISEASES

High yielding varieties with no resistance or tolerance often show suscep-tibility under fields because the seed production is generally done under disease-free environment. This may affect the types of varieties having considerable genetic variation.

11.5.1.8 TECHNIQUES OF PLANT BREEDERS

The variety when release must not have genetic variation such as segrega-tion that is not phenotypically visible. The genetic instabilities need to be check or eliminated to avoid any cytogenetic irregularities prior to release.

11.5.1.9 MAINTENANCE OF GENETIC PURITY DURING THE SEED PRODUCTION

Varietal purity is maintained by following the steps enlisted below (Haan, 1953).

- Seed multiplication using only approved seed.
- Field inspections.
- Roguing

- Seed sampling and prevention of mechanical mixtures.
- Comparison of crops grown from produced stocks and authentic stocks.

Hartman and Kester (1968) also suggested steps for maintenance of genetic purity of seeds as listed below.

- Adequate isolation to avoid natural crossing and mechanical mixtures.
- Rouging of seed production fields before contamination stage such as flowering, harvesting, etc.
- Periodic testing of genetic purity.
- Growing crops in well-suited areas to avoid genetic shifts.
- Seed certification.
- Adoption of the generation system of seed production.
- Grow out tests.

The important factors responsible for genetic purity maintenance during seed production enlisted by Agrawal (1995) are

- control of seed source,
- preceding crop or cropping history of the land,
- isolation,
- rouging,
- seed certification, and
- grow-out testing (GOT).

In recent times, many other alternate laboratory tests for GOT using biochemical and molecular techniques are devised. These are fast and less expensive.

11.5.2 *AGRONOMIC PRINCIPLES*

The agronomic principles followed for general crop production are followed for seed production along with certain specific additional principles. These principles mainly focus on the maintenance of seed quality at various stages of seed production and postharvest stages. These are enlisted below.

- Selection of an agroclimatic region
- Selection of seed plot

- Isolation of seed crops
- Preparation of land
- Selection of variety and seed
- Presowing seed treatment
- Sowing or planting time
- Seed rate
- Sowing methods
- Depth of sowing
- Rouging
- Supplementary pollination
- Weed control
- Disease and insect control
- Nutrition of seed crop
- Irrigation
- Harvesting of seed crops
- Drying of seeds
- Storage of raw seeds

11.6   LEGAL ASPECTS OF SEED QUALITY MANAGEMENT

11.6.1   SEED LEGISLATION

In India, the first and foremost law pertaining to seeds is The Seeds Act, 1966. It was followed by formation and notification of The Seeds Rules in 1968 and the Act was implemented in 1969.

11.6.2   OBJECTIVES

To regulate seed quality of notified kind or varieties for sale and for matters connected to it.

To create an environment in which seed producer or traders could operate effectively and to make good quality seed available to growers.

11.6.3   DETAILS OF PROVISIONS IN THE SEEDS ACT, 1966 AND THE SEEDS RULES, 1968

The list of the events in seed legislation in India is as follows (Table 11.1):

- 1966: The Seeds Act
- 1968: The Seed Rules
- 1972: The Seeds (Amendment) Act
- 1983: The Seeds Control Order
- 1988: New Policy on Seed Development
- 2001: PPV & FRA
- 2004: The Seeds Bill
- 2008: Organization for Economic Co-operation and Development (OECD) member

TABLE 11.1   Details of Provisions in The Seeds Act, 1966 and The Seeds Rules, 1968.

Sr. No.	Section/Rule	Activity/Provisions
1	Section 3	Establishment of Central Seed Committee
2	Section 4	Establishment of central and state seed testing laboratories.
3	Section 5	Notification of kind or varieties
4	Section 6	Power to specify minimum limits of germination and purity
5	Section 7	Regulation of sale of seeds of notified kind/variety
6	Section 8	Establishment of seed certification agency in the state
7	Section 8A	Establishment of seed certification board
8	Section 9	Grant of certificate by a certification agency
9	Section 10	Revocation of certificates
10	Section 11	Appealing against the decisions of seed certification agency
11	Section 12	Seed analysts
12	Section 13	Seed inspector
13	Section 14	Powers of seed inspector
14	Section 15	Procedure to be followed by seed inspector
15	Section 16	Report of seed analyst
16	Section 17	Restriction on export or import of seeds of notified kind/variety
17	Section 18	Recognition of seed certification agencies of foreign countries
18	Section 19	Penalty
19	Section 20	Forfeiture of property
20	Section 21	Offense by companies
21	Section 22	Protection of action taken in good faith
22	Section 23	Power to give directions
23	Section 24	Exemption
24	Section 25	Power to make rules
25	Rule 6(a)	Certifying seeds of notified varieties only

TABLE 11.1 *(Continued)*

Sr. No.	Section/Rule	Activity/Provisions
26	Rule 15	Sowing report – Application
27	Rule 6(d)	Verification of seed source and purchase bill
28	Rule 16	Collection of fees
29	Rule 6(c)	Maintenance of breeder list
30	Rule 6(k)	Inspecting seed farms to assess the field standards
31	Rule 6(b)	Harvesting, sealing and sending to seed processing units
32	Rule 6(f)	Inspecting seed Processing plants
33	Rule 6(e)	Drawing samples and sending for analysis
34	Rule 17-A	Certifying seeds in accordance with IMSC Standards
35	Rule 6(i)	Certifying the quality seeds
36	Rule 17(i)	Affixing tags on Seed containers
37	Rule 17(ii)	Contents of seed certification Tag
38	Rule 9	Affixing labels along with tags on the containers
39	Rule 17	Granting of certificate (Form II)
40	Rule 6(j)	Maintaining Registers and records
41	Rule 17(vi)	Maintaining Registers and records by seed producers
42	Rule 6(g)	Expediting Seed certification works
43	Section 9	Grant of certificates by certification agency
44	Rule 6(h)	Imparting training

11.6.4   SEED CERTIFICATION

Seed certification concept originated in the early 20th century owing to the increased concern for rapid loss of varietal identity in production cycles. Field evaluation of seed crop was initially started by Swedish workers. They started it with the visits of plant breeders and agronomists to the farmers' fields where new varieties have been grown. Field inspection, thus, was started primarily with a view to educate farmers about seed production. Subsequently, it was modified to inspect fields and was found very helpful in maintaining varietal purity in the production chain. In 1919, scientists from USA and Canada met in Chicago and established International Crop Improvement Association that was renamed as Association of Official Seed Certifying Agencies in 1969 and this was the beginning of systematic seed certification in the world.

In India, the need for quality seed was felt with the advent of high yielding varieties of wheat and few other crops that lead to the Green

Revolution. In India, field evaluation and certification of seed crop was started in 1963 with the establishment of National Seeds Corporation. However, seed certification attained the legal status with the enactment of The Seeds Act, 1966 and formulation of Seed Rules, 1968. The Seeds Act, 1966 provided the momentum needed for the establishment of State Seed Certification Agencies. Maharashtra was the first state in India to establish Seed Certifications Agency under the Department of Agriculture as early as 1970. However, Karnataka established the first autonomous Seed Certification Agency in 1974.

Thus, legally sanctioned system for QC, seed multiplication, and production consisting of field inspection, pre- and postcontrol testing and seed quality analysis. In most of the countries, including India, seed certification is voluntary and labeling of seed is compulsory.

11.6.4.1 OBJECTIVES OF SEED CERTIFICATION

- Seed certification focuses on ensuring the minimum standards of seed quality.
- The systematic seed multiplication of improved varieties.
- The identification of new varieties and their rapid multiplication under appropriate and generally accepted names.
- Continuous supply of seed by careful maintenance of quality.

11.6.4.2 PHASES OF SEED CERTIFICATION

This includes seed certification procedures described step by step as described below.

- Receipt and scrutiny of application;
- Seed source verification, class and other requirements of seed to be sown for raising mother seed crop;
- Field inspections to verify compliance to prescribed minimum field standards;
- Supervision of postharvest operations such as processing and packing;
- Verification of conformity to prescribed minimum standards by seed sampling and analysis of genetic purity and/or seed health;
- Issuance of certificate and certification tags, tagging, and sealing.

11.6.4.3   INDIAN MINIMUM SEED CERTIFICATION STANDARDS

IMSCS were formulated and published in 1972 and revised in 2013 to include more crops especially horticultural, plantation and spices, etc. These standards are grouped as general and specific seed certification standards to various crops. The former is applicable to every crop and their varieties eligible for certification, whereas the latter are specifically applicable to field and seed of individual crops.

According to IMSCS, a certified seed must conform to minimum standards of genetic purity. These standards for minimum genetic purity for foundation seed is 99%; for certified seed of varieties, composites, synthetics, and multilines is 98%; for certified hybrid seed is 95%; certified seed of hybrids of cotton, true potato seeds, muskmelon, brinjal, and tomato is 90%; and for hybrid castor is 85%. These standards must be maintained unless crop-specific standards are not separately described.

The crop-specific standards include field and seed standards. Field standards include isolation requirements, limits of off-types, infected plants, and inseparable plants, etc. The seed standards describe limits for pure seed (min.), inert matter (max.), other crop seeds (max.), other distinguishable varieties (max.), weed seeds (max.), germination (min.), moisture content for normal container and vapor-proof containers (max.), etc. The lists of designated diseases and pests, objectionable weeds and cross-compatible crops, and plants are also included. These standards are required strict compliance for production certified seed classes, that is, foundation and certified seeds.

11.6.4.4   TRUTHFUL LABELING

Being limited application of the certification system, there is the provision of other class namely truthfully labeled seed (TLS). The production of TL seed does not require to undergo seed certification procedure, however truthful labeling and compliance to minimum limits of germination and purity need to be fulfilled. This type of seed can be produced to all types of released cultivars of crops irrespective of its notification status. Truthful labeling, unlike certification, is compulsory for all classes of seeds.

11.6.4.5   OECD SEED SCHEME

The OECD, Paris, France was established in 1958 as a multinational organization act as a multilateral forum where policies related to economic and social issues can be discussed, developed, and reformed. Promotion of sustainable economic growth and generation of employment and rising living standard and trade liberalization is the mission of this scheme. It established a framework for certification of seed in international trade. OECD comprises of seven agriculture Seed Schemes listed below.

- Cereal crops
- Maize and sorghum
- Crucifers and other oil or fiber species
- Grass and legume species
- Fodder beet and sugar beet
- Subterranean clover and similar species
- Vegetable crops

The major objectives of these schemes are as follows:

- To encourage use of "quality-guaranteed" seed in member or partici-pating countries of OECD;
- To authorize use of labels and certificates for international trade as per principles for ensuring identity and purity of seed;
- To facilitate overseas seed trade by issuing passports and removal of technical trade barriers;
- To develop guidelines for seed multiplication abroad and for accredi-tation to control activities of private stakeholders.

11.7 MANAGEMENT PRACTICES FOR SEED QUALITY

11.7.1 CROPPING HISTORY

The cropping history of field needs consideration while selecting for seed production to avoid the volunteer plants. Cropping history is inspected in first field inspection of certification program. The cropping history criteria for various seed crops are given in Table 11.2.

11.7.2 SEED SOURCES

The certification process needs one or more relevant evidence to verify the quality of initial seed lot at the time of application scrutiny and/or during

TABLE 11.2 Cropping History Requirements for Seed Production of Various Crops.

Crops	Land requirement criteria
Barley variety and hybrid, rice variety and hybrid, wheat variety and hybrid	1. Preceding one season
Baira variety and hybrid, common millet, barnyard millet, finger millet, Italian millet, Kodo millet, little millet, maize open-pollinated varieties, hybrids, synthetics, composites, Sorghum variety, and hybrid	2. Land free of volunteer plants in previous season
Black gram, Bengal gram, cowpea, green gram, French bean (Rajmash), horse gram, Kesari, lablab, lentil, moth bean, peas, red gram	
Castor variety and hybrid, linseed, Niger, safflower, sesame	
Soybean, Mustard, Niger, Taramira	
Cotton variety and hybrid, jute	
Berseem, Buffelgrass, clover, Dharaf grass, forage sorghum, guinea grass, Lucerne, marvel grass, oats, rice bean, Sudan grass, Napier grass and hybrid, Setaria grass, stylo, teosinte	
Amaranthus, ash gourd, asparagus, beet, bhindi, bitter gourd variety and hybrid, bottle gourd variety and hybrid, broccoli, cabbage, cauliflower, carrot variety and hybrid, celery, chow-chow, cucumber variety and hybrid, chilies, fenugreek, French bean (Rajmash), garlic, Guar, Indian squash, Knol-khol, lettuce, long melon, muskmelon variety and hybrid, onion (aggregate) variety and hybrid, onion variety and hybrid, parsley, peas, pumpkin, variety and hybrid, ridge gourd variety and hybrid, radish variety & hybrid, rattail radish, snake gourd, Snap melon, spinach, sponge gourd variety and hybrid, winter squash variety and hybrid, Yam	
Groundnut	1. Preceding two seasons 2. Land in which crop is grown in Preceding two seasons were of same kind and variety and of equivalent or higher class and are eligible for certification

TABLE 11.2 *(Continued)*

Crops	Land requirement criteria
Bird wood grass, Buffelgrass, Dharaf grass, Dinanath grass, marvel grass, Setaria grass, stylo	1. Preceding five seasons 2. (Foundation stage alone) 3. Land must not be used for cultivation of the same crop
Sunflower variety and hybrid	1. Preceding one year 2. Land in which the crop is grown in preceding year was of same kind or variety and of equivalent or higher class and eligible for certification
Potato, true potato seed	1. Land infested with diseases like wart, brown spot, and common scab must be avoided
Pointed gourd, little gourd, sweet potato, tapioca, taro	1. Land avoided if preceding crop residue is found and drainage from another field planted with same crop. 2. Swampy, low lying, and over shaded areas to be avoided.

Source: Reprinted from IMSCS, 2013.

first inspection. These evidence may be certification tags, seals, labels, seed containers, purchase records, sale records, etc., from producer of certified seed.

11.7.3   ISOLATION AND INTERCROPPING

11.7.3.1   ISOLATION

The minimum isolation prescribed in IMSCS is mandatory to avoid chances of genetic contamination due to the presence of other varieties, impure same variety, diseased plants in some cases, cross-compatible crops, and plants species. The minimum isolation requirements for various crops as per classes of seeds are given in Table 11.3.

11.7.3.2   INTERCROPPING

Intercropping is seed production is, in general, not recommended. However, in certified seed production of oilseeds and pulses intercropping is allowed with the following conditions (IMSCS, 2013).

- Intercropping is applicable to certified seeds class of pulses and oilseeds. The foundation seed crop should strictly be a single crop.
- Any other types of cropping system or pattern are not permitted.
- The crops selected for intercropping should have a different genus and preferably different maturity.
- Only basic crop pertaining to oilseeds or pulses can be registered for certification and companion crop cannot be certified.
- The plating ratio of seed crop and companion crop must be uniform throughout the field.
- Certification agencies will prepare a list of crop combinations for respective states taking into account the following factors while selecting any crop combinations.

   a) The companion crop should not hamper intercultural operation required for a seed crop.
   b) It should not compete for nutrients and moisture or starve seed crop.
   c) It should not mature simultaneously with seed crop or should not carry weed seeds that may mix with seed crop.

TABLE 11.3 Isolation Distance for Certified Seeds of Major Crops

Distance (meters)	Crops (Fields from which seed crop must be separated are provided within brackets)	
3	Cereals and Millets	Barley, millets (Common, Fingert, Italian, Kodo, Little, Barnyard), oats, rice, triticale, wheat
5	Oilseeds	Groundnut, soybean
	Pulses	Black gram, Bengal gram, cowpea, green gram, horse gram, Kesari, lablab, lentil, moth bean
	Fiber crops	Cotton hybrid (between parent plots), jute (other species)
	Vegetables	Cluster bean, French bean, (Rajmash), fenugreek, garlic, lesser yam, multiplier onion, pea, potato, sweet potato, tapioca
10	Forages	Buffel grass, Dharaf grass, Dinanath grass, Guinea grass, marvel grass, Napier grass
20	Forage legumes	Rice bean
	Vegetables	Coccinia, pointed gourd
25	Oilseeds	Linseed, Mustard (self-compatible types)
	Forages	Indian clover, stylo
	Vegetables	Lettuce, tomato
30	Fiber crops	Cotton variety and hybrids, jute
50	Oilseeds	Mustard (self-compatible types), Sesame, Taramira
	Vegetables	True potato seed
100	Cereals and millets	Barley hybrids, rice hybrids, sorghum, wheat hybrids
	Pulses	Red gram variety and hybrid
	Vegetables	Brinjal, tomato hybrids
	Cereals and millets (seed crop infected by loose smut)	Barley variety and hybrid (loose smut infection), oats (loose smut infection), wheat variety and hybrids (loose smut infection)
150	Cereals and millets	Bajra variety and hybrids, maize hybrids, composites, synthetics, sorghum hybrids

TABLE 11.3 *(Continued)*

Distance (meters)	Crops (Fields from which seed crop must be separated are provided within brackets)	
200	Oilseeds	Niger, safflower, sunflower
	Forages	Setaria grass
	Vegetables	Amaranthus, brinjal hybrids, bhindi, capsicum
300	Cereals and millets	Maize hybrids (different kernel color)
	Oilseeds	Castor variety and hybrids
	Vegetables	Asparagus, celery, celeriac, parsley
400	Cereals and millets	Maize inbred, maize single cross, sorghum (Johnson grass, Forage sorghum)
	Oilseeds	Sunflower hybrids
500	Vegetables	Pumpkin, summer squash, winter squash, cucumber, pointed gourd, ridge gourd, snake gourd, sponge gourd, wax gourd, bitter gourd, bottle gourd, Chayote, Indian squash, Long melon, snap melon, muskmelon, watermelon, onion (OP variety and hybrids)
600	Cereals and millets	Maize inbred (different kernel color, texture)
800	Vegetables	Carrot variety and hybrids
1000	Vegetables	Bitter gourd hybrid, bottle gourd hybrid, broccoli, cabbage, cauliflower, Chinese cabbage, cucumber hybrid, garden beet, Knol-khol, muskmelon hybrid, pumpkin hybrid, ridge gourd hybrid, radish, rat-tail radish, sponge gourd hybrid, spinach, summer squash hybrid, seedless hybrid watermelon, sugar beet, turnip, watermelon hybrid, winter squash hybrid
1600	Vegetables	Broccoli hybrid, cabbage hybrid, cauliflower hybrid, Chinese cabbage (fields of other varieties of same species and same genera), Knol-khol hybrid, radish hybrids, turnip hybrids

Source: Reprinted from IMSCS, 2013.

   d) Companion crop should not have same pests and diseases
   e) It should not interfere or create hindrances in the certification
       process.

11.7.4   ROGUING AND WEEDING

Off-type or rogue is a plant that deviates morphologically from varietal
characteristics described by breeder. Off-types and rogues play an important
role in genetic purity maintenance. Removal of off-types and rogues from
seed field before flowering is must to avoid cross-pollination (Table 11.4).
Similarly, presence of cross-compatible weeds also deteriorates genetic
quality. The weeding at appropriate stages is must to avoid cross-pollination.

11.7.5   IRRIGATION

Irrigation plays an important role in determining the physiological quality of
seed. The proper irrigation of mother crop is an essential requirement of the
seed crop. The critical irrigation stages of the crop must be identified to have
better yield and quality of seed harvested.

11.7.6   NUTRITION

The viability and vigor are mainly dependent upon the nutrition of mother
crop. Proper fertilizer application schedule must be followed as per recommendations based on soil tests. Improper nutrient application in terms
of quantity and stage of the crop may result in nutritional imbalance and
disorder affecting seed yield and quality.

11.7.7   BIOTIC STRESS MANAGEMENT

The seed crops, like the commercial crop, are prone to many diseases and
pests and their management need to be done to have healthy crop and
harvest. In seed crop, particularly, seed-borne diseases and pests impose a
serious problem. There are designated diseases of seed crops listed under
IMSCS that need to be kept under control. The list of designated diseases is
given in Table 11.5.

TABLE 11.4 Prescribed Days for Seed Crop Inspection

Sr. No.	Crop	Specifications	Vegetative	Flowering	Flowering, pod, earhead, boll formation stages	Maturity and harvest stages
1.	Rice	a) Short duration	–	85	–	95
		b) Medium duration	–	105	–	120
		c) Long duration	–	120	–	135
2.	Hybrid millets	a) Bajra	40	50	60	80
		b) Maize	45	60	70	90
		c) Sorghum	45	60	70	90
3.	Variety millets	a) Bajra	40	60	–	80
		b) Maize	45	70	–	90
		c) Parental maize	45	70	–	90
		d) Sorghum	45	70	–	90
		e) Finger millet	–	70	–	90
4.	Cotton	a) Suvin	–	75	–	105
		b) TNB 1	–	75	105	125
		c) Parental cotton	–	65	75	115
		d) Hybrid	45	65	105	125
5.	Pulses	a) Black gram	–	40	–	55
		b) Green gram	–	40	–	55
		c) Cowpea	–	45	–	75
		d) Cowpea P152	–	45	–	65
		e) Red gram short duration	–	80	–	100
		f) Long duration	–	120	–	150
		g) Horse gram	–	55	–	70
		h) Bengal gram				
6.	Oilseeds	a) Groundnut	–	60	–	90

TABLE 11.4 *(Continued)*

Sr. No.	Crop	Specifications	Vegetative	Flowering	Flowering, pod, earhead, boll formation stages	Maturity and harvest stages
		b) Sesame	40	60	–	75
		c) Sunflower	40	60	–	75
		d) Castor	–	50	–	90
		e) Mustard	35	45	–	65
		f) Soybean	–	50	–	90
		g) Sunflower hybrid	40	55	65	80
		h) Castor hybrid	40	50	70	90
7.	Vegetable	a) Tomato variety	50	70	–	90
		b) Tomato hybrid	45	60	70	90
		c) Brinjal variety	50	70	–	90
		d) Brinjal hybrid	50	70	80	90
		e) Bhindi	40	60	–	70
		f) Chilies-K2	65	95	–	105
		g) Chilies	80	115	–	125
		h) Beans	–	50	–	70
		i) Pumpkin	60	80	–	100
		j) Ash gourd	60	80	–	100
		k) Bottle gourd	60	80	–	100
		l) Snake gourd	45	60	–	75
		m) Bitter gourd	45	60	–	75
		n) Ribbed gourd	45	60	–	75

Note: 1. These dates are given for general guidance.

2. Considering the age of variety, the difference in agroclimatic conditions and other relevant factors, Assistant Director of Agriculture (Seed Certification) can alter and fix suitable inspection dates.

Source: Reprinted from IMSCS, 2013.

TABLE 11.5 Designated Diseases of Major Seed Crops

Crop		Designated diseases	Causal organisms	Max permitted (No./10000 plants)	
				Foundation Seed	Certified Seed
Cereals					
1.	Triticale	Loose smut	*Ustilago tritici*	10	
		Ergot	*Claviceps purpurea*	2	4
2.	Wheat variety and hybrid	Loose smut	*Ustilago tritici*	10	50
Millets					
1.	Bajra	Grain smut	*Tolyposporium penicillarie*	5	10
		Green ear	*Tolyposporium sengalense*	5	10
		Ergot	*Claviceps microcephala*	5	10
2.	Barley	Loose smut	*Ustilago nuda*	10	50
3.	Oats	Loose smut	*Ustilago avenae*	10	50
4.	Sorghum	Grain smut/kernel smut	*Sphaceotheca sorghi*	5	10
		Head smut	*Sphaceotheca reiliana*	5	10
Pulses					
1.	Cowpea	Ashy stem blight	*Macrophomia phaseoli*	10	20
		Anthracnose	*Colletotrichum lindemuthianum*	10	20
		Ascochyta blight (for hill regions only)	*Ascochyta* sp.	10	20
2.	Green gram	Halo blight	*Pseudomonas phasiolicola*	10	20
Oilseeds					
1.	Sesame	Leaf spot	*Cercospora sesami*	50	100
2.	Sunflower	Downy mildew	*Plasmopara halstedii*	5	50

TABLE 11.5 *(Continued)*

Crop		Designated diseases	Causal organisms	Max permitted (No./10000 plants)	
				Foundation Seed	Certified Seed
Forage sorghum					
1.	Forage sorghum	kernel smut/grain smut	*Sphaceotheca sorghi*	5	10
		Clinton and head smut	*Sphaceotheca reiliana*	5	10
Vegetables					
1.	Brinjal	Phomopsis blight	*Phomopsis vexans*	10	50
2.	Cabbage	Black leg	*Leptosphaeria maculans*	10	50
		Black rot	*Xanthomonas campestris pv. Campestris*	10	50
		Soft rot	*Erwinia carotovora*	10	50
3.	Capsicum/chilies	Anthracnose/die back/ ripe rot	*Colletotrichum capsici*	10	50
4.	Cauliflower	Leaf blight	*Alternaria solani*	10	50
		Black leg	*Leptosphaeria maculans*	10	50
		Black rot	*Xanthomonas campestris pv. Campestris*	10	50
		Soft rot	*Erwinia carotovora*	10	50
5.	Celery	Leaf blight	*Alternaria solani*	10	50
		Root rot	*Phoma apiicola*	10	50
6.	Chinese cabbage	Blackleg	*Leptosphaeria maculans*	10	50
		Black rot	*Xanthomonas campestris pv. Campestris*	10	50
		Soft rot	*Erwinia carotovora*	10	50
7.	Cluster bean	Anthracnose	*Colletotrichum* sp.	10	20
		Ascochyta blight (for hilly areas only)	*Ascochyta* sp.	10	20

TABLE 11.5 *(Continued)*

Crop		Designated diseases	Causal organisms	Max permitted (No./10000 plants)	
				Foundation Seed	**Certified Seed**
8.	French bean (Rajmash)	Bacterial blight	*Xanthomonas cyamopsidis*	10	20
		Bean mosaic	*Macrosiphum pisi*	10	20
		Anthracnose	*Colletotrichum lindemuthianum*	10	20
		Bacterial blight	*Xanthomonas* sp.	10	20
		Ascochyta blight	*Ascochyta phaseolorum*	10	20
9.	Knol-khol	Black leg	*Phoma lingum*	10	50
		Black rot	*Xanthomonas campestris*	10	50
10.	Tomato	Early blight	*Alternaria solani*	10	50
		Tobacco mosaic virus	TMV	10	50
		Leaf spots	*Stemphylium solani*	10	50
11.	Potato	Brown rot	*Pseudomonas solanacearum*	none	3/ha
		Leafroll virus	Potato Virus 1	200	300
		Soft rot	*Erwinia carotovora*	75	100
		Virus	*Solanum virus 14*	200	300
		Mild mosaic	*Solanum virus 1, virus X, Potato latent virus and Potato mottle virus*	200	300
12	Yam	Brown rot/ bacterial wilt	*Pseudomonas solanacearum*	None	None

Source: Reprinted from IMSCS, 2013.

11.7.8 HARVESTING

Best quality of seed can be harvested just after attaining physiological maturity. The maturity indices should be fine-tuned to maximize yield and quality of harvested seed.

11.7.9 THRESHING

Threshing is separation of seeds from plant or fruit on which it is borne. It is critical operation as it may cause physical injuries to seed and may affect germination and yield as well. Threshing can be done manually and mechanically.

11.7.10 SEED PROCESSING

Seed processing determines the final physiological and physical quality. Seed processing comprises of cleaning, drying, grading, treating, and other operations that improve seed quality. The screens are specific to different crops as per the size and shape of seeds. Typical contaminants namely, weed seeds, undersized seeds, damaged seeds, broken and shriveled seeds, straw, chaff, leaves, twigs, stones, soil particles, etc., are removed. The crop-specific screen aperture sizes are enlisted in Table 11.6.

TABLE 11.6 Top and Bottom Aperture Size and Shape of Screen for Seed Processing of Various Crops.

S. No.	Crop	Screen aperture size (mm) and shape	
		Top screen	**Bottom screen**
1	2	3	4
Cereal crops			
1.	Barley:		
	2-rowed	6.50 r	2.30 s
	6-rowed	6.50 r	2.10 s, 2.20 s
2.	Paddy:		
	Coarse grain or bold type	2.8s, 9.0 r	1.85 s
	Medium slender	2.8s, 9.0 r	1.80 s
	Fine or superfine	2.8s, 9.0 r	1.70 s

TABLE 11.6   *(Continued)*

S. No.	Crop	Screen aperture size (mm) and shape	
		Top screen	Bottom screen
1	2	3	4
3.	Wheat:		
	T. aestivum	6.00 r	1.80 s, 2.10 s, 2.30 s
	T. durum	6.00 r	2.10 s, 2.30 s
4.	Triticale	6.00 r	2.10 s
		7.00 r	2.30 s
Millets			
1.	Maize (other than popcorn)	10.50 r, 11.00 r	6.40 r, 7.00 r
2.	Popcorn	8.75 r	4.25 r, 4.75 r
3.	Sorghum	4.75 r	2.10 s, 3.50 r
4.	Pearl millet	3.25 r	1.30 r, 1.30 s, 1.40 r,
			1.40 s, 1.60 r, 1.90 r
5.	Barnyard millet	3.25 r	1.40 s, 1.80 r
6.	Common millet	3.80 r	1.60 s
7.	Finger millet	3.25 r	1.40 s
8.	Italian millet	3.25 r	1.20 s, 1.30 r
9.	Kodo millet	3.80 r	1.60 s, 2.00 r
10.	Little millet	2.50 r	1.60 r
Pulses			
1.	Black gram	5.00 r	2.80 s
2.	Bengal gram	9.00 r, 10.00 r	5.00 r, 5.50 r, 6.00 r
3.	Cowpea	7.00 r	3.50 r, 4.00 r
4.	Green gram	5.50 r	2.80 s, 3.20 s
5.	Indian bean (Sem)	8.75 r	4.75 s
6.	Lentil	7.00 r	3.20 s, 4.00 r, 4.75 r
7.	Pigeon pea (Arhar)	9.50 r	3.20 s, 4.00 r, 4.75 r
8.	Rajmash (French bean)	11.0 r	4.75 s
Oilseeds			
1.	Castor	13.50 r	4.40 s, 6.00 r
2.	Rapeseed and mustard	2.75 r, 3.00 r, 3.25 r	0.90 s, 1.00 s, 1.10 s, 1.40 r
3.	Linseed	4.00 r	2.00 r
4.	Niger	3.20 r	1.20 s

TABLE 11.6 *(Continued)*

S. No.	Crop	Screen aperture size (mm) and shape	
		Top screen	Bottom screen
1	2	3	4
5.	Rocket salad	3.20 r	1.10 s, 1.20 s
6.	Safflower	7.25 r	1.20 s
7.	Sesame	2.40 r	1.60 r, 1.90 r
8.	Soybean	8.00 r	4.00 s
9.	Sunflower	9.00 r	2.40 s
Fibers			
1.	Cotton:		
	Fuzzy	14.30 r	5.20 s
	Delinted	7.20 r	3.90 s
2.	Jute:		
	Capsularis	2.40 r	1.20 r, 1.60 r
	Olitorius	2.00 r	0.80 r, 1.00 r
Forages			
1.	Berseem:		
	Diploid	2.00 r	1.00 s
	Tetraploid	2.40 r	1.20 s
2.	Forage sorghum	4.00 r, 4.75 r	2.10 s
3.	Cluster bean	6.00 r	1.80 s
4.	Guinea grass	2.10 r	2.40×0.65 m
5.	Indian clover	2.10 r	2.40×0.80 m
6.	Lucerne	2.50 r	0.70×0.70×0.70 m
7.	Oats	7.50 r	2.00 s
8.	Setaria grass	2.40 r	1.90 s
9.	Sudangrass	4.00 r	1.20 s, 1.30 s
Vegetable crops			
Cucurbits			
1.	Ash gourd	9.50 r	6.40 r
2.	Bitter gourd	11.00 r	6.50 r
3.	Bottle gourd	11.00 r	6.50 r
4.	Cucumber	8.00 r	2.00 r, 2.50 r
5.	Indian squash	9.50 r	6.40 r
6.	Long melon	5.00 s	1.00 r

TABLE 11.6 *(Continued)*

S. No.	Crop	Screen aperture size (mm) and shape	
		Top screen	Bottom screen
1	**2**	**3**	**4**
7.	Muskmelon	5.00 s	1.00 r
8.	Pumpkin	11.00 r	6.50 r
9.	Ridge gourd	9.50 r	6.40 r
10.	Snake gourd	9.50 r	6.40 r
11.	Snap melon	5.00 s	1.00 r
12.	Sponge gourd	9.50 r	6.40 r
13.	Summer squash	8.00 r	2.00 r
14.	Watermelon	6.00 r	1.80 s
Fruit vegetables			
1.	Brinjal	4.00 r	0.80 s, 2.10 r
2.	Capsicum (sweet pepper)	4.00 r	0.80 s, 2.10 r
3.	Chili (hot pepper)	4.00 r	0.80 s, 2.10 r
4.	Okra	6.00 r	4.30 r
5.	Rat-tail radish	4.50 r	2.00 r
6.	Tomato	4.00 r	0.80 s, 2.10 r
Greens/leafy vegetables			
1.	Asparagus	6.00 r	2.40 r
2.	Celery	1.80 r	0.40 s, 0.64×0.64 m
3.	Fenugreek (Methi):		
	Large and medium	3.25 r	1.20 s
	Small	2.10 r	0.69 x 0.69 m
4.	Lettuce	2.30 r	0.80 r
5.	Parsley	2.75 r	0.75 s
6.	Spinach beet	5.50 r	1.80 s, 1.85 s, 2.25 r
7.	Spinach:		
	Round seeded	5.00 r	2.75 r
	Sharp seeded	8.00 r	2.50 r
8.	Coriander (All varieties)	4.25 r	2.5 s
Cole crops			
1.	Cabbage	2.75 r	0.90 s
2.	Cauliflower	2.75 r	1.10 s
3.	Broccoli	2.75 r	1.10 s

TABLE 11.6   *(Continued)*

S. No.	Crop	Screen aperture size (mm) and shape	
		Top screen	Bottom screen
1	2	3	4
4.	Chinese cabbage (both heading and nonheading)	2.75 r	0.90 s
5.	Knol-kohl	2.75 r	1.10 s
Bulbs crops			
1.	Onion	3.80 r	2.00 r
Root crops			
1.	Carrot	2.30 r	1.00 r
2.	Celeriac	1.80 r	0.40 s, 0.65×0.65 m
3.	Sugar beet:		
	Monogerm	9.00 r	3.00 r
	Multigerm	9.00 r	2.50 s
4.	Garden beet	9.00 r	3.00 r
5.	Radish	4.50 r	2.00 r
6.	Turnip	1.80 r	1.20 r

r: round aperture; s: slotted or oblong aperture; m: sieves with wire mesh.

Source: Reprinted from IMSCS, 2013.

The cleaned seeds are to be brought down to optimum moisture content, that is, 8–10% for the majority of the crops. In general, seeds are dried shade at about 15°C and 10–15% relative humidity with good air recirculation. At the commercial level, seed driers having provisions for air circulation, temperature, and RH control.

Seed is a carrier and prone to various seed-borne diseases and pests. Under the certification program, there is provision for mandatory seed treatments to manage pathogens that are seed-borne in nature. Such treatments are mandatory before granting seed certification. If presowing seed treatment is required, the desired quantity of chemical must be placed inside seed container packed separately and complete information about treatment (IMSCS, 2013). As per IMSCS (2013), treated seed containers must be inscribed with the following instructions:

- Statement of indication that seed is treated;
- The chemical name of substance used; and
- Caution statement like "Do not Use for Food, Feed or Oil Purposes" must be inscribed on the label if applicable. The caution for mercurial

and other toxic substances must be written as "POISON" and prominently displayed on label in red color.

11.7.11 PACKING

The low-volume seed having small size and low seed rate is generally packed in moisture-proof packs. There are automatic machines to pack and seal the desired quantity of seed. However, the high-volume seeds are packed in cloth or gunny bags with or without polythene lining on the inner side. Such packs are not moisture-proof.

11.7.12 LABELING

Labeling is compulsory as per legal requirement. There are different kinds of label or tag for different classes. The class-wise description of seed tags is given below.

The breeder seed tag is golden yellow (ISI No. 356; IS-1978) with a dimension of 12 cm in length and 6 cm in width. The foundation seed tag (both stage I & II) is white in color with dimensions 157.5 cm. The certified seed tag (both stage I & II) is azure blue (ISI No. 104) in color having dimensions 157.5 cm. Likewise, the truthfully labeled seed tag is Opel green (ISI No. 275) in color with dimensions 157.5 cm in dimensions.

The dimensions can be proportionally altered depending upon size of seed packet or container.

11.7.13 STORAGE OF SEEDS

Seeds can be classified into two categories based on their minimum moisture limit and storage potential, that is, orthodox and recalcitrant seeds. The storage potential of orthodox seeds improves with reduction in moisture content to certain label under ambient conditions, such as all cereals, millets, pulses, oilseeds, forages, vegetables, ornamentals, and most leguminous trees, etc. On the contrary, the storage potential of recalcitrant seeds reduces with the reduction in moisture content at ambient condition, for example, avocado, araucaria, chow-chow, cocoa, coconut, durian, Jack fruit, mango, polyalthia, potato, rubber, and tea, etc.

11.8 SUMMARY

Seed, being vital for agriculture, deserves the utmost attention among all other inputs. Seed quality determines magnitude and quality of harvest and productivity of other inputs required for crop production. Quality of seed is, however, determined by quality of crop on which seed is borne. Hence, it is the management of seed crop that plays a pivotal role in quality and productivity of subsequent crop raised. Understanding seed quality, its components, and factors affecting individual component form basis of quality seed production. Moreover, being a commodity of trade, there are certain legislative mechanisms for QC. These mechanisms must be followed to have compliance to minimum field and seed standards. Thus, management of seed crop requires comprehensive understanding of basic principles of seed production, seed quality, QC mechanisms, legal aspects of production and trade, and of course the practical skills of crop husbandry. The postharvest management needs critical attention in determining final quality of harvested seed that reaches end-user.

KEYWORDS

- **crops**
- **legislation**
- **management**
- **principles**
- **production**
- **quality**
- **seed**

REFERENCES

Agarwal, R. L. *Seed Technology*; Oxford & IBH Publishing Co.: New Delhi, India. 1995; p 842.
Bateman, A. J. Contamination of Seed Crop –II. *Heredity* **1947,** *1,* 235–246.
Fieistrizer, W. P. *Cereal Seed Technology.* A Manual on Cereal Seed Production, Quality Control and Distribution, FAO, UN, 1975, p 238.
Haan, H. D. Maintaining Varieties of Self-fertlised Crop Plants. *Euphytica* **1953,** *2* (1), 37–45.

Hartmann, H. T.; Kester, D. E. *Plant Propagation: Principles and Practices*; Prentice Hall Inc.: New Jersey, USA, 1968.

IMSCS. Indian Minimum Seed Certification Standards. CSCB, Ministry of Agriculture, New Delhi, 2013.

Kadam, B. S. Deterioration of Varieties of Crops and the Task of the Plant Breeder. *Indian J. Gen. Plant Breed.* **1942,** *2,* 159–172.

Nema, N. P. *Principles of Seed Certification and Testing*; Allied Publishers: New Delhi, India. OECD, 1985.

Ramamoorthy, K.; Sivasubramaniam, K.; Kannan, A. *Seed Legislation in India*; Agrobios (India): Jodhpur, Rajasthan, India, 2006.

Ramamoorthy, K.; Sivasubramanium, K. *Seed Technology Readyreckoner*; Agrobios: Jodhpur, Rajasthan, India, 2006, p 119.

Thompson, J. R. *An Introduction to Seed Technology*; Leonard Hill: London, UK, 1979.

CHAPTER 12

Effect of Irrigation Frequency on Tree Seedling Production

VALASIA IAKOVOGLOU*

Department of Forestry and Natural Environment Management, Technologiko Ekpedeftiko Irdyma Anatolikis Makedonias and Thrakis (EMaTTech) Drama 66100, Greece

Corresponding author. E-mail: viakovoglou@yahoo.com

ABSTRACT

Mediterranean ecosystems are of particular ecological importance, but they are facing restoration problems, mainly due to their prevailing semi-arid climate. The increased predicted temperatures associated with climate change pose greater obstacles to restoration efforts. This chapter aims to report on species responses, specifically, *Quercus pubescens*, under different irrigation frequencies and address their ability to successfully regenerate sites through research through tools like the root growth potential (RGP). The hypothesis was that seedlings that experience reduced irrigation frequency have a greater RGP. Based on the experimental procedure, under field conditions, seedlings were exposed to five irrigation frequencies and by the end of the month were evaluated based on characteristics (morphological and physiological). Continually, the seedling pre-exposed to the irrigation treatments were placed in an RGP growth chamber under regular irrigation and were evaluated at the end of the month. The results indicated that for the species of *Quercus pubescens* one watering per week was adequate to retain its normal growth while it increased their RGP ability. The water potential and the leaf characteristics were good indicators on the growth status of the seedlings. Overall, the study provided substantial insights on preconditioning seedlings to increase their potential transplanting success while saving water; a substantial advantage for semi-arid ecosystems.

12.1 INTRODUCTION

Mediterranean ecosystems are of high importance, mainly due to their increased biodiversity levels. However, these ecosystems are subjected to frequent and intense disturbances that relate to natural phenomena such as fires and floods. Based on research on climatic alterations induced by the predicted increased temperatures will further enhance the severity and frequency of these phenomena (Xoplaki et al., 2005; Lionello et al., 2006; IPCC, 2013). Further, anthropogenic interference associated with practices such as land-use alterations and overgrazing also induces further biodiversity loss (Thirgood, 1981).

Consequently, due to the importance of these ecosystems, their immediate restoration after a disturbance event is a priority for the forest nurseries. However, the prevailing semi-dry climatic conditions (Lionello et al., 2006; Mendoza et al., 2009; Rudel, 2007; Scarascia-Mugnozza et al., 2000) reduce restoration success. Prevailing drought growth conditions that the plants experience after transplanting, particularly during hot summers, are a determining factor for their growth and survival (Marañón et al., 2004; Salvador et al., 1999).

Therefore, the quality of the produced seedlings by the forest nurseries is a priority, since better-equipped seedlings favor the success of the restoration efforts. Research has indicated that seedlings with larger root systems are better equipped to survive under adverse outdoor growth conditions, especially under reduced water availability. This relates to the increased ability of the seedlings for water and nutrients exploitation that enhances the transplanting success (Puértolas et al., 2003; Villar-Salvador et al., 2008).

Prior to seedling transplant, preconditioning nursery practices reduce transplanting shock (van den Driessche, 1992; Kozlowski and Pallardy, 2002). The preconditioning involves the exposure of the seedlings to a water stress period by reducing the irrigation frequency/quantity. This triggers signals that increase biomass allocation to the roots resulting to seedlings with greater ability to produce new root system; a characteristic that helps seedlings to cope and overcome the transplant stress usually associated with water deficit conditions (Iakovoglou and Halivopoulos, 2016).

Proper irrigation frequency that suits each species provides substantial benefits. It enables the production of qualitatively better-equipped seedlings (e.g., larger root systems) that result in the more successful restoration of highly disturbed sites. It also results in greater water saving that is of substantial value for semi-arid areas where water availability is limited particularly during dry summer periods. Therefore, the associated cost of producing seedlings is smaller, since proper irrigation allows the production of a better quality of planting material (greater root potential) with a reduced amount of water.

Irrigation protocols combined with research tools that help assess the quality of the produced seedlings enables to determine the ideal irrigation frequency for each species. Such tools help in evaluation of the RGP that relates to the root dynamics in developing new roots for further nutrients and water exploitation (Mattsson, 1986; Ritchie and Tanaka, 1990). The evaluation of root growth potential has been used to assess the transplanting ability for conifer species in the North America (Jenkinson, 1980; Larsen et al., 1986). Research for the species of *Fraxinus excelsior* L. (O'Reilly et al., 2002) and *Quercus* spp. (Wilson and Jacobs, 2006) have shown that greater RGP was directly associated with the increased viability of plants under field conditions. Based on the so far cited literature, no research has been conducted on the combined effect of irrigation frequency and the RGP ability of the seedlings. Preliminary research has been carried out for *Pinus halepensis* Mill. where the most stressed plants had the greatest growth potential (Syropli et al., 2014).

One of the native forest species that thrives in the Mediterranean Greek ecosystems is *Quercus pubescens* Willd. (pubescent oak). This species has strategies and survival mechanisms associated with the ability to develop vigorous root systems (Dillaway et al., 2007; Mendoza et al., 2009). It is a highly valuable timber species that also provides food and shelter for many animals. Therefore, it is one of the main species that is highly used by forest Greek nurseries for reforestation purposes.

This study aimed to provide insights on the abilities of *Quercus pubescens* seedlings to produce new roots as evaluated by the RGP under irrigation frequencies. The hypothesis was that seedlings that have experienced reduced irrigation frequency will have a greater ability to produce new roots (greater RGP). Ultimately, the irrigation frequency that provides the best RGP provides better quality seedlings for reforestation efforts that promise greater transplanting success. The finding of this research will help assess the quality of the produced plant material prior to transplant with tools like the RGP for the most successful restoration.

12.2 MATERIAL AND METHODS

The experimental seedlings were *Quercus pubescens* that were grown for three years under field nursery conditions with daily irrigation and weekly fertilization frequency during the summer months at the Forest nursery of

Chalkidona, Greece (41°52′17″ E, 45°167′05″ N). The seedlings were grown in containers of 55 cm × 60 cm × 160 cm (QuickPot QP 24T/16) with a standard nursery soil mixture of 1-part of perlite and 3-parts of peat.

Before the experiment, there was an acclimation period for the seedlings where they were exposed to daily irrigation and no fertilization for a month. The experiment took place during August that is considered the hottest summer month for Greece and was composed of two experimental parts. The first experimental part of the irrigation treatments was tested under field conditions, while at the second experimental part the pretreated seedlings were placed in controlled growth chamber conditions of regular irrigation and evaluated for their RGP.

12.2.1   FIRST EXPERIMENTAL PART

After the acclimation period, the seedlings were placed under outdoor shed conditions to fully control the irrigation of the seedlings from unexpected rainfall events. Further, the seedlings were treated with five irrigation frequencies: watering three times every week (3I/1w), watering twice every week (2I/1w), watering once every week (1I/1w), watering once every two weeks (1I/2w) and watering once every four weeks (1I/4w), for a month. For each irrigation treatment, five seedlings were randomly harvested for evaluation. Further, for the second experimental part, five pretreated seedlings were also used.

12.2.2   SECOND EXPERIMENTAL PART

Seedlings that experienced the five irrigation treatments (first experimental part) were transferred in a growth chamber (Fig. 12.1A) designed for estimating the RGP (Mattsson, 1986). The chamber retained controlled growth conditions with 18 h of light duration (altered with 6 h of dark) under high-pressure sodium lamps (SON T 400 W, General Electric) and controlled air and water bath temperatures of $20 \pm 2\,°C$.

The seedlings were transplanted in stainless steel trays filled with a volumetric soil mixture of 1-part peat and 1-part sand that enabled the development of a new root system (Fig. 12.1B). Continuously, the stainless trays were merged in the water bath of $20 \pm 2\,°C$. The seedlings were grown under the controlled growth conditions for one more month. They were watered three times a week with the excess water being pumped out of the stainless containers with a vacuumed-pipe to avoid anoxic growth conditions.

At the end of the month, the seedlings were harvested. Particularly, the newly developed roots were carefully washed and removed to estimate the ability of each species to grow new roots (Fig. 12.1C).

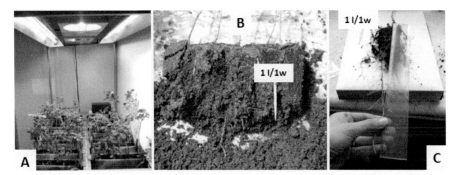

FIGURE 12.1 (A) Presentation of the growth chamber designed to estimate the Root Growth Potential (RGP). (B) Indication of the soil mixture placed in the stainless-steel trays where the seedlings were grown in the growth chamber. (C) The development of the new roots (RGP) for the treatment of one-irrigation per week (1l/1w).

12.2.3 STUDIED VARIABLES

By the end of the month for each experimental part, five seedlings were harvested and evaluated. Specifically, the height and the diameter of the root collar were measured through the use of a digital caliber. The Portable Leaf Area meter (LI-3000C) was used to evaluate the leaf area. The number of leaves, the number of branches, and the number of lateral roots were also determined. The Specific Leaf Area (SLA = leaf area/leaf dry weight) was also estimated (Garnier et al., 2001; Wilson et al., 1999). Further, the dry weights were measured by a digital analytical balance after placing the samples in an oven for three days at the $80 \pm 2 \, ^{\circ}C$. Specifically, for each seedling, the dry weight of the leaves, the stem, the branches, the tap root, and the lateral roots were evaluated. Also, the total above-ground seedling dry weight parts (dry weight of leaves + stem + branches) was estimated. The total dry weights of the below ground seedling parts were estimated as the partitioning of the dry weight of the tap and lateral roots, while the total dry weight of the seedlings was the partitioning to the above and below seedling dry weight parts. The root-to-shoot ration was also estimated. Also, the soil moisture content (Theta Meter type HH1) and the water potential (WP4 Dew Potential Meter) of the seedlings were evaluated prior to seedling harvesting. For the "second experimental part," in addition to the above variables, the

RGP as defined by the dry weight of new roots and their maximum root length were also evaluated.

The statistical analysis of the data was conducted by using the ANOVA with the SPSS® statistical software, version 15.0 (SPSS, 2006) with the data been tested for normality and homogeneity. The mean differences were tested with the Tuckey's multiple range tests at significance levels of $p < 0.05$.

12.3   RESULTS AND DISCUSSION

12.3.1   FIRST EXPERIMENTAL PART

Based on the results of the first experimental part, the reduced irrigation frequency revealed that the 3-year-old *Quecus pubescens* seedlings could tolerate with no apparent negative impacts on their growth was one watering per week. Figure 12.2 provides a visual presentation of the seedlings for each irrigation frequency as indicated by the appearance of the leaves by the end of the experimental month. This was also supported by the water potential measurements, where the 3I/1w, 2I/1w, 1I/1w, and 1I/2w irrigation frequencies retained higher values when compared to the 1I/4w. Although the moisture content had similar values for the 1I/1w and 1I/2w, the water potential was substantially different. This indicates that for the species of *Quercus pubescens* one watering every seven days was adequate to maintain its physiological growth status under field hot summer conditions. Similar results were also reported for the species of *Myrtus cummunis* L. (Iakovoglou and Kokkinou, 2017).

Based on the seedlings' characteristics, it seems that for the majority of the studied variables the irrigation treatments did not differ (Fig. 12.3). This means that the seedlings retained similar characteristics within the period of the experimental month under the irrigation treatments, indicating that those seedlings had the same potential in regards to their irrigation response. Nonetheless, some of the characteristics showed differences among treatments suggesting that those variables could be used as surrogates to address early the seedling respond under the irrigation treatments.

Specifically, the frequency of 3I/1w had the least number of lateral roots (Fig. 12.3), while their dry weights did not retain the smallest mean value (Fig. 12.4). Further, based on the dry weight of tap root, the total dry weight of the below and above ground seedling part was greater for the irrigation frequency of 2I/1w and least for the 1I/4w. Reduced seedling biomass was also observed for the species of *Pistacia lentiscus* L. under reduced irrigation frequency (Cortina et al., 2008). Similarly, for the leaf dry weight, the 2I/1w had the highest mean value with the 1I/2w had the least. Although the irrigation treatment was only for the period of one month, the negative impacts of reduced water availability were apparent for those variables, particularly for the leaf characteristics (Figs. 12.1 and 12.3). Specifically, the seedlings lost part of their leavesto alleviate water stress conditions related to the increased transpiration demand under the hot summer field conditions. This indicates an avoidance mechanism for *Quercus pubescens* associated with leaf abscission to withstand water deficit conditions (McDowell et al., 2008).

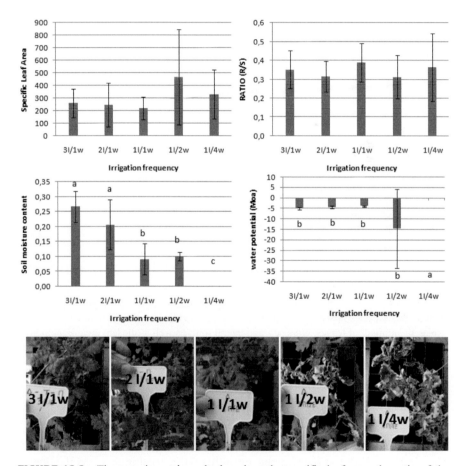

FIGURE 12.2 The experimental results based on the specific leaf area, the ratio of the root-to-shoot, as well as the characteristics of the soil moisture content and the physiological response of the seedlings as reflected by the water potential. Bars indicate the standard deviation of the mean value for each irrigation frequency, while letters indicate the level of statistical difference at the $p < 0.05$.

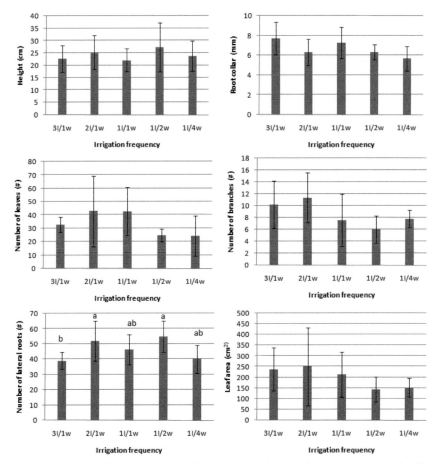

FIGURE 12.3 Seeding characteristics for *Quercus pubescens* that were grown under field conditions for each irrigation frequency. Specifically, seedling height, the diameter of the root collar, the number of leaves, branches, and lateral roots as well as the leaf area. Bars indicate the standard deviation of the mean value for each irrigation frequency, while letters indicate the level of statistical difference at the $p < 0.05$.

12.3.2   SECOND EXPERIMENTAL PART

Based on the results of the second experimental part, the seedling feature that indicated alterations on the growth of the seedlings were the leaves (Fig. 12.5). Specifically, the number of leaves as well as their leaf area of the seedlings decreased as the irrigation frequency reduced, with the 1l/2w and 1l/4w having the least mean values. Similarly, the leaf dry weight also decreased as the irrigation frequency reduced, suggesting a negative impact

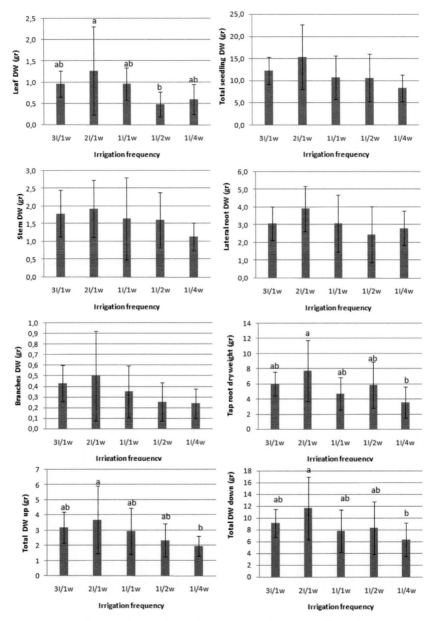

FIGURE 12.4 Biomass characteristics for *Quercus pubescens* seedlings that were grown under field conditions for each irrigation frequency. Specifically, the dry weight of the leaves, stem, branches, tap, and lateral roots, as well as, the total dry weight of the upper and down part of the seedling height and the total seedling dry weight. Bars indicate the standard deviation of the mean value for each irrigation frequency, while letters indicate the level of statistical difference at the $p < 0.05$.

of irrigation frequency of 1I/2w and 1I/4w (Fig. 12.6). Specifically, the seed-lings that were watered only once within the period of one month had no leaves (Fig. 12.7). Although the species of *Quercus pubescens* is character-ized by its ability to retain its leaves, to tolerate water deficit conditions, leaf abscission is one of its physiological responses to tolerate those adverse growth conditions (Ryan, 2011). Similarly, the total dry weight of the above seedling parts reduced as the irrigation frequency reduced, while the number and dry weight of the branches and the total seedling dry weight did not show a specific pattern with reduction in the irrigation frequency.

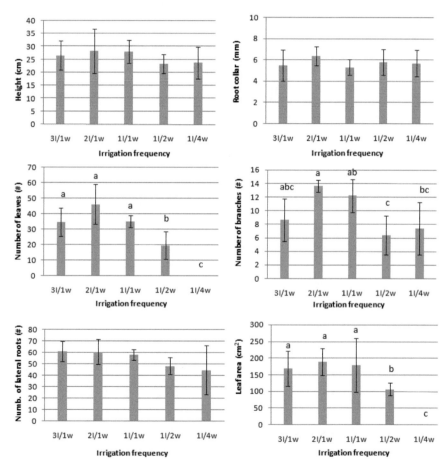

FIGURE 12.5   Characteristics of pretreated seedlings (seedling height, root collar diameter, the number of leaves, branches, and lateral roots as well as the leaf area) based on irrigation frequencies when grown for a month under controlled chamber growth conditions and frequent irrigation. Bars indicate the standard deviation of the mean for each irrigation frequency, while letters indicate the level of statistical difference at the $p < 0.05$.

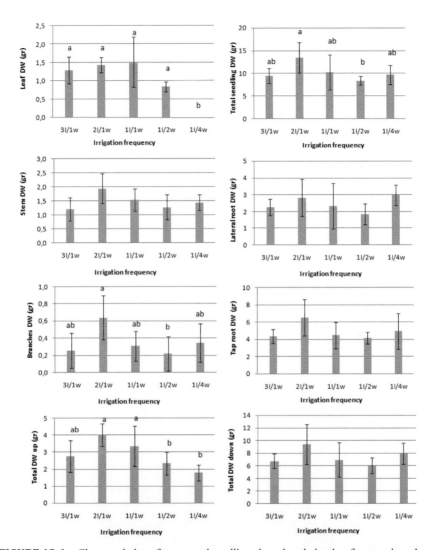

FIGURE 12.6 Characteristics of pretreated seedlings based on irrigation frequencies when grown for a month under controlled chamber growth conditions and frequent irrigation. Specifically, the dry weight of the leaves, stem, branches, tap, and lateral roots, the total dry weight of the upper and down part of the seedling height, and the total seedling dry weight. Bars indicate the standard deviation of the mean value for each irrigation frequency, while letters indicate the level of statistical difference at the $p < 0.05$.

Based on the root-to-shoot ratio, the irrigation frequencies of 2I/1w and 1I/1w had greater allocation to the root systems (Fig. 12.7). That was also supported by the greater ability of those irrigation treatments to grow new roots.

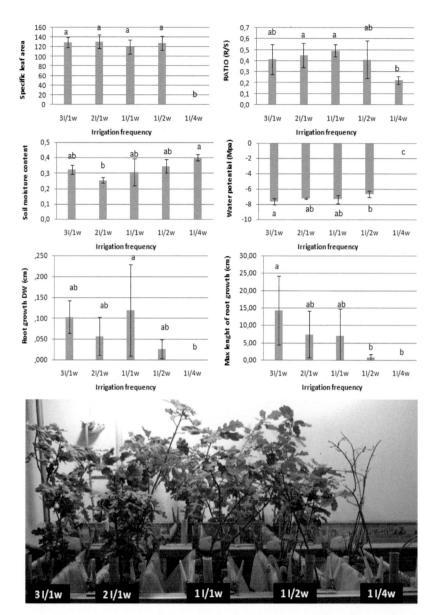

FIGURE 12.7   Characteristics of pretreated seedlings based on irrigation frequencies when growth for a month under controlled chamber growth conditions and frequent irrigation. Specifically, the specific leaf area, the ratio of the root-to-shoot, as well as the characteristics of the soil moisture content, and the physiological response of the seedlings as reflected by the water potential and the root growth potential and their maximum length. Bars indicate the standard deviation of the mean value for each irrigation frequency, while letters indicate the level of statistical difference at the $p < 0.05$.

Consequently, reducing the frequency of water supply induced a shift in the carbon allocation toward greater root systems (Iakovoglou and Halivoloulos, 2016). So, based on the results on the development of new roots, the 1I/1w had the greater RGP that was followed by the other treatments. Similar results were also obtained for the species of *Pinus halepensis* were watering once every two weeks resulted in greater root growth potential (Syropli et al., 2014). For the species of *Quercus pubescens* this suggests that, the irrigation pretreatment frequency of once per week for a month was adequate to trigger allocation for further root growth; a characteristic that promises greater transplanting success in the reforestation efforts while saving water (Chiantante et al., 2006).

This information is of vital importance particularly for ecosystems that experience water scarcity conditions. Although the majority of the species is morphologically and physiologically well equipped, future increased temperatures might pose greater difficulty in reforestation efforts. Nurseries could benefit from these irrigation preconditioning practices and produce seedlings ready to outgrow adverse field conditions by their increased ability to produce new roots that enhance their ability for further nutrients and water exploitation.

12.4 CONCLUSIONS

Based on the results, the species of *Quercus pubescens*, under field conditions (first experimental part) showed an increased ability to tolerate water scarcity conditions as low as irrigating only once every week. This indicates the increased ability of this species not only tolerate water scarcity conditions, but also being able to save water by the reduced water frequency. Further, those seedlings had increased ability to grow new roots (second experimental part). That is an important characteristic for the seedlings since it helps overcome transplanting stress. Nonetheless, further research on other species could further enlighten on species responses on the effects of irrigation frequency in accordance to their ability to grow new roots. This will potentially increase the transplanting success while saving water for ecosystems that experience growth periods of water scarcity conditions similar to those of the Mediterranean region.

ACKNOWLEDGMENTS

This research work was funded under the Project "Research & Technology Development Innovation Projects"-AgroETAK, MIS 453350 in the framework of the operational program "Human Resources Development." It is co-funded by the European Social Fund through the National Strategic Reference Framework (Research Funding Program 2007–2013) coordinated by the Hellenic Agricultural Organization—DEMETER, Forest Research Institute.

KEYWORDS

- **climate change**
- **ecophysiology**
- **regeneration**
- **preconditioning**
- **seedling production**
- **semi-arid**

REFERENCES

Chiantante, D.; Di Iorio, A.; Sciandra, S.; Scippa, G. S.; Mazzoleni, S. Effect of Drought and Fire on Root Development in *Quercus pubenscens* Willd. and *Fraxinus ornus* L. Seedlings. *Environ. Exp. Bot.* **2006,** *56*, 190–197.

Cortina, J.; Green, J. J.; Baddeley, J. A.; Watson, C. A. Root Morphology and Water Transport of Pistacia Lentiscus Seedlings under Contrasting Water Supply: A Test of the Pipe Stem Theory. *Environ. Exp. Bot.* **2008,** *62*, 343–350.

Dillaway, D. N.; Stringer, J. W.; Rieske, L. K. Light Availability Influence Root Carbohydrates, and Potentially Vigor, in White Oak Advance Regeneration. *For. Ecol. Manag.* **2007,** *250*, 227–233.

Garnier, E.; Shpley, B.; Roumet, C.; Laurent, G. A Standardized Protocol for the Determination of Specific Leaf Area and Leaf Dry Matter Content. *Funct.Ecol.* **2001,** *15*, 688–695.

Iakovoglou, V.; Kokkinou, E. Response of *Myrtus communis* Seedlings under Irrigation Frequencies. *Int. J. Bio-resour. Stress Manag.* **2018,** *9*, 069–074.

Iakovoglou, V.; Halivopoulos, G. Ecophysiology Responses of Preconditioning of Forest Species. A Review. *J. Eng. Sci. Technol. Rev.* **2016,** *9*, 7–11.

Jenkinson, J. L. *Improving Plantation Establishment by Optimizing Growth Capacity and Planting Time of Western Yellow Pines*; USDA For. Serv. PSW, 1980.

IPCC. *Climate Change 2013. The Physical Science Basis;* Intergovernmental Panel on Climate Change, Cambridge University Press: Cambridge, UK, 2013.

Kozlowski, T. T.; Pallardy, S. G. Acclimation and Adaptive Responses of Woody Plants to Environmental Stresses. *Bot. Rev.* **2002,** *68*, 270–334.

Larsen, H. S.; South, D. B.; Boyer, J. M. Root Growth Potential, Seedling Morphology and Bud Dormancy Correlate with Survival of Loblolly Pine Seedlings Planted in December in Alabama. *Tree Physiol.* **1986,** *1* (3), 253–263.

Lionello, P.; Rizzoli, M.; Boscolo, R.; Alpert, P.; Artale, V.; Li, L.; Luterbacher, J.; May, W.; Trigo, R.; Tsimplis, M.; Ulbrich, U.; Xoplaki, E. The Mediterranean Climate: An Overview of the Main Characteristics and Issues. *Dev. Earth Environ. Sci.* **2006,** *4,* 1–26.

Lloret, F.; Casanovas, C.; Penuelas, J. Seedlings Survival of Mediterranean Shrubland Species in Relation Root: Shoot Ratio, Seed Size and Water and Nitrogen Use. *Funct. Ecol.* **1999,** *13* (2), 210–216.

Marañón, T.; Zamora, R. R.; Villar, M. R.; Zavala, M. A.; Quero, P. J. L.; Pérez, R. I. M.; Mendoza, S. I.; Castro, G. J. Regeneration of Tree Species and Restoration under Contrasted Mediterranean Habitats: Field and Glasshouse Experiments. *Int. J. Ecol. Environ. Sci.* **2004,** *30,* 187–196.

Mattsson, A. Seasonal Variation in Root Growth Capacity During Cultivation of Container Grown *Pinus sylvestris* Seedlings. *Scand. J. For. Res.* **1986,** *1* (1–4), 473–482.

McDowell, N.; Pockman, W. T.; Allen, C. D.; Breshears, D. D.; Cobb, N.; Kolb, T.; Plaut, J.; Sperry, J.; West, A.; Williams, D. G.; Yepez, E. A. Mechanisms of Plant Survival and Mortality During Drought: Why do Some Plants Survive While Others Succumb to Drought? *New Phytol.* **2008,** *178,* 719–739.

Mendoza, I.; Zamora, R.; Castro, J. A Seedling Experiment for Testing Tree Community Recruitment under Variable Environments: Implications for Forest Regeneration and Conservation in Mediterranean Habitats. *Biol. Conserv.* **2009,** *142* (7), 1401–1499.

O'Reilly, C.; Harper, C.; Keane M. Influence of Physiological Conditions at the Time of Lifting on the Cold Storage Tolerance and Field Performance of Ash and Sycamore. *Forestry* **2002,** *75* (1), 1–12.

Puértolas, J.; Gil, L.; Pardow, J. A. Effects of Nutritional Status and Seedling Size on Field Performance of *Pinus halepensis* Planted on Former Arable Land in the Mediterranean Basin. *Forestry* **2003,** *76* (2), 159–168.

Ritchie, G. A.; Tanaka, Y. Target Seedling Concepts: Height and Diameter. In *Target Seedling Symposium: Proceedings of the Meeting of the Western Forest Nursery Association, Roseburg, OR, USDA Forest Service General Technical Report, RM-200, Fort Collins, CO;* Rose, R., Campbell, J., Landis, T.D., Eds.; 1990; pp 37–52.

Rudel, Ph. Mediterranean Climate Ecosystems. *Encycl. Biodivers.* **2007,** *3,* 1–15.

Ryan, M. G. Tree Responses to Drought. *Tree Physiol.* **2011,** *31,* 237–239.

Salvador, P. V.; Ocana, L.; Penuelas, J.; Carrasco, I. Effect of Water Stress Conditioning on the Water Relations, Root Growth Capacity, and the Nitrogen and Non-structural Carbohydrate Concentration of *Pinus halepensis* Mill. (Aleppo pine) Seedlings. *Ann. For. Sci.* **1999,** *56* (6), 459–465.

Scarascia, M. G.; Oswald, H.; Piussic, P.; Radoglou K. Forests of the Mediterranean Region: Gaps in Knowledge and Research Needs. *For. Ecol. Manag.* **2000,** *132,* 97–109.

SPSS. *200 SPSS,. Rel. 15.0,* SPSS: Chicago, 2006.

Syropli, Aik.; Iakovoglou, V.; Radoglou, K.; Zaimes, G. N. In *Growth of Pinus halepensis Under Controlled Watering Conditions.* 5° Environmental Conference of Macedonia. Thessaloniki, Greece (in Greek), 2014.

Thirgood, J. V. *Man and the Mediterranean Forest;* Academic Press: London, 1981; p 194.

van den Driessche, R. Changes in Drought Resistance and Root Growth Capacity of Container Seedlings in Response to Nursery Drought, Nitrogen, and Potassium Treatments. *Can. J. For. Res.* **1992,** *22* (5) 740–749.

Villar, S. P.; Valladeres, F.; Dominguez, L. S.; Ruiz, D. B.; Fernandez, P. M.; Delgado, A.; Penuelas, J. L. Functional Traits Related to Seedling Performance in the Mediterranean Leguminous Shrub *Retama sphaerocarpa*: Insights from a Provenance, Fertilization, and Rhizobial Inoculation Study. *Environ. Exp. Bot.* **2008,** *64* (2) 145–154.

Wilson, B. C.; Jacobs, D. F. Quality Assessment of Temperate Zone Deciduous Hardwood Seedlings. *New For.* **2006,** *31,* 417–433.

Wilson, J. P.; Thomson, K.; Hodson, G. J. Specific Leaf Area and Leaf Dry Matter Content as Alternative Predictors of Plant Strategies. *New Phytol.* **1999,** *143,* 155–162.

Xoplaki, E.; Luterbacher, J.; Paeth, H.; Dietrich, D.; Steiner, N.; Grosjean, M.; Wanner, H. European Spring and Autumn Temperature Variability and Change of Extremes Over the Last Half Millennium. *Geophys. Res. Lett.* **2005,** *32* (15) 1–4.

CHAPTER 13

Saline Soils: Strategies and Perspective to Counteract Salt Stress in Crops

CINZIA FORNI*

Dipartimento di Biologia, Università di Roma Tor Vergata, Via della Ricerca Scientifica, 00133 Rome, Italy.

Corresponding author. E-mail: forni@uniroma2.it

ABSTRACT

Salinization of soil is increasing with a perspective to lose arable lands. The presence of salt in the soil can damage seriously the crops, causing considerable losses in their yields. To solve this critical issue, the improvement of the knowledge about the response mechanism in plants exposed to salinity is necessary to better select tolerant genotypes that can be used in breeding programs.

This paper recapitulates some aspects of plant response to salinity and the current perspective in solving the problem related to the improvement of plant tolerance to salinity. An overview of salt tolerance studies in *Brassica* is presented.

13.1 INTRODUCTION

Salt-affected soils are spread in several countries with different extent and severity (Ruan et al., 2010). Soils containing excess salts occur naturally in arid and semiarid climates and coastal lagoon systems, that is, natural or primary salinity, whereas secondary salinization is related to inappropriate land management and agricultural practice, like irrigation systems that use water containing trace amounts of sodium chloride (NaCl) and seawater (Tester and Davenport, 2003; Munns, 2005). In saline soils, NaCl can be considered the most prevalent salt but the presence of other soluble salts has been also reported (Munns and Tester, 2008).

Electrical conductivity (ECe) of the soil is commonly considered as an important indicator: A soil is classified as saline when ECe is 4 dS/m or more, which corresponds to 40 mM NaCl (Munns and Tester, 2008). According to FAO (www.FAO.org), a soil with ECe higher than 8 dS/m has to be considered strongly saline, whereas the threshold of ECe for saline soil has been reported to a reference value of 15 dS/m by World Soil Resources Reports (IUSS Working Group WRB, 2007). Depending on the values of ECe of the soils, the crop cultivation ranges from restriction to many crops (moderately saline) to only a few tolerant crops (strongly saline land).

Excess of salts hinders plant growth by affecting the soil–water balance, thus affecting plant nutrient availability and both crop suitability and yields. In agriculture the sensitivity of crops to stress is usually related to losses in yield (Dolferus, 2014); therefore, species with an improved salt tolerance represent a key component in keeping the yields at a good level to sustain food and biofuel production. In saline land, the activity and biodiversity of soil micro-organisms are also affected influencing key soil processes (Canfora et al., 2014).

13.2   PLANTS AND SALINE STRESS

The presence of salt in the soil elicits a stress, that has a negative impact on plant physiology by impairing metabolic processes and decreasing the photosynthesis. Plants try to cope with stress by activating different genes, thus reprogramming their metabolism (Forni et al., 2017). The efficacy of these responses is the basis of plant tolerance to salinity, a rather complex character that shares common traits with the response to other stress (Forni et al., 2017). Intense efforts have been dedicated to elucidating the complicated regulatory mechanisms of plant salt tolerance. The tolerance is also based on the limitation of the take up of salts by the roots or on controlling its concentration and distribution within the plant organs. The network and the regulation of transcription of genes involved in stress response have been well described and reviewed by Balderas-Hernández et al. (2013) and Denlein et al. (2014).

Plant species can be divided into two groups: (1) halophytes, that is, plants tolerant to salinity that naturally grow in saline soils; (2) glycophytes, that is, very sensitive plants whose growth can be severely inhibited by 100–200 mmol/L NaCl (Mahajan and Tuteja, 2005; Zhu, 2007). Variability in salt tolerance has been detected within the species and even genotypes. The major effects of salt on plant morphology and physiology have been described and reviewed by several authors (Munns 2002, 2005; Denlein et al., 2014; Forni et al., 2017). The results obtained in the different experiments have evidenced that the plant response to salinity can depend on the phenological stage, the severity and the length of exposure.

Time frame plays a role in the response to salinity, being very important for the screening of genotypes for tolerance. Salt acclimation or gradual step acclimation (Sanchez et al., 2008) can be induced by gradual exposure to saline conditions (Zhu 2001; Bartels and Sunkar, 2005). This approach can induce salt tolerance in sensitive genotypes, suggesting that the latter may possess a genetic program for tolerance to some extent. The dynamism of acclimation in salt response has been highlighted by the data of Skirycz et al. (2010, 2011), that is, leaves exposed to mannitol, an elicitor of osmotic stress, showed temporally dynamic genetic and morphological changes, depending upon the developmental stage and length of treatment. Vice versa, salt shock is the extreme form of salt stress, when plants are suddenly exposed to a high level of salinity. Salt shock is rare in agriculture or in natural ecosystems, where usually plant exposure to salinity occurs gradually. According to Shavrukov (2013), in experimental condition, the more gradual application of NaCl would result in the more closely mimic of the salt stress response of plants in saline field conditions.

The effects of salts on plants are in some cases shows common traits to other stress, for example, drought. In plants, salt exposure induces osmotic shock or plasmolysis, mostly in the root cells (Munns, 2002). In fact, root is the first target organ where the water uptake decreases with increased salt concentrations. The expression of 5590 genes was found to be related to salt regulation in roots of *Arabidopsis* seedlings, mainly in cortex cells (Geng et al., 2013). After salt exposure, root growth can decrease together with changes of growth direction in the attempt to avoid highly salinity; such directional change is based on an active redistribution of auxin in the root tip. This phenotype, defined as halotropism, has been detected in different species (Galvan-Ampudia et al., 2013).

For the resistance to salt stress, Na^+ and K^+ membrane transporters play a pivotal role (Schroeder et al., 2013). When Na^+ and Cl^- are taken up in large amounts by the root, where Na^+-influx pathways are located, they negatively affect growth by impairing metabolic processes and decreasing the photosynthesis.

Osmotic stress, caused by salt, may induce a water removal from the cytoplasm, thus, reducing cytosolic and vacuolar volumes; the organelle proteins may have decreased activity or even undergo to complete denaturation (Bartels and Sunkar, 2005). Component of stress response, like autophagy, can be the extreme consequence of osmotic stress (Kroemer et al., 2010). Genes involved in autophagocytosis (ATG genes, AuTophaGy-related genes) are functioning in response to salt stress in *Arabidopsis* (Slavikova et al., 2008). Moreover, in barley roots the strong salt shock-induced apoptosis-like cell death (Katsuhara, 1997).

The leaf growth is quite sensitive to osmotic stress; the changes in this organ are quite rapid with the increasing of salinity (Bartels and Sunkar, 2005; Munns, 2002). The reduction of water content and stomata conductance reduce the rate of transpiration, impacting on photosynthetic rate. Therefore, the reduced leaf size, a process known as leaf area adjustment, is considered beneficial. In the meantime, the roots continue to grow, leading to a change in the ratio shoot/root.

The decreased photosynthetic efficiency is caused by salt injury in young photosynthetic leaves that may lead to the acceleration of their senescence (Forni et al., 2017). Moreover, photosynthesis decline and reactive oxygen species (ROS) production result in a decrease of plant growth. In fact, ROS overproduction damages thylakoid membranes and photosystems reduces the concentration of chlorophyll and carotenoids and changes the ratio of chlorophyll a and b (Parida and Das, 2005).

13.3   PLANT RESPONSE TO SALINITY

According to Munns (2002), plant response to salinity can be divided into two phases. The presence of salt outside the roots elicits the first water stress or osmotic phase. Growth reduction is probably regulated by hormone signals from the roots and during this phase, plant needs to adjust the water potential and turgor to reach osmotic homeostasis, usually, this process is rather quick (within hours or 1 day). The second phase, that is, ionic stress component of salinity stress, is longer and becomes more severe within time. Cell injury is caused by the toxic levels of salt concentration in transpiring leaves, that exceed the ability of the cells to locate them in the vacuoles. During the second phase, the growth in younger leaves is reduced and consequently the supply of carbohydrates to the growing tissues.

Salt tolerance mechanism is principally based on plant attempts to minimize the entry of salt at organ and at cellular level (Munns, 2002). Halophytes can perform both, whereas some glycophytes, even though they exclude efficiently salt, are unable to compartmentalize the up taken salt in the vacuole.

Some mechanisms of salinity response have been clarified by the use of overexpression/loss of function lines, obtained mainly in the model plant

Arabidopsis (Denlein et al., 2014; Forni et al., 2017). Two sensory modalities have been evidenced: (1) sensing of the hyperosmotic component, (2) sensing of the ionic Na^+ component of the stress. Therefore, successful coping with salt stress depends on the ability of the plants to sense both components of the stress.

Osmotic stress detected after Na^+ accumulation in the cytosol is due to the impairment of ionic balance (Denlein et al., 2014). To cope with hyperosmotic inner environment and Na^+ component of the stress, signaling plays an important role in eliciting a cascade of responses and in evoking mechanisms counteracting stress (Huang et al., 2012).

After the exposure, the increase of concentration of Ca^{2+} is detected in different root cell types; it is likely that Ca^{2+} channels are coupled with plant hyperosmotic sensor is (Knight et al., 1997) calcium-dependent protein kinases, calcineurin B-like proteins (CBLs), with CBL-interacting protein kinases are the protein activated downstream of Ca^{2+}.

The transcription factors (TFs), activated by Ca^{2+}/calmodulin, are calmodulin-binding transcription activators (Pandey et al., 2013), GT-element-binding like proteins (Weng et al., 2012) and MYBs (Li et al., 2015). Moreover, Ca^{2+} signaling is linked to the activity of salt overly sensitive (SOS) genes (Zhu, 2002). SOS pathway has three major components: (1) SOS3, acting as a Ca^{2+} sensor (Ishitani et al., 2000); (2) SOS2, a serine/threonine-protein kinase; (3) SOS1, a plasma membrane Na^+/H^+ antiporter (Türkan and Demiral, 2009). However, although the increased level of Ca^{2+} can be considered a hallmark in stress response, it cannot be excluded from the presence of Ca^{2+} independent osmotic sensory mechanisms. In the response to salinity cytoskeleton play a role, that is, depolymerization and reorganization of microtubules and stabilization of actin filaments are important in successful withstanding salt stress (Wang et al., 2011). Moreover, involvement of the cytoskeleton in Ca^{2+} influx and in SOS pathway has been reported.

Other second messengers are induced by salt exposure, that is, ROS (Deinlein et al., 2014; Forni et al., 2017). ROS are important molecules acting in signal transduction and mediating cell response to stress. In salt exposed cells, the imbalance between ROS production and scavenging leads to the overproduction of ROS (Miller et al., 2010), a condition that is harmful to cell components, due to the onset of oxidative stress situations damaging severely proteins, lipids, and nucleic acids. To counteract the high level of ROS and to overcome oxidative stress situation, plants have evolved different antioxidant systems, induced by abscisic acid (ABA)-dependent or ABA-independent pathways (Vital et al., 2008).

Plants react to the detrimental effects of the elevated ROS levels through the activation of antioxidant enzymes and the synthesis of molecules with antioxidant properties (e.g., phenolic compounds). Several enzymes are reported to be involved in ROS scavenging (Noctor and Foyer, 1998; Türkan and Demiral, 2009; Di Cori et al., 2013; Forni et al., 2017) whose coordinated activity is fundamental to obtain efficiently a balance between the rate of formation and scavenging of ROS and important in maintenance of hydrogen peroxide at the levels needed for cell signaling (Munns and Tester, 2008).

Production of specific secondary metabolites, possessing antioxidant activity, can be increased or decreased as consequence of ionic and osmotic stress (Mahajan and Tuteja, 2005). Enhanced synthesis of phenolic compounds after salt treatment has been detected barley (Ahmed et al., 2015) in *Brassica napus* (Forni, unpublished results) and other species (Parida and Das, 2005). Increased levels of anthocyanins were detected as response to salt treatment (Parida and Das, 2005), vice versa in salt-sensitive species a decreased concentration of these pigments was determined (Daneshmand et al., 2010).

The reprogramming of metabolic activities involves the fundamental role of different TFs and cis-elements intolerant response, as evidenced in several studies (Balderas-Hernández et al., 2013; Deinlein et al., 2014; Elfving et al., 2011; Golldack et al., 2011; Li et al., 2015; Nakashima et al., 2009; Nuruzzaman et al., 2013; Sakuraba et al., 2015). The overexpression or suppression of these genes can lead to an improvement of plant tolerance to stress conditions.

Tuteja et al. (2014a, 2014b) reported that DEAD-box RNA helicases are differentially regulated not only during development but also in stress response. At posttranscriptional level, small noncoding micro-RNAs can control and modulate the expression of responsive genes in plant exposed to environmental stress (Jeong and Green, 2013). Under this condition, the activation of osmotic stress-responsive (OR) genes has been detected (Kreps et al., 2002; Seki et al., 2002). The OR genes, usually silent under normal conditions, protect the cells from stress through the synthesis of important metabolic proteins and regulation of the downstream genes involved in signal transduction.

The decrease of water potential, caused by the osmotic component, is counteracted by the upregulation of genes relevant for inorganic ion uptake (Mahajan and Tuteja, 2005) and the synthesis of osmolytes. Enhancement of the synthesis of different osmolytes, such as glycine-betaine, proline, sugar alcohols, polyamines, and proteins from the late embryogenesis abundant, has been reported in species exposed to stress conditions (Aziz et al., 1998;

Nawaz and Ashraf, 2010). They help the cell in overcoming the osmotic stress, allowing the re-establishment of homeostasis (Shinozaki and Yamaguchi-Shinozaki, 1997; Zhu, 2002). The hydroxyl group of sugar alcohols can substitute the OH group of water, mechanism that leads to the preservation of membrane structural integrity, especially the thylakoids (Mahajan and Tuteja, 2005; Yokoi et al., 2002).

Studies on transgenic lines have shown that the expression of genes involved in osmolytes biosynthesis is associated with an enhancement of tolerance to different stresses (Bohnert and Jensen, 1996; Zhu, 2001). Trehalose is reported to act in stabilization of dehydrated proteins and lipid membranes and also in protecting biological structures from damage during desiccation (Redillas et al., 2012); transgenic rice, producing high level of this molecule, showed an improved tolerance to both drought and salt stress (Redillas et al., 2012).

Proline and glycine-betaine are the molecules mostly involved in osmoprotection. The accumulation of glycine-betaine has been related to the protection of plants against abiotic stress via osmoregulation or osmoprotection (for review see Giri 2011). Pyrroline-5-carboxylase synthase is the main proline biosynthetic gene; it has been utilized to increase proline level in transgenic plants in order to improve stress tolerance (Verbruggen and Hermans, 2008; Su and Wu, 2004). However, salt tolerance cannot be always related to significant changes of osmolyte synthesis (Di Cori et al., 2013). Therefore, we can hypothesize that the protective role of the osmolyte depends on different factors, like species, cultivar, growth conditions and developmental stage of the plants, and besides these to mechanism of action, different from osmoregulation or osmoprotection (Ashraf, 2004; Giri, 2011).

The regulation of gene transcription also involves the dynamic changes in hormone biosynthesis. Several hormones are involved in the response to abiotic stress, that is, salicylic acid (SA), ethylene (ET), jasmonates (JAs), cytokinins (CK), brassinosteroid (BR) and gibberellic acid (GA) (Deinlein et al., 2014; Forni et al., 2017; Ryu and Cho, 2015). In stress conditions, cross-talk among these hormones have been suggested by different authors (reviewed by Peleg and Blumwald, 2011).

The most studied plant stress-signaling hormones are ABAs. In plants, there are ABA-responsive TFs, which expression is induced by different stresses. The stress response can be divided ABA dependent (Takahashi et al., 2004; Geng et al., 2013; Golldack et al., 2014; Yoshida et al., 2014; Tuteja, 2007) and ABA independent (Yamaguchi Shinozaki and Shinozaki, 2006; Tuteja, 2007). Both pathways regulate OR genes expression (Yoshida et al., 2014); while a reduction of water loss via transpiration is obtained by

ABA-inducible gene expression, that causes stomatal closure (Yamaguchi-Shinozaki and Shinozaki, 2006; Wilkinson and Davies, 2010).

An important role in plant development and response to environmental conditions has been ascribed to CKs and CK receptors (Tran et al., 2010; Nishiyama et al., 2011; Nishiyama et al., 2012). During growth, as wells as adaptation to environmental stress, CK and ABA may exert antagonistic activities (Javid et al., 2011).

JA and its active derivates share a positive role in salt tolerance (Qiu et al., 2014; Zhao et al., 2014). JA enhances the activities of antioxidant enzymes (Qiu et al., 2014), pathogenesis-related proteins and salt stress-responsive proteins (Moons et al., 1997). Furthermore, the application of methyl JA elicits the production of antioxidants, even though the response is species-specific and depends on the concentration of the molecule (Ahmad et al., 2016).

Stress response may induce the production of ET and SA (Mahajan and Tuteja, 2005). Exogenous application of SA promotes photosynthetic rate enhancement, thus, improving tolerance (reviewed by Hayat et al., 2010).

Different stress conditions elicit stress ethylene production (Forni et al., 2017). Salt imposition causes enhancement of ET evolution from the leaves (Dodd and Pérez-Alfocea, 2012). ET can cross-talk with auxin, since members of 1-amino-cyclopropane-1-carboxylate synthase gene family (ACS), encoding rate-limiting enzymes in ET biosynthetic pathways, are regulated by auxin (Tsuchisaka and Theologis, 2004). Improved salt tolerance was related to lower level of ET. In fact, inoculation of plants with bacteria strain containing 1-aminocyclopropane-1-carboxylate (ACC) deaminase gene that reduces stress ET synthesis ameliorates the plant performance in saline conditions (reviewed by Forni et al. 2017).

BR, mainly by exogenous application, induces the expression of stress-related genes; thus, BR helps the keeping of photosynthetic efficiency, the activation of antioxidant enzymes, the synthesis of osmolytes, and other hormone responses (Divi and Krishna, 2009).

Accumulation of auxin, named auxin maxima, is related to cell elongation, organogenesis, and another physiological process (Lau et al., 2008). Reduced level of auxin has been reported in salt-stressed tomato (Dunlap and Binzel, 1996). *Arabidopsis* mutants, defecting in auxin transport, are more sensitive to salt; moreover, inhibition of biomass production was determined in mutants with defects in transcription/receptors involved in the auxin response (Afzal et al., 2005; Liu et al., 2015). These results suggest the important role of auxin in the behavior of the plants exposed to salinity.

13.4 APPROACHES TO SOLVE THE PROBLEM OF SALINITY

The use of good land management practice and the association of plants with plant growth-promoting bacteria (PGPB) or breeding and molecular biology have been considered very promising approaches to solve the problems related to salinity.

In saline land, the adequate maintenance of the physical/chemical characteristics of soil is a fundamental goal that can be reached by rational use of good quality water, even though not always applicable, and the wise use of fertilizers together with appropriate cultural practices. Lakhdar et al. (2009) emphasize the effectiveness of the use of composted municipal solid waste in salt-affected soil, suggesting this practice as a valid alternative to counteract the negative effects of salt exposure on plants. However, compost quality needs to be very carefully checked in order to do not enhance the risk due to the presence of either pollutants or pathogenic organisms in the compost.

Considering the achievement of salt tolerance in plants, a note of caution is necessary since most of the results, obtained so far, come from laboratory and greenhouse experimental conditions. Thus, we do not know yet the limitations and challenges that may be encountered when these approaches will be transferred to the field. Hydroponics is the most popular growth condition applied in these studies with respect to the utilization of soil mixture (reviewed by Shavrukov et al. 2012; Shavrukov, 2013) but plant response to salinity in hydroponics and in soil may be different (Tavakkoli et al., 2010) and a soil-based system is needed to simulate the field responses. Saline soils usually contain different salts, beside NaCl, that can be also harmful. Moreover, most of the studies are focused on the plant response to single stress, even though in field conditions the plants may be challenged by concurrent different stresses.

To obtain a better crop performance, plant acclimation can be considered, as also reported above, both gradual exposure and low-salt level can activate processes leading to an enhancement of tolerance to salinity in different species, providing an improvement in survival, growth, and yield (Pandolfi et al., 2016).

Exogenous applications of hormones or polyamine or the establishment of association with bacteria/mycorrhizal fungi may ameliorate plant tolerance to salinity. Some of the adverse effects of salt can be diminished by exogenous application of hormones (Afzal et al., 2005; Liu et al., 2015). For example, the positive effect of exogenous application of CK has been described and ascribed to its antioxidant activity related to purine breakdown protection (Javid et al., 2011). According to Ghanem et al. (2011), the enhanced synthesis of CK in the root offers the possibility to improve both shoot hormonal and ion status, thus, decreasing the effects of salinity on growth. However, controversy still exists in the literature about the positive role of CK, since CK-deficient mutants showed improved salt and drought tolerance (Nishiyama et al., 2011; Nishiyama et al., 2012).

Exogenous application of polyamines has been suggested (Gill and Tuteja, 2010), basing on the possible relation between the enhanced amount of polyamine concentration and improvement of salt tolerance (Zapata et al., 2004; Alcázar et al., 2010). However, plant response can be highly variable depending on the organ developmental stage that influences the transport, cytoplasmic accumulation, metabolization, and functional expression (Pandolfi et al., 2010).

Associations of crops with rhizospheric/endophytic bacteria and mycorrhizal fungi have also been suggested as an alternative and environmentally sustainable strategy to increase crop yields in salt-affected field (Dodd and Pérez-Alfocea, 2012; Egamberdieva, 2009; Forni et al., 2017; Gamalero et al., 2010). The production of different plant hormones by PGPB improves the growth of the plants (Glick et al., 2007; Forni et al., 2017). Moreover, PGPB can alleviate the symptoms and protect the plants from stress by several mechanisms that confer salt tolerance, for example, through the modulation of the level of the plant hormones, involved in stress response, or osmolyte production (Glick et al., 2007; Glick, 2012; Forni et al., 2017; Mayak et al., 2004).

Screening for tolerant cultivars is important to select genotypes to be used in breeding programs. The existence of wide variability in the responsiveness of crop plants to abiotic stresses and in the control of the response by gene networks with epistatic interactions is well-known (Dolferus, 2014). Salt tolerance is a quantitative trait that is quite difficult to study and requires efficient means to evaluate the level of tolerance. Nevertheless, the identification of germplasm, helps to maintain the biomass production under different stress conditions, needs to be foreseen (Dolferus, 2014).

Because of the long-time required in obtaining salt-tolerant cultivars by conventional breeding programs, alternative approaches have been considered in parallel. Today, the available techniques and tools allow the study of gene expression in plants exposed to different stress, including salinity (Takahashi et al., 2004). Up- and downregulated genes responding to stress have been identified (reviewed by Xiong and Zhou, 2002; Jamil et al., 2011; Shavrukov, 2013; Deinlein et al., 2014; Cabello et al., 2014). Based on the results of these studies, the biotechnology seeks the possibility of manipulation of stress-responsive genes (Munns, 2005; Denlein et al., 2014;

Cabello et al., 2014). In this perspective, the identification of candidate genes for plant salt tolerance improvement can become easier by quantitative trait locus (QTL) analyses coupled with marker-assisted selection (Ashraf and Foolad, 2013).

Several genes can be the possible candidate for genetic engineering as suggested by numerous authors (Munns, 2005; Ji et al., 2013; Cabello et al., 2014; Wang et al., 2016). Results of the experiments, related to these topics, are summarized and reviewed by Munns (2005), Denlein et al. (2014), and Cabello et al. (2014). In the perspective of genetic engineering, the expression of inducible promoters should be preferred to the constitutive ones, since they do not affect growth, while in the meantime they can increase tolerance when stress is applied (Munns and Tester, 2008).

13.5 CASE REPORT: BRASSICA SPP.

The Brassicaceae family includes a wide range of horticultural crops with more than 30 species and several varieties and hybrids (Rakow, 2004). Some of them have economic significance in agriculture as a source of food, vegetable oil (Wanasundara, 2011), medicinal products (Pagliaro et al., 2015), and possible utilization in phytoremediation projects (Szczyglowska et al., 2011; Mourato et al., 2015). There are six economically important species: *B. juncea* L. (Indian mustard, target of several phytoremediation works) (Mourato et al., 2015), *B. oleracea* L. (varieties of this species include vegetables used as food), *B. rapa* L. and *B. nigra* (L.) W. D. J. Koch (used for the oil content of the seeds) (Kopsell et al., 2007), *B. napus* L. (oilseed rape, canola, a globally important oil crop worldwide, used in human nutrition and industry as lubricant and biodiesel) (Hua et al., 2012). The seeds of the latter species are a fundamental source of oil for human consumption and have a protein content between 20 and 35% of dry weight (Wanasundara, 2011).

Abiotic stresses, such as drought, cold, and high salinity, can frequently affect the yield and quality of these important crops. Overall, the data collected on tolerance to salinity in different *Brassica* species show a significant interspecific and intraspecific variation in the level of salt tolerance within the genus (Kumar et al., 2009).

Chakraborty et al. (2016), by evaluating and comparing the role of plasma membrane transporters in salt tolerance in *B. juncea, B. oleracea* and *B. napus,* considered the latter as the most tolerant species.

In *B. juncea,* the experiments by Fatma et al. (2016) showed that in the presence of salt stress the combined application of NO and S (100 µM NO and 200 mg S/ kg soil, respectively) decreased the negative effects of salt on stomatal behavior, photosynthetic activity, and growth. The enzymatic activities of ATP-sulfurylase, catalase (CAT), ascorbate peroxidase (APX), and glutathione reductase (GR) and optimized NO generation reduced the oxidative stress caused by salt exposure.

The effectiveness of the activity of some antioxidant enzymes, polyphenol oxidase, APX and CAT, in minimizing oxidative stress is also confirmed by the data obtained in our work (unpublished results), where an enhancement of the activities was observed in *B. napus* cv Edimax Cl plants, exposed either gradually or directly to salt for 28 and 35 days.

Proteomic analyses have been also applied to determine differentially expressed proteins in plants of *Brassica* exposed to salt. Jia et al. (2015) reported changes in protein patterns in leaves of *B. napus* exposed to 200 mM NaCl for 24 h, 48 h, and 72 h. The proteins differentially expressed were those associated with protein metabolism, damage repair, and defense response, which contribute to alleviate the salt detrimental effects on chlorophyll biosynthesis, photosynthesis, energy synthesis, and respiration in oilseed rape leaves.

Seedlings of the same species, pretreated with 245 mM NaCl (salt treatment) or 25% polyethylene glycol 6000 (drought treatment) (Luo et al., 2015), showed significant decreases in water content and photosynthetic rate, whereas compatible osmolytes were accumulated; oxidative damage was also observed. The proteomic profiles of family proteins, related to stress response, were changed in treated plants (Luo et al., 2015).

A study on the transcriptome profiles was performed on canola roots at the germination stage, that is, up to 24 h after H_2O (control) and NaCl treatments. Changes in the expression of genes involved in the metabolism of proline, inositol and carbohydrates, and in oxidation–reduction processes were detected, thus, evidencing the importance of these genes in stress response at this growth stage (Long et al., 2015).

To ameliorate salt tolerance in *Brassica*, several studies have been focused on the identification of candidate genes to be used in molecular breeding for salt tolerance (Kumar et al., 2015; Yong et al. 2015; Lang et al., 2017). The data provided by the QTL analyses represent valuable information for studying the genetic control of salt tolerance in this genus, and they will be very useful in marker-based breeding. Progress has been made in this field, even though few salt-tolerance cultivars and lines have been obtained so far because of the difficulties of transferring stress-tolerant traits from interspecific and intergeneric sources (reviewed by Zhang et al., 2014).

Plant transformation with gene of bacterial origin may be also helpful to obtain enhancement of salinity tolerance. The canola cv. Westar was transformed to express a bacterial ACC deaminase (EC 4.1.99.4) gene under the control of different promoters (Sergeeva et al., 2006). Transformed and nontransformed plants were treated with 0–200 mM NaCl, and the fresh and dry weights of plants, leaf proteins, and chlorophyll concentrations were determined. In the transgenic canola lines, the activity of ACC deaminase lowered the synthesis of stress ET and improved salt tolerance.

13.6   CONCLUSIONS

In the latest years, the increasing number of papers published on salinity confirms the importance of this issue. Even though the researches dealing with salt stress have clearly revealed the physiological responses to this stress and the metabolic pathways involved, we have still to make the leap on the response of plants to salinity in field conditions, where more than one stressor can be present. Molecular biology tools provide new data on crops that could be helpful in molecular breeding. Strong bottleneck for successful breeding is the complexity of the tolerance mechanisms and the variability of response within the species. However, the adoption of emerging strategies for ameliorating plant salt tolerance will offer and pave the pathway for the rationale design and development of new salt-tolerant varieties.

ACKNOWLEDGMENT

Apologies are due to colleagues whose relevant work I was not able to cite due to space limitations.

KEYWORDS

- **abiotic stress**
- ***Brassica***
- **crop**
- **salinity**
- **soil**

REFERENCES

Afzal, I.; Basra, S.; Iqbal, A. The Effect of Seed Soaking with Plant Growth Regulators on Seedling Vigor of Wheat Under Salinity Stress. *J. Stress Physiol. Biochem.* **2005,** *1* (1), 6–14.

Ahmad, P.; Rasool, S.; Gul, A.; Sheikh, S. A.; Akram, N. A.; Ashraf, M.; Kazi, A. M.; Gucel, S. Jasmonates: Multifunctional Roles in Stress Tolerance. Front. *Plant Sci.* **2016,** *15,* 813.

Ahmed, I. M.; Nadira, U. A.; Bibi, N.; Cao, F.; He, X.; Zhang, G.; Wu, F. Secondary Metabolism and Antioxidants are Involved in the Tolerance to Drought and Salinity, Separately and Combined, in Tibetan Wild Barley. *Environ. Exper. Botany.* **2015,** *111,* 1–12.

Alcázar, R.; Altabella, T.; Marco, F., Bortolotti, C.; Reymond, M.; Koncz, C.; Carrasco, P.; Tiburcio, A. F. Polyamines: Molecules with Regulatory Functions in Plant Abiotic Stress Tolerance. *Planta 231* **2010,** *231,* 1237–1249.

Ashraf, M. Some Important Physiological Selection Criteria for Salt Tolerance in Plants. *Flora* **2004,** *199,* 361–376.

Ashraf, M.; Foolad, M. R. Crop breeding for Salt Tolerance in the Era of Molecular Markers and Marker-assisted Selection. *Plant Breed.* **2013,** *132,* 10–20.

Aziz, A.; Martin, T. J.; Larher, F. Stress-induced Changes in Polyamine and Tyramine Levels can Regulate Proline Accumulation in Tomato Leaf Discs Treated with Sodium Chloride. *Physiol. Plant.* **1998,** *104,* 195–202.

Balderas, H. V. E.; Alvarado, R. M.; Fraire, V. S. Conserved Versatile Master Regulators in Signaling Pathways in Response to Stress in Plants. *AoB Plants* **2013,** *5,* plt033. doi: 10.1093/aobpla/plt033.

Bartels, D.; Sunkar, R. Drought and Salt Tolerance in Plants. *Crit. Rev. Plant Sci.* **2005,** *24,* 23–28.

Bohnert, H. J.; Jensen, R. G. Strategies for Engineering Water Stress Tolerance in Plants. *Trends Biotechnol.* **1996,** *14* (3) 89–97.

Cabello, J. V.; Lodeyro, A. F.; Zurbriggen, M. Novel Perspective for the Enineering of Abiotic Stress Tolerance in Plants. *Curr. Opin. Biotechnol.* **2014,** *26,* 62–70.

Canfora, L.; Bacci, G.; Pinzari, F.; Lo Papa, G.; Dazzi, C.; Benedetti, A. Salinity and Bacterial Diversity: To What Extent Does the Concentration of Salt Affect the Bacterial Community in a Saline Soil? *PLoS One* **2014,** *9* (9). e106662.(https://doi.org/10.1371/journal.pone.0106662).

Chakraborty K., Bose J., Shabala L.; Shabala S. Difference in Root K^+ Retention Ability and Reduced Sensitivity of K^+-permeable Channels to Reactive Oxygen Species Confer Differential Salt Tolerance in Three Brassica Species. *J. Exp. Bot.* **2016,** *67,* 4611–4625.

Daneshmand, F.; Arvin, M. J.; Kalantari, K. M. Physiological Response to NaCl Stress in Three Wild Species of Potato *in vitro. Acta Physiol. Plant.* **2010,** *32,* 91–101.

Deinlein, U.; Stephan, A. B.; Horie, T.; Luo, W.; Xu, G.; Schroeder, J. I. Plant Salt-tolerance Mechanisms. *Trends Plant Sci.* **2014,** *19,* 371–379.

Di Cori, P.; Lucioli S.; Frattarelli A.; Nota P.; Tel-Or E.; Benyamini E.; Gottlieb H.; Caboni E.; Forni C. Characterization of the Response of In Vitro Cultured *Myrtus communis* L. Plants to High Concentrations of NaCl. *Plant Physiol. Biochem.* 2013, *73,* 420–426.

Divi, U. K.; Krishna, P. Brassinosteroid: a Biotechnological Target for Enhancing Crop Yields and Stress Tolerance. *New Biotechnol.* **2009,** *26,* 131–136.

Dodd, I. C.; Pérez A. F. Microbial Amelioration of Crop Salinity Stress. *J. Exp. Bot.* **2012,** *63,* 3415–3428.

Dolferus, R. To Grow or not to Grow: a Stressful Decision for Plants. *Plant Sci.* **2014,** *229,* 247–261.

Dunlap, J.; Binzel, M. NaCl Reduces indole-3-acetic Acid Levels in the Roots of Tomato Plants Independent of Stress Induced Abscisic Acid. *Plant Physiol.* **1996,** *112,* 379–384.

Egamberdieva, D. Alleviation of Salt Stress by Plant Growth Regulators and IAA Producing Bacteria in Wheat. *Acta Physiol. Plant.* **2009,** *31,* 861–864.

Elfving, N.; Davoine, C.; Benlloch, R.; Blomberg, J.; Brännström, K.; Müller, D.; Nilsson, A.; Ulfstedt, M.; Ronne, H., Wingsle, G.; Nilsson, O.; Bjrklund, S. The *Arabidopsis thaliana* Med25 Mediator Subunit Integrates Environmental Cues to Control Plant Development. *Proc. Nat. Acad. Sci. USA* **2011,** *108,* 8245–8250.

Fatma, M.; Masood, A.; Per, T. S.; Khan, N. A. Nitric Oxide Alleviates Salt Stress Inhibited Photosynthetic Performance by Interacting with Sulfur Assimilation in Mustard. *Front. Plant Sci.* **2016,** *7,* 521. doi: 10.3389/fpls.2016.00521.

Forni, C.; Duca, D.; Glick, B. R. Mechanisms of Plant Response to Salt and Drought Stress and Their Alteration by Rhizobacteria. *Plant Soil.* **2017,** *410,* 335–356.

Galvan, A. C. S.; Julkowska, M. M.; Darwish, E.; Gandullo, J.; Korver, R. A. Brunoud, G.; Haring, M. A.; Munnik, T.; Vernoux, T.; Testerink, C. Halotropism is a Response of Plant Roots to Avoid a Saline Environment. *Curr. Biol.* **2013,** *23,* 2044–2050.

Gamalero, E.; Berta, G.; Massa, N.; Glick, B. R.; Lingua, G. Interactions Between *Pseudomonas putida* UW4 and *Gigaspora rosea* BEG9 and Their Consequences on the Growth of Cucumber Under Salt Stress Conditions. *J. Appl. Microbiol.* **2010,** *108,* 236–245.

Geng, Y.; Wui, R.; Wei Wee, C.; Xie, F.; Wei, X.; Yeen Chan, P. M.; Than, C., Duan, L.; Dinneny, J. R. A Spatio-temporal Understanding of Growth Regulation During Salt Stress Response in *Arabidopsis*. *Plant Cell.* **2013,** *25,* 2132–2154.

Ghanem, M. E.; Albacete, A.; Smigocki, A. C.; Frébort, I.; Pospisilova, H.; Martinez, A. C.; Acosta, M.; Sánchez, B. J.; Dodd, I. C.; Pérez, A. F. Root-Synthesized Cytokinins Improve Shoot Growth and Fruit Yield in Salinized Tomato (*Solanum lycopersicum* L.) Plants. *J. Exp. Bot.* **2011,** *62,* 125–140.

Gill, S. S., Tuteja N. Polyamines and Abiotic Stress Tolerance in Plants. *Plant Signal. Behav.* **2010,** *5,* 26–33.

Giri J. Glycinebetaine and Abiotic Stress Tolerance in Plants. *Plant Signal. Behav.* **2011,** *6,* 1746–1751.

Glick, B. R. Plant Growth-promoting Bacteria: Mechanisms and Applications. *Scientifica* (Article ID 963401), **2012.** http://dx.doi.org/10.6064/2012/963401.

Glick, B. R.; Cheng, Z.; Czarny, J., Duan, J. Promotion of Plant Growth by ACC Deaminase-containing Soil Bacteria. *Eur. J. Plant Pathol.* **2007,** *26,* 329–339.

Golldack, D.; Lüking, I.; Yang, O. Plant Tolerance to Drought and Salinity: Stress Regulating Transcription Factors and Their Functional Significance in the Cellular Transcriptional Network. *Plant Cell Rep.* 2011, *30* (8), 1383–1391.

Golldack, D.; Li, C.; Mohan, H.; Probst, N. Tolerance to Drought and Salt Stress in Plants: Unraveling the Signaling Networks. *Front. Plant Sci.* **2014,** 5, 1–10.

Hayat, Q., Hayat, S.; Irfan, M.; Ahmad, A. Effect of Exogenous Salicylic Acid Under Changing Environment: A Review. *Environ. Exp. Bot.* **2010,** *68* (1) 14–25.

Hua, W.; Li, R. J.; Zhan, G. M.; Liu, J.; Li, J.; Wang, X. F.; Liu, G. H.; Wang, H. Z. Maternal Control of Seed Oil Content in *Brassica napus*: The Role of Silique Wall Photosynthesis. *Plant J.* **2012,** *69,* 432–444.

Huang, G. T.; Ma, S. L.; Bai, L. P.; Zhang, L.; Ma, H.; Jia, P.; Liu, J.; Zhong, M.; Guo, Z.-F. Signal Transduction During Cold, Salt, and Drought Stresses in Plants. *Molec. Biol. Rep.* **2012,** *39,* 969–987.

Ishitani, M.; Liu, J.; Halfter, U.; Kim, C. S.; Shi, W.; Zhu, J. K. SOS3 Function in Plant Salt Tolerance Requires N-myristoylation and Calcium Binding. *Plant Cell* **2000,** *12,* 1667–1678.

IUSS Working Group WRB, 2007. World Reference Base for Soil Resources 2006, First Update. 2007. World Soil Resources Reports No. 103. FAO, Rome.

Jamil, A.; Riaz S.; Ashraf, M.; Foolad, M. R. Gene Expression Profiling of Plants Under Salt Stress. *Crit. Rev. Plant Sci.* **2011,** *30,* 435–458.

Javid, M. G.; Sorooshzadeh, A.; Moradi, F., Modarres, S. S. A. M.; Allahdadi, I. The Role of Phytohormones in Alleviating Salt Stress in Crop Plants. *Austral. J. Crop Sci.* **2011,** *5,* 726–734.

Jeong, D. H.; Green, P. J. The Role of Rice microRNAs in Abiotic Stress Responses. *Plant Biol.* **2013,** *56,* 187–197.

Ji, H.; Pardo, J. M.; Batelli, G.; Van Oosten, M. J.; Bressane, R. A.; Li, X. The Salt Overly Sensitive (SOS) Pathway: Established and Emerging Roles. *Mol. Plant* **2013,** *6,* 275–286.

Jia, H.; Shao, M.; He, Y.; Guan, R.; Chu, P.; Jiang, H. Proteome Dynamics and Physiological Responses to Short-term Salt Stress in *Brassica napus* Leaves. *PLoS One* **2015,** *10* (12), e0144808. doi: 10.1371/journal.pone.0144808.

Katsuhara, M. Apoptosis-like Cell Death in Barley Roots Under Salt Stress. *Plant Cell Physiol.* **1997,** *38,* 1091–1093.

Knight, H.; Trewavas, A. J.; Knight, M. R. Calcium Signalling in *Arabidopsis* Thaliana to Drought and Salinity. *Plant J.* **1997,** *12,* 1067–1078.

Kopsell, D. A.; Mc Elroy, J. S.; Sams, C. E.; Kopsell, D. E. Genetic Variation in Carotenoids Concentrations Among Diploid and Amphidiploid Rapid-cycling *Brassica* species. *Hortscience* **2007,** *42,* 461–465.

Kreps, J. A.; Wu, Y.; Chang, H. S.; Zhu, T.; Wang X.; Harper, J. F. H. Transcriptome Changes for *Arabidopsis* in Response to Salt, Osmotic, and Cold Stress. *Plant Physiol.* **2002,** *130,* 2129–2141.

Kroemer, G.; Mariño, G.; Levine, B. Autophagy and the Integrated Stress Response. *Mol. Cell* **2010,** *40,* 280–293.

Kumar, G.; Purty R. S.; Sharma, M. P.; Singla, P. S. L.; Pareek A. Physiological Responses Among *Brassica* species under salinity stress show strong Correlation with Transcript Abundance for SOS Pathway-related Genes. *J. Plant Physiol.* **2009,** *166,* 507–520.

Kumar, M.; Choi, J. Y.; Kumari, N.; Pareek, A.; Kim, S. R. Molecular Breeding in *Brassica* for Salt Tolerance: Importance of Microsatellite (SSR) Markers for Molecular Breeding in *Brassica. Front. Plant Sci.* **2015,** *6,* 668. doi: 10.3389/fpls.2015.00688.

Lakhdar A.; Rabhi M.; Ghnaya T.; Montemurro F.; Jedidi N.; Abdelly C. Effectiveness of Compost Use in Salt-affected Soil. *J. Hazard. Mat.* **2009,** *171,* 29–37.

Lang, L.; Xu, A.; Ding, J.; Zhang, Y.; Zhao, N.; Tian, Z.; Liu, Y.; Wang, Y.; Liu, X.; Liang, F.; Zhang, B.; Qin, M.; Dalelhan, J.; Huang, Z. Quantitative Trait Locus Mapping of Salt Tolerance and Identification of Salt-tolerant Genes in *Brassica napus L. Front. Plant Sci.* **2017,** *8,* 1000. doi: 10.3389/fpls.2017.01000.

Lau, S.; Jürgens, G.; De Smet, I. The Evolving Complexity of the Auxin Pathway. *Plant Cell* **2008,** *20,* 1738–1746.

Li, C.; Ng, CK.-Y.; Fan, L.-M. MYB Transcription Factors, Active Players in Abiotic Stress Signaling. *Environ. Exper. Bot.* **2015,** *114,* 80–91.

Liu, W.; Li R. J.; Han, T. T.; Cai, W.; Fu, Z. W.; Lu, Y. T. Salt Stress Reduces Root Meristem Size by Nitric Oxide-mediated Modulation of Auxin Accumulation and Signaling in *Arabidopsis. Plant Physiol.* **2015,** *168,* 343–356.

Long, W.; Zou, X.; Zhang, X. Transcriptome Analysis of Canola (*Brassica napus*) Under Salt Stress at the Germination Stage. *PLoS One* **2015,** *10* (2), e0116217. https://doi.org/10.1371/journal.pone.0116217.

Luo, J.; Tang, S.; Peng, X.; Yan, X.; Zeng, X.; Li, J.; Li, X.; Wu, G. Elucidation of Cross-talk and Specificity of Early Response Mechanisms to Salt and PEG Simulated Drought Stresses in *Brassica napus* Using Comparative Proteomic Analysis. *PLoS One* **2015,** *10* (10), e0138974. doi: 10.1371/journal.pone.0138974.

Mahajan, S.; Tuteja, N. Cold, Salinity and Drought Stresses: An Overview. *Arch. Biochem. Biophys.* **2005,** *444,* 139–158.

Mayak, S., Tirosh, T., Glick, B. R. Plant Growth-promoting Bacteria that Confer Resistance in Tomato to Salt Stress. *Plant Physiol. Biochem.* **2004,** *42* (6), 565–572.

Miller, G.; Suzuki, N.; Ciftci Yilmaz, S.; Mittler, R. Reactive Oxygen Species Homeostasis and Signaling During Drought and Salinity Stresses. *Plant Cell Environ.* **2010,** *33,* 453–467.

Moons, A.; Prinsen, E.; Bauw, G.; Montagu, M. V. Antagonistic Effects of Abscisic Acid and Jasmonates on Salt Stress Inducible Transcripts in Rice Roots. *Plant Cell* **1997,** *9,* 2243–2259.

Mourato, M. P.; Moreira, I. N.; Leitão, I.; Pinto, F. R.; Sales, J. R.; Martins, L. L. Effects of Heavy Metals in Plants of the Genus Brassica. *Int. J. Molec. Sci.* **2015,** *16,* 17975–17998.

Munns, R. Comparative Physiology of Salt and Water Stress. Plant Cell Environ. **2002,** 25, 239–250.

Munns, R. Genes and Salt Tolerance: Bringing them Together. *New Phytol.* **2005,** *167,* 645–663.

Munns, R.; Tester, M. Mechanisms of Salinity Tolerance. *Ann. Rev. Plant Biol.* **2008,** *59,* 651–681.

Nakashima, K.; Ito, Y.; Yamaguchi, S. K. Transcriptional Regulatory Networks in Response to Abiotic Stresses in *Arabidopsis* and Grasses. *Plant Physiol.* **2009,** *149,* 88–95.

Nawaz, K.; Ashraf, M. Exogenous Application of Glycine Betaine Modulates Activities of Antioxidants in Maize Plants Subjected to Salt Stress. *J. Agron. Crop Sci.* **2010,** *196,* 28–37.

Nishiyama, R.; Watanabe, Y.; Fujita, Y.; Le, D. T.; Kojima, M.; Werner, T.; Vankova, R.; Yamaguchi-Shinozaki, K.; Shinozaki, K.; Kakimoto, T. Analysis of Cytokinin Mutants and Regulation of Cytokinin Metabolic Genes Reveals Important Regulatory Roles of cytokinins in Drought, Salt and Abscisic Acid Responses, and Abscisic Acid Biosynthesis. *Plant Cell.* **2011,** *23* (6), 2169–2183.

Nishiyama, R.; Le, D. T.; Watanabe, Y.; Matsui, A.; Tanaka, M.; Seki, M.; Yamaguchi, S. K.; Shinozaki, K.; Tran, L. S. Transcriptome Analyses of a Salt-tolerant Cytokinin-deficient Mutant Reveal Differential Regulation of Salt Stress Response by Cytokinin Deficiency. *PLoS One* **2017,** *7* (2), e32124. doi:10.1371/journal.pone.0032124.

Noctor, G.; Foyer, C. H. Ascorbate and Glutathione: Keeping Active Oxygen Under Control. *Ann. Rev. Plant Physiol. Plant Mol. Biol.* **1998,** *49,* 249–279.

Nuruzzaman, M.; Sharoni, A. M.; Kikuchi, S. Roles of NAC Transcription Factors in the Regulation of Biotic and Abiotic Stress Responses in Plants. *Front. Microbiol.* **2013,** *4,* 248. doi: 10.3389/fmicb.2013.00248.

Pagliaro, B.; Santolamazza, C.; Simonelli, F.; Rubattu, S. Phytochemical Compounds and Protection from Cardiovascular Diseases: A State of the Art. *BioMed Res. Int.* **2015,** *918069.* doi: 10.1155/2015/918069.

Pandey, N., Ranjan, A., Pant, P., Tripathi, R. V., Ateek, F., Pandey, H. P., Patre, U. V.; Sawant S. V. CAMTA 1 Regulates Drought Responses in *Arabidopsis thaliana*. *BMC Genomics* **2013,** *14,* 216.

Pandolfi, C.; Pottosin, I.; Cuin, T.; Mancuso, S., Shabala, S. Specificity of Polyamine Effects on NaCl-induced ion Flux Kinetics and Salt Stress Amelioration in Plants. *Plant Cell Physiol.* **2010,** *51,* 422–434.

Pandolfi, C.; Azzarello, E.; Mancuso, S.; Shabala, S. Acclimation Improves Salt Stress Tolerance in *Zea mays* Plants. *J. Plant Physiol.* **2016,** *201,* 1–8.

Parida, A. K.; Das, A. B. Salt Tolerance and Salinity Effects on Plants: A Review. *Ecotoxicol. Environ. Saf.* 2005, *60,* 324–349.

Peleg, Z.; Blumwald, E. Hormone Balance and Abiotic Stress Tolerance in Crop Plants. *Curr. Opinion Plant Biol.* **2011,** *14,* 1–6.

Purty, R. S.; Kumar, G.; Singla, P. S. L.; Pareek, A. Towards Salinity Tolerance in *Brassica*: An Overview. *Physiol. Mol. Biol. Plants* **2008,** 14, 39–49.

Qiu, Z.; Guo, J.; Zhu, A.; Zhang, L.; Zhang, M. Exogenous Jasmonic Acid can Enhance Tolerance of Wheat Seedlings to Salt Stress. *Ecotoxicol. Environ. Saf.* **2014,** *104,* 202–208.

Rakow, G. Species Origin and Economic Importance of *Brassica*. In *Brassica*; Pua, E.-C., Douglas, C., Eds.; Springer: Berlin,Heidelberg, Germany, 2004; Vol. 64, pp 3–11.

Redillas, M. C. F. R.; Park, S. H.; Lee, J. W.; Kim, Y. S.; Jeong, J. S.; Jung, H.; Bang S. W.; Hahn T. R.; Kim J. K. Accumulation of Trehalose Increases Soluble Sugar Contents in Rice Plants Conferring Tolerance to Drought and Salt Stress. *Plant Biotechnol. Rep.* **2012,** *6,* 89–96.

Ruan, C. J.; da Silva, J. A. T.; Mopper, S.; Qin, P.; Lutts, S. Halophyte Improvement for a Salinized World. *Crit. Rev. Plant Sci.* **2010,** *29,* 329–359.

Ryu, H.; Cho, Y. G. Plant Hormones in Salt Stress Tolerance. *J. Plant Biol.* **2015,** *58,* 147–155.

Sakuraba, Y.; Kim, Y. S.; Han, S. H.; Lee, B. D.; Paek N. C. The *Arabidopsis* Transcription Factor NAC016 Promotes Drought Stress Responses by Repressing AREB1 Transcription Through a Trifurcate Feed-forward Regulatory Loop Involving NAP. *Plant Cell* **2015,** *27,* 1771–1787.

Sanchez, D. H.; Lippold, F.; Redesting, H.; Hannah, M. A.; Erban, A.; Krämer, U.; Kopka, J.; Udvardi, M. K. Integrative Functional Genomics of Salt Acclimatization in the Model Legume *Lotus japonicus*. *Plant J.* **2008,** *53,* 973–987.

Schroeder, J. I.; Delhaize, E.; Frommer, W. B.; Guerinot, M. L.; Harrison, M. J.; Herrera E. L.; Horie T.; Kochian L. V.; Munns R.; Nishizawa N. K.; Tsay Y. F.; Sanders D. Using Membrane Transporters to Improve Crops for Sustainable Food Production. *Nature* **2013,** *497,* 60–66.

Seki, M.; Narusaka M.; Ishida, J.; Nanjo, T.; Fujita, M.; Oono, Y.; Kamiya, A.; Nakajima, M.; Enju, A.; Sakurai, T.; Satou, M.; Akiyama, K.; Taji, T.; Yamaguchi, S. K.; Carninci, P.; Kawai, J.; Hayashizaki, Y.; Shinozaki, K. Monitoring the Expression Profiles of 7000 *Arabidopsis* Genes Under Drought, Cold and High-salinity Stresses Using a Full-length cDNA Microarray. *Plant J.* **2002,** *31,* 279–292.

Sergeeva, E.; Shah, S.; Glick, B. R. Growth of Transgenic Canola (*Brassica napus* cv. Westar) Expressing a Bacterial 1-aminocyclopropane-1-carboxylate (ACC) Deaminase Gene on High Concentrations of Salt. *World J. Microbiol. Biotechnol.* **2006,** *22,* 277–282.

Shavrukov, Y.; Genc, Y.; Hayes, J. The Use of Hydroponics in Abiotic Stress Tolerance Research. In *Hydroponics - A Standard Methodology for Plant Biological Researches*; Asao, T., ed.; InTech, 2012; pp 39–66.

Shavrukov, Y. Salt Stress or Salt Shock: Which Genes are we Studying? *J. Exp. Bot.* **2013,** *64*, 119–127.

Shinozaki, K.; Yamaguchi, S. K. Gene Expression and Signal Transduction in Water-stress Response. *Plant Physiol.* **1997,** *115*, 327–334.

Skirycz, A.; De Bodt, S.; Obata, T.; De Clerq, I.; Clayes, H.; De Rycke, R.; Andriankaya, M.; Van Aken, O.; Van Breusegem, F.; Fernie, A. R.; Inzé, D. Developmental Stage Specifity and the Role of Mitochondrial Metabolism in the Response of *Arabidopsis* Leaves to Prolonged Mild Osmotic Stress. *Plant Physiol.* **2010,** *152*, 226–244.

Skirycz, A.; Clayes, H.; De Bodt, S.; Oikawa, A.; Shinoda, S.; Andriankaja, M.; Maleux, K.; Barbosa Eloy, N.; Coppens, F.; Yoo, S. D.; Saito, K.; Inzé, D. Pause-and-stop: The Effects of Osmotic Stress On Cell Proliferation During Early Leaf Development in Arabidopsis and a Role for Ethylene Signalling in Cell Cycle Arrest. *Plant Cell* **2011,** *23*, 1876–1888.

Slavikova, S.; Ufaz, S.; Avin, W. T.; Levanony, H.; Galili, G. An Autophagy-associated Atg8 Protein is Involved in the Responses of *Arabidopsis* Seedlings to Hormonal Controls and Abiotic Stresses. *J. Exp. Bot.* **2008,** *59*, 4029–4043.

Su, J.; Wu, R. Stress Inducible Synthesis of Proline in transgenic Rice Confers Faster Growth Under Stress Conditions Tan that with Constitutive Synthesis. *Plant Sci.* **2004,** *166*, 941–948.

Szczyglowska, M.; Piekarska, A.; Konieczka, P.; Namieśnik, J. Use of Brassica Plants in the Phytoremediation and Biofumigation Processes. *Int J. Mol. Sci.* **2011,** *12*, 7760–7771.

Takahashi, S.; Seki, M.; Ishida, J.; Satou, M.; Sakurai, T.; Narusaka, M.; Kamiya, A.; Nakajima, M.; Enju A.; Akiyama, K. Monitoring the Expression Profiles of Genes Induced by hyperosmotic, High Salinity, and Oxidative Stress and Abscisic Acid Treatment in *Arabidopsis* Cell Culture Using a Full-length cDNA Microarray. *Plant Mol. Biol.* **2004,** *56*, 29–55.

Tavakkoli, E.; Rengasamy, P.; Mcdonald, G. K. The Response of Barley to Salinity Stress Differs Between Hydroponics and Soil Systems. *Functional Plant Biol.* **2010,** *37*, 621–633.

Tester, M.; Davenport R. Na+ Tolerance and Na+ Transport in Higher Plants. *Ann. Bot.* **2003,** *91*, 503–527.

Tran, L. S.; Shinozaki, K.; Yamaguchi, S. K. Role of Cytokinin Responsive Two-component System in ABA and Osmotic Stress Signaling. *Plant Signal. Behav.* **2010,** *5*, 148–150.

Tsuchisaka, A.; Theologis, A. Unnique and Overlapping Expression Patterns Among the Arabidopsis 1-amino-cyclopropane-1-carboxylate Synthase Gene Family Members. *Plant Physiol.* **2004,** *136*, 2983–3000.

Türkan, I.; Demiral, T. Recent Development in Understanding Salinity Tolerance. *Environ. Exp. Bot* **2009,** *67*, 2–9.

Tuteja, N. Mechanisms of High Salt Tolerance in Plants. *Methods Enzymol.* **2007,** *428*, 419–438.

Tuteja, N.; Banu, S. A.; Huda, K. M. K.; Gill, S. S.; Jain, P.; Pham, X. H.; Tuteja, R. A pea p68, a DEAD-box Helicase, Provides Salinity Stress Tolerance in Transgenic Tobacco by Reducing Oxidative Stress and Improving Photosynthesis Machinery. *PLoS One* **2014,** *9* (5), e98287. doi: 10.1371/journal.pone.0098287.

Tuteja, N.; Tarique, M.; Banu, M. S.; Ahmad, M.; Tuteja, R. *Pisum sativum* p68 DEAD-box Protein is ATP-dependent RNA Helicase and Unique Bipolar DNA Helicase. *Plant Mol. Biol.* **2014,** *85*, 639–651.

Verbruggen, H.; Hermans, C. Proline Accumulation in Plants: A Review. *Amino Acids* **2008**, *35*, 753–759.

Vital, S. A.; Fowler, R. W.; Virgen, A.; Gossett, D. R.; Banks, S. W.; Rodriguez, J. Opposing Roles for Superoxide and Nitric Oxide in the NaCl Stress-induced Upregulation of Antioxidant Enzyme Activity in Cotton Callus Tissue. *Environ. Exp. Bot.* **2008**, *62*, 60–68.

Wan, H.; Chen, L.; Guo, J.; Li, Q.; Wen, J.; Yi, B.; Ma, C.; Tu, J.; Fu, T.; Shen, J. Genome-wide Association Study Reveals the Genetic Architecture Underlying Salt Tolerance-related Traits in Rapeseed (*Brassica napus* L.). *Front. Plant Sci.* **2017**, *8,* 593. doi: 10.3389/fpls.2017.00593.

Wanasundara, J. P. D. Proteins of Brassicaceae Oilseeds and their Potential as a Plant Protein Source. *Crit. Rev. Food Sci. Nutrition.* **2011**, *51*, 635–677.

Wang, C.; Zhang, L. J.; Huang, R. D. Cytoskeleton and Plant Salt Stress Tolerance. *Plant Signal. Behav.* **2011**, *6*, 29–31.

Wang, H.; Wang, H.; Shao, H.; Tang, X. Recent Advances in Utilizing Transcription Factors to Improve Plant Abiotic Stress Tolerance by Transgenic Technology. *Front. Plant Sci.* **2016**, 7, 67.

Weng, H.; Yul, Y. C.; Gosney, M. J.; Hasegawa, P. M.; Mickelbart, M. V. Poplar GTL 1 is a Ca^{2+}/calmoldulin-binding Transcription Factor that Functions in Plant Water Use Efficiency and Drought Tolerance. *PLoS One* 2012, *7* (3), e32925. doi: 10.1371/journal.pone.0032925.

Wilkinson, S.; Davies, W. J. Drought, Ozone, ABA and Ethylene: New Insights from Cell to Plant to Community. *Plant Cell Environ.* **2010**, *33*, 510–525.

Xiong, L.; Zhu, J. K. Molecular and Genetic Aspects of Plant Responses to Osmotic Stress. *Plant Cell Environ.* **2002**, *25*, 131–139.

Yamaguchi, S. K.; Shinozaki, K. Transcriptional Regulatory Networks in Cellular Responses and Tolerance to Dehydration and Cold Stresses. *Ann. Rev. Plant Biol.* **2006**, *57*, 781–803.

Yokoi, S.; Bressan, R. A.; Hasegawa, P. M. Salt Stress Tolerance of Plants. JIRCAS *Work. Rep.* **2002**, *23*, 25–33.

Yong, H. Y.; Wang, C.; Bancroft, I.; Li, F.; Wu, X.; Kitashiba, H., Nishio T. Identification of a Gene Controlling Variation in the Salt Tolerance of Rapeseed (*Brassica napus* L.). *Planta* **2015**, *242*, 313–326.

Yoshida, T.; Mogami, J.; Yamaguchi, S. K. ABA Dependent and ABA-Independent Signaling in Response to Osmotic Stress in Plants. *Curr. Opin. Plant Biol.* **2014**, *21*, 133–139.

Zapata, P. J.; Serrano, M.; Pretel, M. T.; Amoros A.; Botella M. A. Polyamines and Ethylene Changes During Germination of Different Plant Species Under Salinity. *Plant Sci.* **2004**, *167*, 781–788.

Zhang, X.; Lu, G.; Long, W.; Zou, X.; Li, F.; Nishio T. Recent Progress in Drought and Salt Tolerance Studies in *Brassica* crops. *Breed. Sci.* **2014**, *64*, 60–73.

Zhao, Y.; Dong, W.; Zhang, N.; Al X.; Wang, M.; Huang, Z.; Xiao, L.; Xia, G. A Wheat Allene Oxide Cyclase Gene Enhances Salinity Tolerance via Jasmonate Signaling. *Plant Physiol.* **2014**, *164*, 1068–1076.

Zhu, J. K. Plant Salt Tolerance. *Trends Plant Sci.* **2001**, *6*, 66–71.

Zhu, J. K. Salt and Drought Stress Signal Transduction in Plants. *Ann. Rev. Plant Physiol. Plant Mol. Biol.* **2002**, *53*, 247–273.

Zhu, J. K. Plant Salt Stress. *Encyclopedia of Life Science*, Wiley, 2007, pp 1–3.

CHAPTER 14

Biopesticides for Sustainable Crop Protection and Improvement

M. MADHAVI[1*], CH. ARUNA KUMARI[1], V. RAM REDDY[2],
B. LAXMI PRASANNA[2], K. MANOHAR[3], and A. NAVATHA[4]

[1]Department of Plant Pathology, Agricultural College,
Professor Jayashankar Telangana State Agricultural University,
Jagtial 505529, India

[2]Department of Genetics and Plant Breeding, Agricultural College,
Professor Jayashankar Telangana State Agricultural University,
Jagtial 505529, India

[3]Plant Pathologist, College of Agriculture, Rajendranagar,
Hyderabad 500030, India

[4]Agricultural College, Administration Section, Professor Jayashankar
Telangana State Agricultural University, Jagtial 505529, India

*Corresponding author. E-mail: madhagonii@gmail.com

ABSTRACT

The chapter deals about the biopesticides which are natural substances to control different biotic stresses in an ecofriendly manner.

It discusses briefly with the strategies of biological control, impact of synthetic pesticides on environment, different components of integrated pest and disease management, concepts, development, usefulness of biopesticides, different types and success of biopesticides in controlling the economically important pests, and pathogens as an integral component in sustainable agriculture.

14.1 INTRODUCTION

In recent years, and production of agricultural crops are greatly hampered because of many biotic and abiotic factors; besides these the changes in climatic/weather conditions have still worsened the productivity.

The farmers, who are helpless against natural conditions like climatic factors, focus on biotic stress to save the crop for increasing the yield and productivity. As a part of this, disregarding the future ill effects, farmers started using chemical pesticides. From the past decades, over and extensive usage of these synthetic organic chemicals led to a number of adverse long term environmental problems including extinct of natural flora, fauna, and so on. The conventional chemical pesticides though enhanced the food production, have adversely affected the environment and nontarget organisms.

Continuous accumulation of chemical fertilizers and pesticides in the environment is resulting in increase of pollution and harming the ecosystem. Many of the pesticides being used today are remaining within the plants for long duration and these residues are entering food chain, as they are also persistent as residues in soil and ecosystem. Therefore, in the present situation high priority may be given to adopt the usage of biopesticides in an ecofriendly manner for sustainable crop production. Biopesticides are a powerful tool in creating new generation sustainable agricultural products.

They are best alternative against few of the most problematic synthetic pesticides that are currently in use. In nature, several organisms including predators, parasitoids, microbial agents act as natural enemies to various pest infestations. Variety of insects belonging to arthropod taxa namely, ladybird beetles, ground beetles, spiders, and lace wings act as predators and are polyphagous. Parasitoids have specialized life styles that allows them in finding their host and thereby attacking/killing, though the host specific parasites are variable, parasites may attack only one life cycle of a host (egg or larva).

14.2 APPROACHES OF BIOLOGICAL CONTROL

These are the three biological pest control strategies—importation, augmentation, and conservation.

14.2.1 IMPORTATION

Introduction of an exotic or co-evolved biological control agent for permanent and long term control of the pest (Eilenberg et al., 2001). It includes introducing a pest natural enemies into new localities where their presence is lacking. Generally, the government authorities will be practicing this type of approach.

Few splendid importation programs are cited below.

1. The pest cottony cushiony scale *Icerya purchasi*, which devastated citrus industry in California, was totally checked with the instigation of *Rodolia cardinalis*, a predatory insect pest and also by a parasitoid fly that was introduced from Australia in late 19th century.

2. After 20 years of introduction of natural enemies nearly 75% of alfalfa weevil *Hypera postica* population was brought down in Northeastern United States.

3. From China, a wasp *Trichogramma ostrininae* was introduced for the control of *Ostrinia nubilalis* a European corn borer, the most destructive pest of North America. (4) During 1920s under classical bio-control program the population levels of *Levuana iridescens* an important serious coconut pest was controlled.

Important exotic pests of India:

1. Two Parasitodis *(Acerophagus papyae, Pseudleptomastix mexicana)* imported from Puerto Rico USDA and quarantined at NBAH were used for the control of Paracoccus marinates, the mealy bug of papaya that caused serious damage in economically important crops and standing crop of mulberry in Coimbatore.

2. During the year 2009–2010, the parasite *Quadrastichus mendeli* was introduced from Australia and released in Bangalore and nearby areas of Karnataka and Orissa for the control of Eucalyptus gall wasp *Leptocybe invasa* a pest introduced from southeast Asia in 2006 which later became established as a serious pest in South India, Uttar Pradesh, and New Delhi.

3. Parasitoids *Eurytoma erythrinaea* and *Aprostocetus exertus* were introduced during 2008 from South Africa to control Erythrina gall wasp *Qudastichus erythrinae* which produces galls in different plant parts of Erythrina sp (coral tree) in Karnataka and Tamil Nadu. The classical biocontrol approach is mostly effective against exotic insect pests.

The drawback for failure though not thoroughly understood they might be attributed to the poor adaptation of natural enemies to the introduced environmental conditions and locations, lack of appropriate syncing between the life cycle of the pest and natural enemy.

14.2.2   AUGMENTATION

The two perspective of augmentation biological control are namely, (1) Inundation, and (2) Inoculation

1. Inundation biological control: it utilizes living organisms in the control of pests by the introduced organisms itself (Eilenberg et al., 2001). When the pest population crosses the economic injury level, then the bioagents are released in huge amounts for early control of the pest. If, once after release, the population of pest has further increased, after over a period the bioagents will be reintroduced. The timescale is weeks or months as the events are often limited to one cropping season.

    Ex. Predators such as Lacewings, lady bird beetles and parasitoids *Trichogramma* are released more frequently in large number.

2. Inoculation biological control: intentional release of biocontrol agent that multiplies and control the pest in an extended period of time (Eilenberg et al., 2001). The underlying objective is to let the natural enemy to increase their population size and may control the pest in due course of time. Different events of biological control are limited to one cropping period. The greenhouse White fly and the spotted spider mite were controlled with the periodical release of *Encarsia formosa* (parasitoid) and *Phytoseiulus persimilis* (predatory mite).

3. Conservation: conservation refers to enhancing and maintaining of natural enemies that are already present in the landscape. Various methods namely, alteration of the management practices, adoption of strip cropping or polyculture, provision of hosts to get predators through times of lack of food, provision of nonhost foods like sugar, nectar sources as crucial sources for attracting and retaining most of the parasites and predators, and so on.

Examples of successful biological control agents of India are briefly mentioned below:

1. Control of cottony cushion scale, *Icerya purchasi* on fruit trees by its predatory vedalia beetle *Rodalia cardinalis* in Nilgiris which was

imported from California (1929) and from Egypt (1930). The predatory was multiplied under in vitro and when released had effectively
checked the pest within one year period.

2. During 1983–84, the water fern *Salvinia molesta* in Bangalore
was biologically suppressed by the weevil *Cyrtobagous salviniae*
imported from Australia (1982).

3. For control of Water hyacinth (*Eicchornia crassipes*) three exotic natural
enemies namely, *Neochetina eichhorniae* and *N. bruchi* and *Orthoga-
lumna terebrantis* were introduced from South America in 1982.

4. The apple wooly aphis, *Eriosoma lanigerum* was controlled in
Coonor area with the introduction of parasitoid *Aphelinus mali*. The
egg parasitoid v. *Trichogramma australicum* @ 50,000/ha/wk was
released for 4–5 weeks from one month after planting for the control
of shoot borers of sugar cane, cotton boll worms, stem borers of
paddy, and sorghum.

5. *Cryptolaemus montrouzieri* was effective in suppression of *Centro-
coccus isolitus* on brinjal, *Pulvinaria hirsutus* on grape, and *Pseudo-
coccus carymbatus* on citrus.

14.3   BIOPESTICIDES HISTORY

The earliest agricultural biopesticides were the plant extracts wherein, the
history says the natural insecticides rotenone (roots of derris plant), pyre-
thrum (flower heads of chrysanthemum) and nicotine (leaves of tobacco)
were used before 1940s to control various pests and diseases. Later, during
1940s use of synthetic chemicals was started for pest control.

In 18th and the beginning of 19th centuries, the theme of biological control
was to use birds and entomophagous insects; where microbes were properly
not known during that time. The wider aspects of microbe-based biological
control were known with discovery of *Bacillus thuringiensis* (Bt) bacteria
(Aronson et al., 1986; Martin and Traverse, 1989; Siegel and Shadduck, 1990;
Marrone, 1994; Joung and Cote, 2000).

The Japanese biologist, Shigetane Ishiwata isolated Bt from diseased
silk worm. The bacteria *B. thuringiensis* (Spores) was the first widely used
biopesticide developed during 19th century. Later, Ernst Berliner, a German
biologist rediscovered it from diseased caterpillar of flour moth. In 1911,
Bt is classified as type species, that is, *B. thuringiensis*. The main concept
of microbial pest control, its selective action on specific pest attracted the
attention of many researchers.

In France, early in 1920s Bt was used as biological insecticide and have developed Sporeine, the first commercial Bt product, in 1938. In the United States, extensive usage of biopesticides began in the 1950s and also, they have even published the research studies on Bt efficacy and soon registered Thuricide the first commercial Bt product in 1961 (USEPA, 1998). Since then, different subspecies, varieties, strains of Bt were identified that are effective against various insect pests (Gonzales et al., 1982; Carlton, 1988). Thereafter, Bt has covered nearly 90% of biopesticide market (Chapple et al., 2000; Chattopadhyay et al., 2004; Romeis et al., 2006), and at present several Bt strains have registered as biopesticides globally (Glare and O Callaghan, 200). During 19th century usage of mineral oils have started as plant protectants among the biological control experiments and by 20th century, soil microbiology and ecological studies had led in identifying different soil microbes which are antagonist to pathogens and insects pests, by different mechanisms (antagonism or hyper parasitism or antibiosis or competition etc).

Even though most of them have proven under field conditions, only few of them were commercially developed which could sustain the situation at that point of time against usage of synthetic pesticides.

During mid of 20th century, there was a predominant adoption of toxic chemical insecticides in different crop ecosystems because of which the research and developmental activities of biological control were come down. However, during this period the utilization of new products developed were restricted to niche markets only where the synthetic chemicals were not economical. As a first viral insecticide, Heliothis NPV has received Elcar label in the year 1975.

The biocontrol pathogen, *B. thuringiensis* var. *israelensis* discovered in 1977 was toxic against flies and the strain *tenebrionis* against beetles in 1983. During 1979, U.S. EPA registered first insect pheromone to mass trap Japanese beetles. In early 1990s, research studies were started on kaolin clay as an insect repellent in organic fruit orchards and made available in commercial form in organic systems. Similar transformation was seen in Biopesticides development and their usage for the control and management of plant diseases.

During 1980 and 1990, success stories on commercial basis was seen from the products containing *Agrobacterium radiobacter* against crown gall of woody crops, *Pseudomonas fluorescens* against fire blight in orchard crops wherein the over usage of streptomycin had resulted in development of resistant pathogen populations. In greenhouses and pot mixing industries, products with variety of microbes with suppressive nature against soil borne pathogens were introduced into the market. Increased cost on over usage of chemical pesticides has led in resurgence of academic and industrial research for biopesticides development.

The organic agriculture had rapidly expanded from the past decade, thus there was a prompt increase in adoption rates and paved a way for the increase in development of new biopesticides during mid-1990s. Under U.S. EPA Biopesticides division, nearly 100 biopesticides active ingredients were registered and available commercially in different products.

The pioneer workers all the world who has worked on biopesticides has stated that the antagonistic microbes can be used as an alternative to synthetic chemical pesticides in the control of crop pests (Le Conte, 1874; McCoy et al., 1988). Later, these pioneer Works and further researches had become breakthrough for the development of microbe-based pesticides (Sundheim and Tronsmo, 1988). The pioneer workers who have worked on biopesticides had stated use of antagonistic microbes is a best alternative against synthetic pesticides for the control of insect pest. Boverin, (*Beauveria bassiana*) the first fungal product developed in 1965 from former Union of Soviet Socialist Republics (USSR) for control of Colorado potato beetle and also the codling moth (De Faria and Wright, 2007). Heliothis nuclear polyhedrosis virus (NPV) is the first viral biopesticide declared in 1973 (Szewczyk et al., 2011).

14.4 ENVIRONMENTAL IMPACT OF CHEMICAL PESTICIDES

The usage of chemical pesticides increased several folds since 1940s for control of different insect pests and diseases.

Several environmental issues have aroused in recent past regarding the usage of these pesticides with due concern of the public health particularly the children. Many of the pesticides which are under usage for controlling the pests are highly toxic pesticides that can harm not only the humans but even environment. Increased environmental concern as they are nonbiodegradable, attention is directed toward the use of certain natural chemicals which are both effective and ecofriendly. Importance was felt to incorporate these as key elements in the insect management programs to minimize harmful effect on environment.

Several incidences are stating the poisonous effect of DDT as quoted by Hill and Robison (1945), Tschirley (1973), Longnecker et al. (1997), Conis et al. (2010), and Qiu (2013). The farmworkers, people residing near to agricultural areas, small children, and so on, are the victims of hazardous effects of organophosphates (Landrigan et al., 1999; Eskenazi et al., 1999; Fenske et al., 2000; McCauley et al., 2001; Quandt et al., 2004; Eskenazi et al., 2008). Acute toxicity of organophosphates and carbamates is a severe problem in under developed countries, ignorance about their hazards and lack of information has led to many deaths among agricultural workers (Konradsen et al., 2003).

Intensified usage of synthetic pesticides in agriculture had changed ecological conditions that had affected soil fauna (Edwards and Thompson, 1973; Tripathi and Sharma, 2005; Frampton et al., 2006; Bezchlebov et al., 2007). The population of beneficial insects (bees, wasps, and other) involved in pollination had been drastically reduced due to the increased application of pesticides in most of the agriculturally important crops (Gill et al., 2012).

On high pesticide exposure, there is a decline in frog population (Bruhl et al., 2013) Even several species of birds have wiped out or are on the verge of it because of pesticides. The synthetic pesticides have showed devastating effects on ecosystems, due to lack of alternative and it was impossible to diminish their utility and effects (Wu and Chen, 2004; Aktar et al., 2009).

14.5   FACTORS FOR THE EMERGENCE OF BIOPESTICIDE MARKET

Increased conscious on environment safety, hike in price of chemical insecticides and increased resistance of insects to these products, to decrease the toxic residual effects of synthetic chemicals in foodstuffs, especially in export markets there aroused a need to their emergence. At an impressive rate of 20%, the consumption of biopesticides is growing globally.

At present the biopesticides cover 2% in the world pesticide market and its share is going to increase tremendously in coming years.

Majority of the consumers have become more health conscious and prefer for organic food. Following are the reasons for which the usage of biopesticides are likely to increase at higher rate: increase in demand for organic food, increasing in number of insects developing resistance to existing chemicals, and increase in cost of developing new chemical pesticides.

14.6   FUNDAMENTAL COMPONENTS OF IPM

Sustainable agriculture mainly focus on protecting the environment, public health in addition to animal welfare. It integrates the economic profitability and social equity to cater the needs of future generations. In recent past, most of the growers are working to create sustainable agriculture system as their forefront toward the beneficial organisms.

Generally, an IPM program combines cultural practices, biological controls (i.e., predatory insects, micro-organisms) and chemical control to keep pest populations low and therefore it became a key factor of sustainable agriculture. However, under severe conditions, chemical control may be opted. Most of the biopesticides are environmentally friendly, target specific, enhance the crop growth and also confer resistance to different pests and diseases.

They sustainably balance and maintain the microbial environment and habitat. Thus, they can be integrated as one of the component in IPM program and as such in sustainable agriculture system. There is an urgent requirement for alternative tactics to help make crop protection more sustainable.

14.7   BIOPESTICIDES CONCEPT

The inconsistency raised at global level in understanding the term biopesticide given by USEPA, the International Biocontrol Manufactures Association (IBMA) and the International for Biological Control (IOBC, 2008) had promoted to use the term biocontrol agents (BCAs) to biopesticide (Guillon, 2003).

According to IBMA, the BCAs are classified into four groups: (1) macrobials, (2) micorbials, (3) natural products, and (4) semiochemicals. Many of the agricultural crops and other vegetation are susceptible to insect pest and disease infestations. These naturally occurring chemicals or materials are effective and ecofriendly were designated as biopesticides. In other words they are the management tools with beneficial microbial origin, fungi, nematodes, viruses, protozoa, the biologically based active ingredients. The characteristics of commercial ideal biopesticide (Andy Cherry, 2005) are as follows:

a)   It should possess high efficacy.
b)   It should be fast acting with consistent results.
c)   It should exhibit specificity against broad spectrum of pests.
d)   Manufacturable at low cost.
e)   It should possess a shelf life of at least one year.
f)   Should be simple to use.
g)   The biopesticide should be environmentally friendly and provide beneficial profits to grower.

Biopesticides are used successfully for managing the pesticide resistance, used with other products either alone or in mixtures, at early crop growth stage under low pest pressure, late in the season with short preharvest intervals, at critical field events (multiple harvests), and to manage pesticide residue.

The benefits of biopesticides are as follows:

a) Inherently biopesticides are less toxic than conventional synthetic pesticides,
b) Target specific (pest),
c) Requires in small amounts,
d) Quick decomposition and Pollution free,
e) Greatly reduces the usage of chemical pesticides with increased crop yields,
f) Used effectively and safely,
g) They are environment safe,
h) Act as an important pest management tool (pest resistance, environmental concern) limits the use of chemical pesticides, and
i) Resistance development toward these pesticides is difficult.

14.8 DEVELOPMENT OF BIOPESTICIDES

The biopesticides development on commercial basis depends on different fields namely, application technology, operational execution, microbiology, manufacturing and packaging technology, fermentation technology, formulation technology, regulatory, and also the quality control (Andy, 2005).

Biopesticides developed in Africa under public research sector (Andy, 2005):

1. Beauveria and Metarhizium are developed against insect pests namely, Banana weevil (*Cosmopolites sordidus*), Larger grain borer *(Prostephanus truncates)*, Locusts and grasshoppers, Termites (Macrotermes spp. and Odontotermes spp), Coffee berry borer (*Hypothanemus truncates*), Cowpea beetle *(Callosobruchus maculatus)*, Chilo, and Sesamia (stem borers).
2. Viruses: (a). Nucleopolyhedroviruses against cotton bollworm *(Helicoverpa armigera)*, Armyworm *(Spodoptear exempta)*, (b) Granuloviruses developed against Diamondback moth *(Plutella xylostella)*, potato tuber moth *(Phthorimoea opercula)*, (c) Cypoviruese- developed

against Cowpea pod borer *(Maruca testularies)* and Pink borer *(Sesamia xylostella).*

14.9 BROADLY USED BIOPESTICIDES

The strains of bacterium *Bacillus thuringiensis* are the most widely used microbial pesticides which control pests of cabbage and other solanaceous crops. The biofungicides are the microbial biopesticides such as *Trichoderma* spp., *Bacillus subtilis, Pseudomonas fluorescens*, biohericides-*Phytohthora* spp., and bioinsecticides (Bt), and so on, are effective against specific pathogens and insect pests (Gupta and Bikshit, 2010).

14.9.1 UTILITY OF BIOPESTICIDES

From the total biopesticide market inclusive of all types biopesticide products share for, bacterial biopesticides (74%); fungal biopesticides (10%); viral biopesticides (5%); predator biopesticides (8%); predator biopesticides (8%); and others (3%) (Thakore, 2006). By 2008, there were approximately 73 microbial active ingredients that were registered by USEPA which include 35 bacterial products, 15 fungi, 6 nonviable (genetically engineered) microbial pesticides, 8 plant incorporated protectants, 6 viruses and one each for protozoan and yeast (Steinwand, 2008).

14.9.2 MICROBIAL PESTICIDES

14.9.2.1 MODE OF ACTION

Different biopesticides have their distinctive mode of action. They suppress the pests either by synthesizing the toxic metabolites against their target pest or prevent the establishment of pathogens through mechanisms like competition hyperarasitism antibiosis, and so on (Clemson, 2007).

14.9.2.2 MONITORING OF MICROBIAL PESTICIDES

Continuous monitoring of the microbial pesticides is essential for ensuring their ineffectiveness against the nontarget organisms, including humans.

14.10   BIOPESTICIDES SCENARIO IN INDIAN AGRICULTURE

Biopesticides and bio-control agents are used successfully in Indian agriculture (Kalra and Khanuja, 2007). The biocontrol agent *Bacillus thuringiensis* effectively controls diamondback moths (cabbage), Heliothis in cotton, pigeon pea and many of solanacous crops; *Beauveria* against mango hoppers, coffee pod borer and mealy bugs; Products of neem are effective on cotton White fly; NPV against *Helicoverpa* in gram; Trichogramma controls sugarcane borers; while *Trichoderma*-based products against soil borne diseases in different crops.

Biopesticides registered under Insecticide Act of 1968 in India (Gupta and Dikshit, 2010) are as follows:

(1) Bacterial biopesticides—*B. thuringiensis* var. *israelensis, B. rgyeubfuwbaua* var. *galleriae, B. sphaericus, P. fluoresens,* (2) Entomopathogenic fungi—*Beauveria bassiana,* (3) Virus based biopesticides—NPV of *H. armigera,* NPV of *S. litura,* and (4) Botanical biopesticides—Neem based pesticide, Cymbopogan.

14.11   BIOPESTICIDES TYPES

Biopesticides are categorized into three major groups (Kalra and Khanuja, 2007), depending on the nature of active ingredient present. These include:

14.11.1   MICROBIAL PESTICIDES

The pesticides which contain microorganisms namely, bacterium, fungus, virus, or protozoan as active ingredient (a.i) which is specific to its target insect pest (s) and controls different types of pests.

Certain microbial pesticides (fungi) can act against some of the weed species to control and even specific insects. The strains of *B. thuringiensis,* are most widely used for the control of certain insects in crucifers, solanacous, and other vegetable crops. The microbial biopesticides had become an important component in the management of crop diseases. Bt when applied on plant foliage upon feeding shows its toxicity toward the caterpillar or larvae of various insect pests. The specific target insect pest can be determined with the production of that particular Bt which gets binds to larval mid gut and thereby causes death of insect larvae. Several

Bt strains, where few of them were specific against fly larvae and mosquitoes are now developed.

14.11.1.1 BACULOVIRUSES

The target specific viruses that effectively controls lepidopterous pests in cotton, rice and vegetables. They are not commercially available in India (Gupta and Dikshit, 2010).

14.11.1.2 TRICHODERMA SPP

Soil borne saprophytic biocontrol agent effective against soil borne diseases in dry land crops.

Trichogramma spp.: Minute wasps acting as egg parasites and effective against lepidopteran pests such as soothed bollworms, pink bollworm in cotton, vegetable, and fruit pest.

14.11.2 PLANT INCORPORATED PROTECTANTS (PIPS)

These are pesticidal substances obtained by genetic engineering of plants by introducing the genes and proteins into the plant system and make the genetically modified plant to become resistant against certain insects and pathogens. Ex. Bt gene- the modified plant synthesis the substance which is poisonous to pest. EPA will regulate both protein as well as its genetic material, while the plant by itself will not be regulated.

14.11.3 BIOCHEMICAL PESTICIDES

These are the natural substances (plant extracts, pheromones, or fatty acids) which helps in controlling the insect pests by means of nontoxic mechanisms. They include plant materials like corn gluten, garlic oil, black pepper, and so on, which will interfere with mating (insect pheromones), molting, and food-finding reaction. While some the scented plant exudes acts as insect traps. These biopesticides control the insect pests without killing them while, the conventional synthetic pesticides will directly kill or inactivate the pests. Pheromones are commonly used in detecting, monitoring, and sometimes for controlling the insect populations.

14.11.3.1 BOTANICAL BIOPESTICIDES (PLANT PRODUCTS)

Increased global concern of the pesticidal pollution had led to the usage of botanicals in crop protection. Though 2400 plant species were reported with pesticidal properties, neem is the most ecofriendly and reliable authentic source. It affects the reproductive and digestive process of insects.

The biopesticidal characters of neem are wide and its products are more effective against arthropods (350 spp), nematodes (12 spp) fungi (15 spp.), viruses (3) and other insect pests (Nigam et al., 1994). The active ingredient Azadirachtin interrupt the metamorphosis in insects (Tomlin, 2007), while in chickpea, the larval population of *H. armigera*, can be effectively reduced by Neem Seed Kernel Extract (NSKE) (Bhushan et al., 2011).

Neem extracts are found to affect more than 195 species of insects (Sharma and Malik, 2012). The biopesticides of neem are systemic in nature. They also provide long term protection against a number of pests, with adverse effect on beneficial insects and pollinators. Apart from neem several plant extracts are found to have biopesticidal properties. Few of these are specified below.

Centre for Indian Knowledge Systems has tested the efficacy of neem, onion, garlic, Persian lilac, turmeric, tobacco, ginger, pongam, aloe, tulsi, and so on, to control different plant diseases (Kandpal, 2014).

Examples of a few plant products that has registered as biopesticides (Buss and Park Brown, 2002): (1) Limonene and Linalool—effective against aphids, mites, fleas, and so on; (2) Neem—effective against a various types of sucking and chewing pests; (3) Pyrethrum/Pyrethrins—effective against ants, flies, fleas, and so on; (4) Rotenone— against foliage feeding insects (Colorado potato beetle, asparagus beetle, and bean beetles); (5) Ryania— is effective particularly against caterpillars (European corn ear worm, corn borer, and others) and thrips; and (6) Sabadilla—effective against, harlequin bugs, squash bugs, caterpillars, thrips, and so on. Plant extracts having the potentiality of biopesticides (Khandapal, 2014):

1. Pudina kashayam, Adathoda kashayam, and Triphala kashayam— was effective against controlling leaf folder, Helminthosporium leaf spot, bacterial leaf blight.
2. Andrographis kashayam and Sida kashayam effective on Aphids and borers in brinjal, okra
3. Garlic arkam—effective against leaf folder, bacterial leaf blight, Helminthosporium leaf spot:

   a) Botanical Origin Biopesticides: Anosom *(Annona squamosa)*, Derisom *(Pongamia glabra)*, and Margosom *(Azadirachta indica)*.

b) Microbial Origin (based) Biopesticides—(i) Fungal biocontrol agents (biological fungicides): *T. viride, T. harzianum, Fusarium proliferatum;* Bacterial biological control agents: *Pseudomonas fluorescens, Bacillus subtilis;* Entomopathogenic fungi (Biological Insecticides): *Beauveria bassiana, Metarhizium anisopliae, Verticillium lecanii, B. thuringiensis* var *krustaki,* Ha- NPVSL-NPV; Biological Nematicides: *Paecilomyces lilacinus, Bacillus firmus* Mosquito larvicides: *B. thuringiensis* var *israelensis.* (ii) Microbial products: Peptidomimetics—A nonpeptide organic scaffold, that binds to target insectophore and grafts to the back structure for production of peptidomimetic. It is a potential main compound in developing new and novel insecticides, thereby overcoming the bioavailability issues of peptides entering the insect body (Nicholson, 2007) and Pheromone—The chemicals released by a group of microorganisms acting as signal messages in attracting an opposite sex of same species, for example, sex pheromone in codling moth.

Pheromones combined traps can be used for determining different types of insect pests and helps in taking protection measures. Pheromone traps are mainly based on "attract and to kill" technique disrupting the mating of insects. The main concept of mating disruption with pheromone traps was successful in control of several insect pests. In Germany and Switzerland, using this technique, nearly 20% of grape growers produce wine without spraying any insecticides.

While in the United States, the technique was highly effective in the control of pink bollworm, oriental fruit moth, codling moth, grapevine moth, and European grape moth, to name a few. In the western US, for the control of caterpillar nearly 40% of fruit trees were treated with mating disruption. In 1970s, the concept (of Mating disruption) started with "hexalure" the sex attractant to control pink bollworm, *Pectinophora gossypiella* (Saunders) and its discovery in 1973 was known to be first commercial formulation that was successful in 1978 (Baker et al., 1991). The infestations of southern pine beetle, Dendroctonus was suppressed by the inhibitor-based tactic (Saolm et al., 1995).

14.11.3.2 *BIOPESTICIDES ADOPTION*

(1) In general, farmers adopt the usage of biopesticides mainly based on presence of ample evidence available under the field efficacy of biopesticides

to control the crop damages and gives increased yields. (2) Most of the high quality biopesticides products are made available in sufficient quantities and at affordable prices. (3) Strengthening of the supply chain management of biopesticides.

14.11.3.3   DISADVANTAGES OF BIOPESTICIDES

Slow effect, degraded rapidly by ultra violet light, not available easily, lack persistence, and wide spectrum activity.

14.11.3.4   CONSERVATION OF BIOLOGICAL CONTROL AGENTS

Conservation of BCAs may be ascertained by early usage of pesticides; use of nonhost toxic pesticides, avoiding usage of persistent synthetic pesticides, adopting spot sprays; planting variety of flowering species for nectar and pollen sources, providing shelter and moisture sources, and so on.

14.11.3.5   PROMOTION OF BENEFICIALS

A favorable habitat is created to improve the chances of sustenance and multiplication of beneficial organisms through farm scaping and maintenance of food resources, that is, nectar and pollen to the adult parasitoids and predators near to their niches. The Apiaceae members are potential insectary plants, wild carrot, coriander, fennel flowers attracts the parasitoid wasps. Crop residues, organic mulches, mild fluctuations in weather conditions (temperature and moisture) provide concealed places for soil habitat insect predators spiders, rove beetles, and centipedes. Provide wind breaks, hedgerow, strip cultivation of perennial vegetation, prey perching sites, and so on. For harbor of predator pests. Appropriate method of pesticide usage should be followed for minimal exposure of beneficial organisms to the environmental condition.

14.11.3.6   HABITAT MANIPULATION

Grow diversified crops throughout growing season that may flower in different times for the availability of nectar, pollen, and shelter to natural enemies which are well adapted to local conditions and tolerate low populations of plant-feeding insects pests.

14.11.3.7 CONSERVING PARASITES AND PREDATORS

Management strategies adopted to preserve many of the beneficial insects. Certain tips that help in the maximization of value from beneficial insects in and surrounding the fields are:

Use of economic thresholds when they are not available; usage of selective insecticides which targets only a specific group of insects and shows no harm to natural enemies; selective application patterns as spraying only in patches, field edges or in strips; crop rotation that prevents insects in reaching potential levels; providing favorable habitat to the beneficial insects, and so on. Many of the studies have revealed that the beneficial arthropods move through the field margins into crops thus making biological control more intensive toward crop rows that are near to the wild vegetation than in the field centers. Few examples are cited below: (1) parasitism of rape pollen beetle was found to be about 50% at edges of the field than in middle of the field in Germany. (2) In Michigan, the parasitism of ichneumonid wasp *(Eriborus terbrans)* against European corn borer was more toward the periphery of field.

Similarly, it was observed in the Hawaiian sugar cane, nectar bearing plants in the field margins, improved the effectiveness of the sugarcane weevil parasite *Lixophaga sphenophori*. European studies have revealed that creating corridors to natural enemies can be achieved by sowing diversified flowering plants in strips that will cut across fields for every 165–330 feet, so that the beneficial utilize these corridors for circulating and dispersing in field centers.

KEYWORDS

- **synthetic pesticides**
- **environmental impact**
- **microbial pesticides**
- **biopesticides**
- **integrated pest management**
- **development**
- **agriculture**

REFERENCES

Cherry, A. *Biopesticides a Global Perspective. Crop Production Programme*; Natural Resources Institute, University of Greenwich: UK, 2005.

Aktar, M. W.; Sengupta, D.; Chowdhury, A. Impact of Pesticides Use in Agriculture: Their Benefits and Hazards. *Inter Discip. Toxicol.* **2009**, *2*, 1–12.

Aronson, A.; Beckman, W.; Dunn, P. *Bacillus thuringiensis* and Related Insect Pathogens. *Microbiol. Rev.* **1986**, *50*, 1–24.

Baker, T. C.; Staten, R. T.; Flint, H. M. Use of Pink Bollworm Pheromone in the Southwestern United States. In *Behavior Modifying Chemicals for Insect Management*; Ridgeway, R. L., Silverstein, R. M., Inscoe, M. N., Eds.; Marcel Dekker: New York, NY, 1991; pp 417–436.

Bezchlebová, J.; Cernohlávková, J.; Lána, J.; Sochová, I.; Kobeticová, K.; Hofman, J. Effects of Toxaphene on Soil Organisms. *Ecotoxicol. Environ. Saf.* **2007**, *68*, 326–334.

Bhushan, S.; Singh, R. P.; Shanker, R. Bioefficacy of Neem and *Bt* Against Pod Borer, *Helicoverpa armigera* in Chickpea. *J. Biopest.* **2011**, *4*, 87–89.

Brühl, C. A.; Schmidt, T.; Pieper, S.; Alscher, A. Terrestrial Pesticide Exposure of Amphibians: An Underestimated Cause of Global Decline? *Sci. Rep.* **2013**, *3*, 1135.

Buss, E. A.; Park, B. S. G. Natural Products for Insect Pest Management. ENY- 350, 2002.

Carlton, B. Development of Genetically Improved Strains of *Bacillus thuringiensis*. In *Biotechnology for Crop Protection*; Hedin, P., Menn, J., Hollingworth, R. Eds.; American Chemical Society: Washington, DC, 1988; pp 260–279.

Chapple, A. C.; Downer, R. A.; Bateman, R. P. Theory and Practice of Microbial Insecticide Application. In *Field Manual of Techniques in Invertebrate Pathology*; Lacey, L. A., Kaya, H. A. Eds.; Kluwer: Dordrecht, 2000; pp 5–37.

Chattopadhyay, A.; Bhatnagar, N. B.; Bhatnagar, R. Bacterial Insecticidal Toxins. *Crit. Rev. Microbiol.* **2004**, *30*, 33–54.

Clemson, H. G. I. C. *Organic Pesticides and Biopesticides, Clemson Extension, Home and Garden Information Center*; Clemson University: Clemson, 2007.

Conis, E. M. S.; M. J. Debating the Health Effects of DDT: Thomas Jukes, Charles Wurster and the Fate of an Environmental Pollutant. *Public Health Rep.* **2010**, *125*, 337–342.

De Faria, M. R.; Wright, S. P. Mycoinsecticides and Mycoacaricides: A Comprehensive List With Worldwide Coverage and International Classification of Formulation Types. *Biol. Contr.* **2007**, *43*, 237–256.

Edwards, C. A.; Thompson, A. R. Pesticides and the Soil Fauna. *Res. Rev.* **1973**, *45*, 1–79.

Eilenberg, J.; Hajek, A.; Lomer, C. Suggestions for Unifying the Terminology in Biological Control. *Biocontrol* **2001**, *46*, 387–400.

Eskenazi, B.; Bradman, A.; Castorina, R. Exposures of Children to Organophosphate Pesticides and Their Potential Adverse Health Effects. *Environ. Health Perspect.* **1999**, *107*, 409–419.

Eskenazi, B.; Lisa, G. R.; Amy, R. M.; Asa, B.; Kim, H.; Nina, H.; Caroline, J.; Laura, F.; Dana, B. B. Pesticide Toxicity and the Developing Brain. *Basic Clin. Pharmacol. Toxicol.* **2008**, *102*, 228–236.

Fenske, R. A.; Lu, C.; Simcox, N. J.; Loewenherz, C.; Touchstone, J.; Moate, T. F.; Allen, E. H.; Kissel, J. C. Strategies for Assessing Children's Organophosphorus Pesticide Exposures in Agricultural Communities. *J. Expo. Anal. Environ. Epidemiol.* **2000**, *10*, 662–671.

Frampton, G. K.; Jansch, S.; Scott, F. J. J.; Römbke, J.; Van den Brink, P. Effects of Pesticides on Soil Invertebrates in Laboratory Studies: A Review and Analysis Using Species Sensitivity Distributions. *J. Environ. Toxicol. Chem.* **2006**, *25*, 2480–2489.

Gill, R. J.; Rodriguez, O. R.; Raine, N. E. Combined Pesticide Exposure Severely Affects Individual and Colony Level Traits in Bees. *Nature* **2012**, *491*, 105–108.

Glare, T. R.; O'Callaghan, M. *Bacillus thuringiensis: Biology, Ecology and Safety*; Wiley: Chichester, 2000.

Gonzalez, J. M.; Brown, B. J.; Carlton, B. C. Transfer of *Bacillus thuringiensis* Plasmids Coding for δ-endotoxin Among Strains of *B. thuringiensis* and *B. cereus*. *Proc. Natl. Acad. Sci.* **1982**, *79*, 6951–6955.

Gupta, S.; Dikshit, A. K. Biopesticides: An Ecofriendly Approach for Pest Control. *J. Biopest.* **2010**, *3*, 186–188.

Guillon, M. L. Regulation of Biological Control Agents in Europe. In *International Symposium on Biopesticides for Developing Countries*; Roettger, U., Reinhold, M., Eds.; CATIE: Turrialba, 2003; pp 143–147.

Gupta, S.; Dikshit, A. K. Biopesticides: An Ecofriendly Approach for Pest Control. *J. Biopest.* **2010**, *3*, 186–188.

Hill, K. R.; Robinson, G. Fatal D.D.T. Poisoning. *Br. Med. J.* **1945**, *2*, 845–847.

Joung, K. C.; Côte', J. C. A Review of the Environmental Impacts of the Microbial Insecticide *Bacillus thuringiensis* In *Agriculture and Agri-food*; Technical Bulletin: Canada, 2000; p 29.

Kalra, A.; Khanuja, S. P. S. Research and Development Priorities for Biopesticide and Biofertiliser Products for Sustainable Agriculture in India. In *Business Potential for Agricultural Biotechnology*; Teng, P. S., Ed.; Asian Productivity Organisation, 2007; pp 96–102.

Konradsen, F.; Hoekb, C. D. C.; Hutchinson, G.; Daisley, H.; Singh, S.; Eddleston, M. Reducing Acute Poisoning in Developing Countries-Options for Restricting the Availability of Pesticides. *Toxicology* **2003**, *192*, 249–261.

Landrigan, P. J.; Claudio, L.; Markowitz, S. B.; Berkowitz, G. S.; Brenner, B. L.; Romero, H.; Wetmur, J. G.; Matte, T. D.; Gore, A. C.; Godbold, J. H.; Wolff, M. S. Pesticides and Inner-city Children: Exposures, Risks, and Prevention. *Environ. Health Perspect.* **1999**, *107*, 431–437.

Le Conte, J. L. Hints for the Promotion of Economic Entomology. *Am. Assoc. Adv. Sci.* **1874**, *22*, 11–22.

Longnecker, M. P.; Rogan, W. J.; Lucier, G. The Human Health Effects of DDT (Dichlorodiphenyltrichloroethane) and PCBS (Polychlorinated Biphenyls) and An Overview of Organochlorines in Public Health. *Ann. Rev. Public Health* **1997**, *18*, 211–244.

Marrone, P. G. Present and Future Use of *Bacillus thuringiensis* in Integrated Pest Management Systems: An Industrial Perspective. *Biocon. Sci. Technol.* **1994**, *4*, 517–526.

Martin, P. A. W.; Traverse, R. S. Worldwide Abundance and Distribution of *Bacillus thuringiensis* Isolates. *Appl. Environ. Microbiol.* **1989**, *55*, 2437–2442.

Mc Coy, C. W.; Samson, R. A.; Boucias, D. G. Entomogenous Fungi. In *Handbook of Natural Pesticides, Microbial Pesticides Part A, Entomogenous Protozoa and Fungi*; IgnoVo, C. M., Mandava, N. B. Eds.; CRC Press: Boca Raton, 1988; Vol. 5, pp 151–236.

Mc Cauley, L.; Beltran, M.; Phillips, J.; Lasarev, M.; Sticker, D. The Oregon Migrant Farm Workers Community: An Evolving Model for Participatory Research. *Environ. Health Perspect.* **2001**, *109*, 449–455.

Nicholson, G. M. Fighting the Global Pest Problem: Preface to the Special Toxicon Issue on Insecticidal Toxins and their Potential for Insect Pest Control. *Toxicon* **2007**, *49*, 413–422.

Nigam, S. K.; Mishra, G.; Sharma, A. Neem: A Promising Natural Insecticide. *Appl. Bot. Abstr.* **1994**, *14*, 35–46.

Qiu, J. *Organic Pollutants Poison the Roof of the World: Accumulation of DDT in Himalayas exceeds that seen in Arctic*; Nature News, 2013.

Quandt, S. A.; Arcury, T. A.; Rao, P.; Snively, B. M.; Camann, D. E.; Doran, A. M.; Yau, A. Y.; Hoppin, J. A.; Jackson, D. S. Agricultural and Residential Pesticides in Wipe Samples from Farm Worker Family Residences in North Carolina and Virginia. *Environ. Health Perspect.* **2004,** *112*, 382–387.

Romeis, J.; Meissle, M.; Bigler, F. Transgenic Crops Expressing *Bacillus thuringiensis* Toxins and Biological Control. *Nat. Biotechnol.* **2006,** *24*, 63–71.

Salom, S. M.; Grossman, D. M.; Mc Clellan, Q. C.; Payne, T. L. Effect of an Inhibitor-based Suppression Tactic on Abundance and Distribution of Southern Pine Beetle (Coleoptera: Scolytidae) and its Natural Enemies. *J. Econ. Entomol.* **1995,** *88*, 1703–1716.

Sharma, S.; Malik, P. Biopestcides: Types and Applications. *Int. J. Adv. Pharm. Biol. Chem.* **2012,** *1*, 508–516.

Siegel, J. P.; Shadduck, J. A. Clearance of *Bacillus sphaericus* and *Bacillus thuringiensis* ssp. Israelensis from Mammals. *J. Econ. Entomol.* **1990,** *83*, 347–355.

Sundheim, L.; Tronsmo, A. Hyperparasites in Biological Control. In *Biocontrol of Plant Diseases*, Mukerji, K. G., Garg, K. L., Eds.; CRC Press Boca Raton: USA, 1988; Vol. 1, pp 53–70.

Steinwand, B. *Biopesticide Ombudsman (Personal Communication)*; US Environmental Protection Agency: Washington, DC, 2008.

Szewczyk, B.; Lobo de Souza, M.; Batista de, C. M. L.; Moscardi, M. L.; Moscardi, F. Baculovirus Biopesticides. In *Pesticides–Formulations, Effects, Fate*; Stoytcheva, M. Ed.; InTech, 2011.

Thakore, Y. The Biopesticide Market for Global Agricultural Use. *Ind. Biotechnol.* **2005,** *2*, 192–208.

Tripathi, G.; Sharma, M. Effects of Habitats and Pesticides on Aerobic Capacity and Survival of Soil Fauna. *Biomed. Environ. Sci.* **2006,** *18*, 169–175.

Tomlin, C. *The Pesticide Manual*, 11th Ed.; British Crop Protection Council: 49 Downing Street, Farham, Survey GU97PH, UK, 2007.

Tschirley, F. H. Pesticides, Relation to Environmental Quality. *JAMA* **1973,** *224*, 1157–1166.

Vaishali, K. Biopesticides. *Int. J. Environ. Res. Dev.* **2014,** *4*, 191–196.

Wu, C.; Chen, X. Impact of Pesticides on Biodiversity in Agricultural Areas. *Ying Yong Sheng Tai Xue Bao* **2004,** *15*, 341–344.

CHAPTER 15

Morphological Characterization of Phytopathogenic Fungi Isolated from Seeds of Barley Plants (*Hordeum vulgare*) in Mexico

TERESA ROMERO CORTES[1], VÍCTOR HUGO PÉREZ ESPAÑA[1], PABLO ANTONIO LÓPEZ PÉREZ[1], EDUARDO RANGEL CORTÉS[1], MARIO A. MORALES OVANDO[2], MARIO RAMÍREZ-LEPE[3], and JAIME ALIOSCHA CUERVO -PARRA[1*]

[1]*Escuela Superior de Apan-Universidad Autónoma del Estado de Hidalgo, Carretera Apan-Calpulalpan, Km 8, Chimalpa Tlalayote s/n, Colonia Chimalpa, 43900 Apan, Hidalgo, Mexico*

[2]*Universidad de Ciencias y Artes de Chiapas, Sede Acapetahua, Calle central norte s/n entre 4ª y 5ª norte, 30580. Acapetahua, Chiapas, Mexico*

[3]*Unidad de Investigación y Desarrollo en Alimentos, Instituto Tecnológico de Veracruz, Av. Miguel Ángel de Quevedo No. 2779, Colonia Formando Hogar, Veracruz, Ver, Mexico*

Corresponding author. E-mail: jalioscha@gmail.com

ABSTRACT

Worldwide, barley (*Hordeum vulgare* L.) is the fourth most important cereal after wheat, maize, and rice and it is used in the livestock, food, and brewing industry. The main producer of this cereal is the Russian Federation with a production of 18 million tons per year. In Mexico, the barley is planted in an approximate area of 283,386 ha; 83% of this area is located in the States of Hidalgo (44%), Mexico (11%), Puebla (14%), and Tlaxcala (14%). The cultivation conditions depend on rainfall as a unique source of moisture during the summer cycle. Unfortunately, the minimum tillage methods and monoculture of cereals have favored the increase of phytopathogens causing foliar spots, root rot, and fusariosis; which is particularly important because it affects yield and produces toxins in the grain that are harmful to human and animal health. Among the phytopathogenic fungi that cause losses in barley plantations worldwide, *Puccinia striiformis* can be mentioned that causes yellow or linear rust. *Puccinia hordei* that causes leaf rust or brown rust, *Drechslera teres/ Pyrenophora teres* that causes net stain, with losses in yield greater than 50%, to the fungi *Alternaria* spp., *Fusarium* spp., *Epicoccum* sp., which cause the black tip, *Fusarium* spp., which cause fusariosis, *F. graminearum/Gibberela zeae* that causes seedling blight, *Bipolaris sorokiniana/Cochliobolus sativus* that causes seedling blight or blurred spot, *Ustilago nuda* that causes loose smut, and *U. hordei* causing covered smut disease. The yellow rust and the red spot diseases cause the greatest damage to the barley plantations. The phytopathogenic fungi classification of barley worldwide has been based on the use of morphological characters and the relationship with their hosts. Therefore, performing the morphological characterization of fungal isolates from the barley plant in Mexico will allow us to have knowledge about the microorganisms that are present in our country and thus to control those that are harmful to the plant. For that, the aim of this research was the isolate and morphological characterization of fungi associated with diseased barley plants in Mexico.

15.1 INTRODUCTION

Worldwide, barley (*Hordeum vulgare*) is the fourth most important cereal, followed by wheat, maize, and rice. Both the seed and the plant are used in the livestock, food, and brewing industry (Sánchez, 2011). The largest producer of this cereal is the European Union with a production of 859,500,000.00 tons, followed by Russia with a production of 17,000,000 metric tons per year. In the American continent, the main producer is Argentina with 3,400,000 tons per year (PMC, 2017).

In Mexico, the barley is planted in an approximate area of 336,000 ha; where 90% of this area is located among the states of Guanajuato, Hidalgo, Mexico, Puebla, and Tlaxcala (Zamora et al., 2008; SAGARPA, 2017). Based on the United States Department of Agriculture (USDA) estimated, annual production of barley for Mexico will be 735,000 tons, ranking No. 19 globally (PMC, 2017).

The crop is produced under rainfed or seasonal conditions in the summer cycle, depending on rainfall as a single source of irrigation (SAGARPA,

2009). In the Hidalgo state, barley cultivation occupies the second socioeconomic importance after maize, in terms of area sown, production volumes obtained and the number of producers (Gómez et al., 1997). However, this crop is affected by several phytopathogenic fungi responsible for diseases such as rust, foliar spots, root rot, and fusariosis. The latter is of great importance as it affects yield and contaminated grain produces toxins that are harmful to animal and human health (Gilchrist-Saavedra, 2000).

15.1.1 USES OF BARLEY PLANT

In Mexico, barley is a crop of great economic and social importance in the high valleys of the country, because farmers prefer it because their vegetative cycle is short, has resistance to drought, low temperatures, and saline soils. Of which, the states of Guanajuato and Hidalgo are the two main producers of barley grains in Mexico, with 372,167 and 268,595 tons (SAGARPA, 2017).

At present, this cereal is produced in almost all the world, destining it mainly to two types of market: like food for cattle and for the malt production. Particularly in Mexico, approximately 70% of the barley produced is used by the malting industry and the remaining 30% corresponds to varieties that are mainly used for cattle feed.

The consolidation in the domestic and export markets of the two large breweries in Mexico and the good positioning of their products in the world markets has led to the development integrated of a malt production industry in Mexico. This industry has, in turn, developed its own barley grain traders, which enter into contracts with agricultural producers for the production of malt varieties demanded by industry (Espinosa et al., 2003). However, the numerous diseases present in this crop are a strong limitation of production, especially due to the high cost of fungicides and their application (Gilchrist-Saavedra, 2000).

15.1.1.1 PHYTOPATHOGENIC FUNGI AFFECTING BARLEY CULTIVATION

Barley plantations are affected by phytopathogenic fungi that cause losses worldwide, may be mentioned the following: *Puccinia striiformis* causes "yellow or stripe rust" (Gilchrist-Saavedra et al., 2005), *Puccinia hordei* causes "leaf rust" or "brown rust" (Sánchez, 2011), *Drechslera teres* causes "the net blotch," causing losses of up to 50% (Gilchrist-Saavedra, 2000),

Alternaria spp., *Fusarium* spp., and *Epicoccum* sp., cause "the black tip" (Carmona et al., 2011), *Fusarium* spp., they cause "fusariosis" (Zúñiga et al., 2010), *F. graminearum*/*Gibberella zeae* causes "seedling blight," *Bipolaris sorokiniana*/*Cochliobolus sativus* causes "seedling blight" or "blurred spot," *Ustilago nuda* causes "flying coal" (Carmona et al., 2011), and *Ustilago hordei* causes "covered smut of barley" (Zúñiga et al., 2010). Of these diseases, which cause greater damage to the barley plantations are the yellow rust and the red spot (Carmona et al., 2011; Sánchez, 2011). In general, the crop is frequently affected by foliar stains and the different species of pathogenic fungi of the genus *Fusarium* which has been favored by the cultural methods used for the tillage and the retention of the harvest residues, which has favored the increase of the inoculum. The infected grain is the primary inoculum of the vast majority of diseases (Gilchrist-Saavedra et al., 2005).

15.2 METHODOLOGY

Thirteen samples of 500 g of seed per lot from 13 different localities, varieties, and years of cultivation in the upper valleys area were analyzed for the states of Guanajuato, Hidalgo, and Puebla. The general data for the samples studied are specified in Table 15.1 and Figure 15.1.

TABLE 15.1 Origin of Barley Grains Samples.

Lot number	Variety	Origin place	Harvest date
M1	Esmeralda	Apan, Hidalgo	2010
M2	Forrajera	Mijapa, Hidalgo	2011
M3	Forrajera	Tepeapulco, Hidalgo	2013
M4	Esmeralda	Apan, Hidalgo	2012
M5	Adabella	Tepepatlaxco, Hidalgo	2014
M6	Esmeralda	San Felipe, Hidalgo	2009
M7	Esmeralda	Leon, Guanajuato	2013
M8	Esmeralda	Libres, Puebla	2008
M9	Gaviota	Leon, Guanajuato	2013
M10	Adabella	Almoloya, Hidalgo	2013
M11	Josefa	Apan, Hidalgo	2015
M12	Josefa	Apan, Hidalgo	2016
M13	Josefa	Apan, Hidalgo	2017

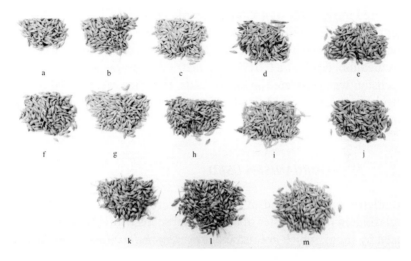

FIGURE 15.1 Morphological characteristics of barley seed samples. M1 (a), M2 (b), M3 (c), M4 (d), M5 (e), M6 (f), M7 (g), M8 (h), M9 (i), M10 (j), M11 (k), M12 (l), M13 (m).

15.2.1 *METHODS OF CULTURING AND ISOLATING FUNGI*

Barley seeds (10 g) were disinfected with 10% sodium hypochlorite solution (NaOCl) for one minute. Subsequently, the seeds were dried at room temperature and potato dextrose agar (PDA) was used for the development of fungal species. Samples were incubated for 7 days at 25°C. Subsequently, they were analyzed with a microscope stereoscopic and in those where fungal colonies were observed, 5 mm diameter discs were cut with the aid of a punch and placed in other Petri dishes with PDA medium for their growth, isolation and subsequent morphological characterization. The isolated strains were incubated for 5 days at 25°C or until all of the culture medium was filled.

15.2.2 *MAINTENANCE AND PROPAGATION OF STRAINS*

For maintenance and propagation of the strains, a spore wash was carried out with a sterile solution of 0.01% Tween 20 (Arévalo et al., 2005) at a concentration of 1×10^6 spores/mL for each isolated phytopathogenic fungus. The spore concentration was performed by the direct total count by the Thoma chamber method. One part of this spore suspension was transferred to another Petri dish, homogeneously distributed, incubated at 25°C for 7 days and stored refrigerated at 4°C under sterile conditions until use. In order to maintain the viable culture, the re-plantings were carried out every 30 days (Alvarez, 2007). After each microorganism was grown in the Petri dish, with PDA medium, 5 mL of a 0.01% Tween 20 solution was added and the spore suspension was recovered in sterile vials, to which were added 5 mL of a 40% glycerol solution and finally, the suspensions of spores were preserved in freezing at −86°C until use.

15.2.3   MICROORGANISMS USED

The microorganisms used in this study were strains of phytopathogenic fungi isolated from samples of barley plant seeds with symptoms of disease caused by fungi, which are listed below: *Drechslera teres*, *Bipolaris sorokiniana*, *Fusarium graminearum*, *Fusarium austroamericanum*, *Fusarium pseudograminearum*, *Rhizopus oryzae*, *Puccinia triticina*, *Puccinia striiformis*, *Puccinia recondita*, *Puccinia hordei*, *Alternaria alternata*, *Penicillium digitatum*, *Penicillium citrinum*, and *Penicillium oxalicum*. The fungal strains were isolated from seeds with characteristics of disease as yellow rust and brown rust from the upper valleys area of the states of Guanajuato, Hidalgo, and Puebla.

15.2.4   MORPHOLOGICAL CHARACTERIZATION

Morphological descriptions were based on comparisons with descriptions of other authors (Ireta and Gilchrist, 1994; Crous et al., 1995; Scudamore and Hetmanski, 1995; Maenetje and Dutton, 2007; Manamgoda et al., 2014; Lawrence et al., 2016), augmented by new observations as noted. PDA medium was the standard growth medium used for the growth rate and the morphological study of the reproductive structures of all fungi. Microscopic observations and measurements of the reproductive structures were made with an optical microscope (ZEIGEN, Model ZB-7100). All strains were stored as conidia and hyphae at −86°C until processed.

15.3   RESULTS AND DISCUSSION

Fungi responsible for causing diseases are a major factor in the low productivity of a crop. In this respect, cereals grains such as barley can easily be colonized by fungal species, which cause their deterioration (Soldevilla et al., 2005). All barley samples in the upper valleys of the states of Guanajuato, Hidalgo, and Puebla that were sampled showed fungal strains. From a total of 13 lots of samples of barley seeds with disease symptoms, 64 strains of phytopathogenic fungi were isolated, of which 27 were recovered from the variety Esmeralda, 13 from the Adabella variety, 11 from the variety Josefa, 9 of the Forrajera variety, and 6 of the Gaviota variety of barley (Table 15.2).

The results obtained in this research are similar to those reported by other authors for other barley-producing areas of the world (Soldevilla et al., 2005; Ocampo et al., 2005; Lowe and Ulmer, 2006; Bolton et al., 2008; García et al., 2012).

In other studies, the presence of *Penicillium* and *Aspergillus* genera as predominant fungi has been reported in barley grains (Scudamore and Hetmanski, 1995; Maenetje and Dutton, 2007). However, our results do not coincide with those reported by these authors because in this study the species isolated from the genus *Penicillium* (Table 15.2) are not predominant fungal genera. This result may be due to the presence of other genera of fungi of greater economic importance for this crop (Fig. 15.2).

Within these important genera that were isolated as predominant is the complex of rust of cereals. Species of this genus have been reported to be responsible for causing diseases such as *P. striiffformis* "4.5%" (Wellings, 2010), and brown rust caused by *P. triticina* "4.5%," *P. hordei* "7.5%," and *P. recondita* "3.0%" (Steffenson et al., 1993; de Vallavieille-Pope et al., 1995; De Wolf et al., 2010; Bolton et al., 2008; Sánchez, 2011). The other predominant fungal genera in this study were *Fusarium* and *Rhizopus* with 18.5 and 15%, respectively. The genus *Fusarium* is responsible for causing fusariosis of the spike, a disease whose importance lies in its low yield and the toxins generated in the affected grains (Gilchrist-Saavedra et al., 2005).

All geographic areas where cereal crops are grown in Mexico present problems against *Fusarium* spp., varying the species at each location and at different times (Ireta and Gilchrist, 1994; CIMMYT, 2004). The losses can vary considerably, many times not being related to the yield, but yes with the content of toxins present in the grains. That is why big companies that use grain to make concentrated animal feed or cereals in flakes, for human consumption, control the content of toxins, imposing limits on their concentration. However, when there is no way to control the toxin content, infected grains become a health problem (Gilchrist-Saavedra, 2000).

In relation to *R. oryzae*, this genus has been reported to cause diseases of fruits of several species, such as strawberry (Farrera et al., 2007), tulipán (Hisaki et al., 2006), cocoa (Cuervo-Parra et al., 2011), and barley

TABLE 15.2 Microorganisms Isolated from Barley Seeds.

Fungal species	Variety of barley					% of total occurrence in isolation[a]
	Adabella (JCPn)	Esmeralda (JCPn)	Gaviota (JCPn)	Forrajera (JCPn)	Josefa (JCPn)	
Drechslera teres	7, 50	2, 10, 19, 51	–	–	16, 57	32.00
Bipolaris sorokiniana	6	3, 12, 30	–	43, 65	14, 44	32.00
Fusarium graminearum	28, 53	1, 34, 55, 62	59	–	15, 64	36.00
Fusarium austroamericanum	–	–	–	40	–	4.00
Rhizopus oryzae	9, 27	0, 20, 29	22	24, 41	18, 45	40.00
Fusarium pseudograminearum	–	–	46	–	47	8.00
Puccinia triticina	8	–	21	–	17	12.00
Puccinia striiformis	26	35	–	–	58	12.00
Puccinia recondita	37	–	–	38	–	8.00
Puccinia hordei	54	48, 61	60	39	–	20.00
Alternaria alternata	–	13, 31, 32, 49, 56	–	25	–	24.00
Penicillium oxalicum	63, 52	11, 4	–	42	–	20.00
Penicillium citrinum	–	5, 33	–	–	–	8.00
Penicillium digitatum	–	36	23	–	–	8.00

[a]Percentage of occurrence for n = de 25 Petri dishes with PDA medium (5 replicates per barley variety).
n: identification number of each strain.

(Romero-Cortes et al., 2016). Although this species is not reported as a pathogen of barley, their rapid growth observed during its isolation would allow it to colonize and destroy the seeds and plants in a very short time, being the first report of this fungus as pathogen for this crop in Mexico.

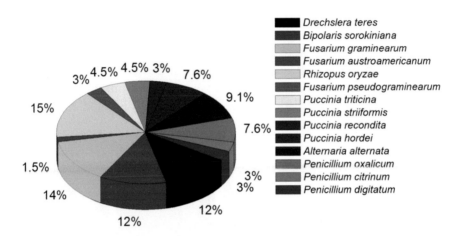

FIGURE 15.2 Percentage of more predominant genera.

The measurements of different morphological structures of phytopathogenic fungi are described below. For *Rhizopus oryzae* the colonies showed a diameter of 75–80 mm, sporangiophore with stipes of more than 1500 μm in length, sporangium of more than 150 μm in diameter and conidia of 5–8 μm in length. For *Drechslera teres* colonies shown 5.1 mm/day growth rate, conidiophores showed different shape (64–79 × 10–17 μm), and conidia being in the range 36–102 × 13–15 μm. In the case of *Bipolaris sorokiniana*, colonies grew on PDA medium showed a diameter of 35–40 mm, abundant sporulation of conidiophores with size of 130–154 × 6–8 μm, conidias are dark olivaceous brown with a size of 77–146 × 15–19 μm. In the case of *Alternaria alternata*, colonies in PDA medium showed a rapid growth with a diameter of 37–40 mm in 7 days. Conidias were small to moderate in size, 20–29 × 8–10 μm.

For *Fusarium graminearum*, *F. austroamericanum*, and *F. pseudoamericanum*, it was observed that their growth was 5, 5.6, and 5.3 μm/day, respectively. In all three species, the presence of macroconidia was observed, ranging from 2.5 × 35–65 μm, with globular chlamydospores of 10–12 μm in diameter. The presence of microconidia was not observed. On the other hand, in the case of the barley rust, it was observed that *Puccinia recondita* showed uredospores of brown color and spherical shape of 16–28 μm in diameter. For *P. striiformis* the uredospores were spherical to ovate in shape, orange colored, and with a size of 23–35 × 20–35 μm. *Puccinia triticina* showed uredospores of brown color and of oval form of around 25–30 × 15–20 μm. Finally, *P. hordei* showed spherical uredospores in shape, orange, and with a size of 13–18 × 10–14 μm. For fungi of the genus *Penicillium* (*P. oxalicum, P. citrinum, P. digitatum*), blue-green conidia with a growth diameter of 35–40 μm were observed at 7 days of growth. The conidia were round to ellipsoidal in *P. oxalicum*, unicellular and observed as chains not branched at the end of the phialide, between 2 and 5 μm in diameter. The morphological characteristics of the fungal species isolated from barley grains are shown in Figures 15.3 and 15.4.

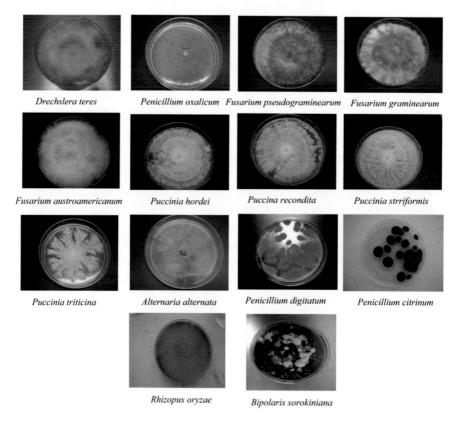

Drechslera teres	*Penicillium oxalicum*	*Fusarium pseudograminearum*	*Fusarium graminearum*
Fusarium austroamericanum	*Puccinia hordei*	*Puccina recondita*	*Puccinia strriformis*
Puccinia triticina	*Alternaria alternata*	*Penicillium digitatum*	*Penicillium citrinum*
	Rhizopus oryzae	*Bipolaris sorokiniana*	

FIGURE 15.3 Macroscopic characteristics of fungal species isolated from barley plant seeds.

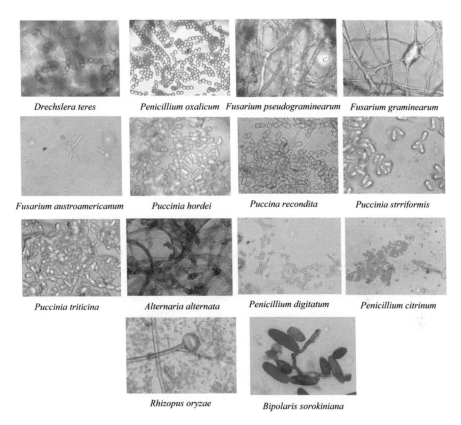

FIGURE 15.4   Microscopic characteristics of fungal species isolated from barley plant seeds.

15.4   CONCLUSIONS

Knowledge of the fungi species present in a particular crop is of utmost importance to be able to implement strategies aimed at the prevention and control of the diseases that these fungal agents can cause in the cultivation of barley. Likewise, the use of reliable techniques for the identification of strains of phytopathogenic fungi is of equal importance to avoid their dispersion within an area.

KEYWORDS

- *hordeum vulgare*
- phytopathogenic fungi
- morphological characterization
- barley
- microorganism

REFERENCES

Alvarez, N. M. Purificación y caracterización parcial de dos celulasas de *Trichoderma harzianum* CINV17. Master's Thesis, Instituto Tecnológico de Veracruz, 2007.

Arévalo, G. E.; Ortiz, B. C.; Zúñiga, C. L.; Gonzáles, V. J. Hoja Técnica No. 51. Selección de plantas de cacao resistentes a la Moniliasis usando savia del floema y fluidos embriónicos de frutos jóvenes. *Manejo Integrado de Plagas y Agroecología (Costa Rica)*. **2005**, *76*, 86–88.

Bolton, M. D.; Kolmer, J. A.; Garvin, D. F. Wheat Leaf Rust Caused by *Puccinia triticina*. *Mol. Plant Pathol.* **2008**, *9*, 563–575.

Carmona, M.; Barreto, D.; Romero A. Enfermedades del cultivo de cebada. Importancia, síntomas y manejo. In: CEBADA CERVECERA: Bases funcionales para un mejor manejo del cultivo; Miralles, D. J., Benech-Arnold, R. L., Abeledo, L. G., Eds.; 2011; pp 133–169.

Centro Internacional de Mejoramiento del Maíz y el Trigo (CIMMYT). *Programa de Maíz del CIMMYT. 2004. Enfermedades del* maíz: una guía para su identificación en el campo; 4th ed., CIMMYT: México, D. F., 2004.

Crous, P. W.; Janse, B. J. H.; Tunbringe, J.; Holz, G. DNA Homology Between *Pyrenophora japonica* and *P. teres*. *Mycol. Res.* **1995**, *99*, 1098–1102.

Cuervo, P. J. A.; Ramírez, S. M.; Sánchez, L. V.; Ramírez, L. M. Antagonistic Effect of *Trichoderma harzianum* VSL 291 on Phytopathogenic Fungi Isolated from Cocoa (*Theobroma cacao* L.) Fruits. *Afr. J. Biotechnol.* **2011**, *10*, 10657–10663.

De Wolf, E.; Paul, P.; Osborne, L.; Trenuta A. *Identificando a las Royas del Trigo y Cebada, USDA-CREES Extension Integrated Pest Management Program Award 2009-41533-05331*; 2010; Vol. 1, pp 1–4.

de Vallavieille, P. C.; Huber, L.; Leconte, M.; Goyeau, H. Comparative Effects of Temperature and Interrupted Wet Periods on Germination, Penetration, and Infection of *Puccinia recondita* f. sp. *tritici* and *P. striiformis* on Wheat Seedlings. *Phytopathology* **1995**, *85*, 409–415.

Espinosa, M.; Nieto, B. J.; Cervantes, M. A.; González, C. M. *Plan Estratégico de Investigación y Transferencia de Tecnología en el Sector Agropecuario y Agroindustrial. Cadena Agroalimentaria de Cebada. Etapa II: Identificación de Demandas Tecnológicas en la Cadena Agroalimentaria de Cebada. Plan Estratégico de Necesidades de Investigación y Transferencia de Tecnología;* Fundación Guanajuato Produce: Querétaro, México, 2003; 20.

Farrera, P. R. E.; Zambrano, V. A. E.; Ortiz, M. F. A. Identificación de hongos asociados a enfermedades del fruto de la fresa en el municipio Jáuregui del estado Táchira. *Rev. Fac. Agron. (LUZ).* **2007,** *24,* 269–281.

García, C.; Palmero, D.; De Cara, M.; Cruz, A.; González, J. M. Microbiota asociada a la enfermedad de la punta negra del trigo duro. Efectos del riego, el abonado nitrogenado y la variedad cultivada en la incidencia de la enfermedad. *ITEA. Inform. Téc. Econ. Agrar.* **2012,** *108,* 343–356.

Gilchrist, S. L.; Fuentes, D. G.; Martínez, C. C.; López, A. R. M.; Duveiller, E.; Singh, R. P.; Henry, M.; García A. *Guía* práctica para la identificación de algunas enfermedades de trigo y cebada; Segunda Edición. México, D. F., Centro Internac. de mejoramiento de Maíz y Trigo (CIMMYT); 2005; 68.

Gilchrist, S. L. I. Problemas Fitosanitarios de los Cereales de Grano Pequeño en los Valles Altos de México. *Rev. Mex. Fitopatol.* **2000,** *18,* 132–137.

Gómez, M. R.; García, S. R.; Pérez, C. J. P. Guía Para Cultivar Cebada Maltera de Temporal en el Estado de *Hidalgo;* Instituto Nacional de Investigaciones Forestales, Agrícolas y Pecuarias, Centro de Investigación de la Región Centro, Campo Experimental Pachuca. Folleto para Productores, 1997; Vol. 8, p 23.

Hisaki, V.; Benva, M.; Wright, E. R.; Morisigue, D. *Podredumbre* húmeda poscosecha de bulbos de tulipán ocasionada *por Rhizopus stolonifer. Jornadas de Enfermedades en Cultivos Bajo Cubierta. Actualización Fitosaniataria en Cultivos Protegidos;* Libro de Resúmenes: La Plata; 2006; 69.

Ireta, J.; Gilchrist, L. *La Roña de la Espiga del Trigo;* Reporte espec. de trigo. No. 21a, CIMMYT; 1994; 25.

Lawrence, D. P.; Rodonto, F.; Gannibal, P. B. Biodiversity and Taxonomy of the Pleomorphic Genus *Alternaria. Mycol. Prog.* **2016,** *15,* 3.

Lowe, D.; Ulmer, H. The Influence of Starter Culture on Barley Contaminated with *Fusarium culmorum* TMW 4.0754. *J. Am. Soc. Brew. Chem.* **2006,** *64,* 158–165.

Maenetje, P. W.; Dotton, M. F. The Incidence of Fungi and Mycotoxins in South African Barley and Barley Products. *J. Environ. Sci. Health* **2007,** *42,* 229–236.

Manamgoda, D. S.; Rossman, A. Y.; Castlebury, L. A.; Crous, P. W.; Madrid, H.; Chukeatirote, E.; Hyde, K. D. The Genus *Bipolaris. Stud. Mycol.* **2014,** *79,* 221–288.

Ocampo, S. I. O.; Jaimez, O. J.; Contreras, L. E.; Carrazana, G. J. Estudio de la Microflora y Contenido de Aflatoxinas Presentes en cebadas Cultivadas y Almacenadas en el Estado de Hidalgo. In *VII Congreso Nacional de Ciencias de los Alimentos y III Foro de Ciencia y Tecnología de Alimentos. 1-3 de junio;* Guanajuato, Gto: México, 2005; pp 245–253.

Producción Mundial Cebada (PMC). Cebada Producción Mundial 2017/2018, 2017.

Romero, C. T.; Ramírez, L. M.; Pérez, E. V. H.; López, P. P. A.; Morales, O. M. A.; Cuervo, P. J. A. *Morphological and Molecular Characterization of Rhizopus oryzae Strains Isolated from Barley Grains. Memoirs of the XX Congreso Nacional de Ingeniería Bioquímica, IX Congreso Internacional de Ingeniería Bioquímica, XIV Jornadas Científicas de Biomedicina y Biotecnología Molecular;* Veracruz, Mexico, 2016; pp 171–179.

SAGARPA. Servicio de Información y Estadística Agroalimentaria y Pesquera, Anuario Estadístico de la Producción Agrícola, 2009.

SAGARPA. Aumenta 33 por ciento producción de cebada en México, 2017.

Sánchez, F. C. F. Evaluación participativa de cuatro líneas y tres variedades de cebada (*Hordeum vulgare* L.), resistentes a sequía, en dos Épocas de siembra y en invernadero, en la Espoch, Riobamba, provincia de Chimborazo. Thesis, Esc. de Ingeniería Agronómica, Riobamba-Ecuador, 2011; 145.

Scudamore, K. A.; Hetmanski, M. T. Nature Occurrence of Mycotoxins and Mycotoxigenic Fungi in Cereals in the United Kingdom. *Food Addit. Contam.* **1995,** *12*, 377–382.

Soldevilla, C.; Vázquez, C.; Patiño, B.; Jurado, M.; González, J. M. T. Hongos toxicogénicos asociados a trigo y cebadas de Castilla y León. *Bol. San. Veg. Plagas.* **2005,** *31*, 519–529.

Steffenson, B. J.; Jin, Y.; Griffey, C. A. Pathotypes of *Puccinia hordei* with Virulence for the Barley Leaf Rust Resistance Gene *Rph7* in the United States. *Plant Dis.* **1993,** *77*, 867–869.

Wellings, C. Threat specific contingency plan, Barley stripe rust (*Puccinia striiformis* f. sp. *hordei*). *Plant Health Aust.* **2010,** 32.

Zamora, D. M.; Solano, H. S.; Gómez, M. R.; Rojas, M. I.; Ireta, M. J.; Garza, G. R.; Ortiz, T. C. Adabella: Variedad de cebada maltera para Valles Altos de la Mesa Central de México. *Agric. Téc. Méx.* **2008,** *34*, 491–493.

Zúñiga, J.; Lezáun, J. A.; Esparza M.; Garnica I. Enfermedades transmitidas por semilla en Trigos y cebadas. *Navar. Agrar.* **2010,** *6*, 29–32.

CHAPTER 16

Assessment of Plant Genetic Resources of Chili Germplasm

ANUPAM DAS, SUBRATA KUNDU, and BISWAJIT GHOSH*

Plant Biotechnology Laboratory, Department of Botany, Ramakrishna Mission Vivekananda Centenary College, Rahara, Kolkata 700118, India

Corresponding author. E-mail: ghosh_b2000@yahoo.co.in

ABSTRACT

The capsicum species, commonly known as chili peppers are pharmaceutically and economically important plants belonging to the Solanaceae family. Although domesticated in the Americas, the peppers have been distributed throughout the world and integrated into the world cuisine and food products. The chili fruits are vital to the human being as they are commonly used as vegetables, spices, and for therapeutic purposes. It possesses a wide range of pharmacologically important secondary metabolites including carotenoids, flavonoids, and vitamins that are beneficial to human health. These compounds have been reported to possess anti-cancer, antioxidant, anti-inflammatory, and antimicrobial properties. The exclusive metabolites present within the capsicum are the alkaloids capsaicinoids that make peppers pungent and are sequestered mainly in the placenta of the fruits. The nutritional content, as well as pungency of pepper, exhibit incredible diversity among different pepper types. The analysis of plethora of genetic resources of capsicum is pivotal for screening beneficial traits present within the enormous size of germplasm as well as for improved utilization in breeding programs. Therefore, in this chapter, we have emphasized on morphological, chemical, genetic, as well as disease diversity in different capsicum species cultivated in diverse geographical locations.

16.1   INTRODUCTION

Chili, a perennial shrub belonging to the Solanaceae family, originated in the tropical South American region and considered as an important dietary component since its domestication (Khan et al., 2014). As per estimates for 2011, about 3.8 million hectares of land was utilized for peppers cultivation, out of which 2.5 m ha is in Asia and 0.8 m ha in Africa (Faostat, 2013). It has been reported that only five genera of capsicum have been cultivated amongst twenty-seven genus (Onus and Pickersgill 2004; Olmstead et al., 2008). The five cultivated species of *Capsicum* are *C. annuum* L., *C. chinense* Jacq., *C. frutescens* L., *C. baccatum* L., and *C. pubescens,* and are recognized as economically important vegetable crops throughout the world due to their multipurpose and advanced application in food and therapeutic industries (Kehie et al., 2012; Kothari et al., 2010). *C. annuum* is found to be widespread, economically important and exploited maximum in commercial breeding programs. The fruit of *Capsicum* has immense ethnopharmacological importance and has been traditionally used throughout the world in cuisine and food products due to its distinctive flavor and color (Andrews, 1995; Kothari et al., 2010). It contains a variety of vital nutrients and bioactive compounds that exhibit a wide array of activities, including free radical scavenging, antimicrobial, antiviral, anti-inflammatory, and anticancer properties (Saidu and Garba, 2011; Luo et al., 2011). Chili possesses unique pharmacologically important secondary metabolite capsaicinoids that is a major class of alkaloid found in chili fruits. More than 22 different capsaicinoids have been reported in chili peppers, capsaicin and dihydrocapsaicin being the most common ones (Bosland and Votava, 2012). Among different capsaicinoids, capsaicin dihydrocapsaicin, nordihydrocapsaicin, homodihydrocapsaicin, and homocapsaicin were found to be predominant (Bosland 1996; Kozukue et al., 2005; Wahyuni et al., 2011; Davis et al., 2007). In the pericarp of chili fruits, capsaicin and dihydrocapsaicin that differ only in the acyl group existed for about 90% of total capsaicinoids (Bernal et al., 1993, Walpole et al., 1996, Kobata et al., 1998). It has been reported that capsaicinoids have versatile pharmaceuticals activities including against mutagenesis or tumorigenesis (Yoshitani et al., 2001, Sanchez et al., 2007), potent antimicrobials (Cichewicz 1996, Careaga et al., 2003), antioxidants (Henderson et al., 1999), and analgesic (Kaale et al., 2002, Caterina et al., 2000). They are found to be effective in the neuronal pain transmission and neurogenic inflammation (Szolcsányi, 2004, Demirbilek et al., 2004) and possess anticancer effect that is closely associated with the prevention of cell proliferation and migration and induction of apoptosis (Luo et al., 2011).

Capsaicin has been proven effective in inhibiting platelet aggregation (Hogaboam and Wallace, 1991) and expansion of cancer cells (Min et al., 2004, Zhang et al., 2008). It has been reported that capsaicin also decreases membrane lipid peroxidation in human erythrocytes exposed to oxidative stress (Luqman and Rizvi, 2006).

The implementation of modern plant breeding resulted in swiping of heterogeneous traditional cultivars by commercial hybrid varieties with consistent yields including various disease resistance traits (Lanteri et al., 2003). This phenomenon led to a significant reduction in genetic diversity in *Capsicum* and leading to the extinction of some important germplasm (Hammer et al., 2003; Votava et al., 2005). Under such circumstances, the evaluation of genetic resources of *Capsicum* spp. is upmost essential to detect important accessions for commercial breeding and development of conservation policies. Therefore, the major objective of the present chapter includes the assessment of morphological, chemical, and genetic diversity corroborated with disease diversity existing in the different *Capsicum* species.

16.2 ASSESSMENT OF MORPHOLOGICAL DIVERSITY

Morphological identification and characterization are the principal phase in the description and classification of germplasm (Smith and Smith 1989). The variation in morphological traits within plant populations could exhibit as adaptations to different selection pressures (Morrison and Weston, 1985, Hageman and Fahselt, 1990). Consequently, methodical classification and assessment of plant genetic resources (PGR) is essential for effective use of germplasm for conventional or modern breeding techniques (Mehmood et al., 2008; Padilha et al., 2016). The future use of the collected germplasm is completely dependent on the proper characterization of PGR. Accurate characterization of the accessions facilitates their conservation and allow their proper utilization in breeding programs (Padilha et al., 2016). According to "The protection of plant varieties and Farmer's Rights" (Government of India, 2001) act, a registrable cultivar needs to qualify the criteria of distinctiveness, uniformity, and stability (DUS) that can be validated by stipulating the characterization of important qualitative traits (Ramanna, 2003). Throughout the world, the grant of Plant Breeders' Rights depends on the qualification of the DUS criteria (Cooke et al., 2003). Characterization of accessions is the only way to stop biopiracy, thereby, helpful in solving many social and ethical issues (Esquinas-Alcázar 2005). The key benefits of phenotypic characterization are quick, easy scoring, and cost efficient (Ganguly et al., 2012). The chili fruit of the wild progenitor was found to be small, red-colored, pungent, and deciduous with soft fleshed but domestication and successive artificial selections resulted in significant discrepancy in size, form, color, and level of pungency (Ortiz et al., 2010; Paran and van der Knaap, 2007). A large phenotypic diversity is exhibited among the cultivated peppers due to human preferences at the diverse regions. The phenotypic variance in chili fruits is measured based on some important morphological characteristics including average yield per plant, number of fruits per plant, average fruit length, fresh weight (g), seeds per fruit, and pulp/seeds ratio. The wide range of distribution in different morphological parameters of chili fruits cultivated in different geographic locations is represented in Table 16.1 and Figure 16.1.

16.3   ANALYSIS OF CHEMICAL DIVERSITY

Several groups of researchers have reported that the interaction between genotype and environment play a significant role in phytochemical constituents in chili fruit (Zewdie and Bosland, 2000; Lee et al., 2005). The major capsaicinoids content among different *Capsicum* accessions varied greatly in different geographical locations (Butcher et al., 2012; Kundu et al., 2015; Zewdie and Bosland, 2000; Islam et al., 2015). It has also been reported that the synthesis of carotenoids and flavonoids in pepper fruits is significantly affected by a discrepancy in environmental factors (Lee et al., 2005; Lee et al., 1995). The nonpungent genotypes showed absence of capsaicinoids but possessed variable amounts of capsinoids, the nonpungent analogs of capsaicinoids (Kobata et al., 1998; Jarret et al., 2014; Zunun-Pérez et al., 2017). Chili fruits are also rich sources of various phenolics and flavonoids; quercetin, catechin, luteolin, apigenin, and their derivatives being the important one (Marín et al., 2004; Wahyuni et al., 2011; Dubey et al., 2015). It has been reported that the phenolic content was found to be in the range from 0.35 to 133.2 mg GAE/g dry weight and can differ according to the genotype, stages of maturity, and geographical locations (Gurnani et al., 2016; Dutta et al., 2016; Conforti et al., 2007; Marín et al., 2004). A wide array of carotenoids including capsanthin, zeaxanthin, β-cryptoxanthin, β-carotene, capsorubin, and anthocyanin are found in *Capsicum* fruits [Rodriguez-Uribe et al., 2014; Carvalho et al., 2015; Topuz and Ozdemir, 2007]. Irrespective of final fruit color these carotenoids are present in most chili fruits and their abundance is also reported to be cultivar-specific (Guzman et al., 2010; Wahyuni et al., 2011; Wall et al., 2001). Among different types of vitamins vitamin

TABLE 16.1 The Wide Range of Distribution of Morphological Characters of Chili Fruits Cultivated in Different Agroclimatic Conditions.

Region of study	No. of accessions	No. of characters studied	*Capsicum* species	Major findings	References
India	30	12	*C. annuum*	Fruit length (cm), 2.9–5.16 Fruit diameter (cm), 0.83–1.97 Plant height (cm), 57.03–71.68 Days to first flowering, 36.07–60.5 No of primary branch/plant, 3.80–6.23 Seed per fruit, 31.48–44.69 Fruit weight (g), 1.01–2.4 Fruit/plant, 44.24–427.95	Yatung et al. (2014)
Brazil	20	12	*C. annuum*	Days to flowering, 66.67–110.00 Days of the first ripe fruit, 138.33–170.67 Plant height (cm), 18.57–46.63 Canopy diameter (cm), 23.12–48.72 Fruit number per plant, 510–890 Fresh fruits weight (g), 0.42–17.33 Dry fruit weight (g), 0.13–2.8 Fruit length (mm), 11.61–70.13 Fruit width (mm), 6.95–25.62 Fruit wall thickness (mm), 0.52–3.31 Yield/plant (g), 845–1350g	Padilha et al. (2016)
Bangladesh	60	27	*Capsicum* sp.	Fruit color at immature stage, green/black/green with blackish blush/dark green Fruit color at mature stage, green/black/green with blackish blush/dark green Fruit shape- Elongate/conical	Rahman et al. (2017)

TABLE 16.1 (Continued)

Region of study	No. of accessions	No. of characters studied	*Capsicum* species	Major findings	References
				Corolla color, white/light yellow/purple with white margin	
				No. of fruits per plant, 1.00–70.50	
				Fruit length (cm), 1.00–7.20	
				Fruit width (cm), 0.54–5.00	
				Individual fruit weight (g), 0.80–3.60	
				Yield/plant (g), 1.09–155.57	
Uganda	37	48	*C. annuum*	Days to flowering, 10–59	Nsabiyera et al. (2013)
				Days to fruiting, 13–63	
				Days to fruit maturity, 60–112	
				Plant height (cm), 49–136	
				Canopy diameter (cm), 42–119	
				Fruits/plant, 4–62	
				Fresh fruits weight (g), 1.3–44.4	
				Fruit length (cm), 2.2–15.2	
				Fruit width (cm), 0.9–3.1	
				Pedicel length (cm), 2.4–5.5	
				Fruit wall thickness (mm), 0.9–3.9	
				Seeds/fruit, 31–148	
				Immature fruit color, white/yellow/green/orange/purple/deep purple	
				Mature fruit color, white/lemon-yellow/pale orange–yellow/orange–yellow/pale orange/orange/light red/red/dark red/purple/brown/black	

TABLE 16.1 *(Continued)*

Region of study	No. of accessions	No. of characters studied	*Capsicum* species	Major findings	References
Brazil	30	10	*Capsicum* sp.	Fruit shape, elongate/almost round/triangular/campanulate/blocky Plant height (cm), 18.00–88.50 Diameter of canopy (cm), 33.66–92.33 Seeds/fruit- 6.00–51.00 Fruit length (cm), 0.71–5.5 Fruit diameter (cm), 0.3–3.7 Fruit shape, elongate/triangular/round/campanulate/square	Bianchi et al. (2016)
Central America, the Caribbean Basin and South America	264	13	*C. chinense*	Immature fruit color, white/yellow/green/purple Mature fruit color, yellow/orange/red/ brown/black/ ivory/salmon Fruit shape, elongate/almost round/triangular/campanulate/blocky Fruit length (mm), 6.27–70.44 Fruit width (mm), 6.83–40.32 Pedicel length (mm), 14.75–44.84 Fruit weight (g), 0.20–14.50 Placenta size, greater than one-fourth to half fruit length/ greater than half fruit length	Bharath et al. (2013)
Central Brazil	30	22	*C. baccatum*	Fruit length (mm), 0 to >100 Fruit width (mm), 0 to >40 Fruit wall thickness (mm), 0.0 to >2.0 Average weight of 10 fruits (g), 0 to >12	Martinez et al. (2017)

TABLE 16.1 (*Continued*)

Region of study	No. of accessions	No. of characters studied	*Capsicum* species	Major findings	References
Nigeria	5	15		Fruit shape, elongate/triangular/round/bell-like	Zhigila et al. (2014)
				Mature fruit color, dark red/red/light red/orange	
			C. annuum var. *abbreviatum*	Fruit length (mm), 42.35–126.69	
			C. annuum var. *annuum*	Fruit width (mm),19.51–65.32	
			C. annuum var. *accuminatum*	Pedicel length (mm), 27.94–44.94	
			C. annuum var. *grossum*	seeds/fruit, 41.43–108.4	
			C. annuum var. *glabriusculum*		
Northwestern Mexico	17	12	*C. annuum* L. var. *glabriusculum*	Height of plant (cm), 53.0–249.0	López-España et al. (2016)
				Length of fruit (mm), 2.7–9.4	
				Width of fruit (mm), 2.4–7.2	
				Weight of fruit (mg), 2.8–130.6	
				Number of seeds per fruit, 1–25	
Nigeria	5	23	*C. annuum, C. frutescens*	Length of fruit (cm), 1.3–2.8	Aziagba (2015)
				Width of fruit (cm), 0.15–2.7	
				Fruit shape, ovoid/linear	
				Seeds/fruit, 4–10	
				Fruit color, yellow/red	
				Leaf length (cm), 5.4–9.9	
				Leaf width (cm), 4.2–5.0	

TABLE 16.1 (*Continued*)

Region of study	No. of accessions	No. of characters studied	*Capsicum* species	Major findings	References
India	9		*C. annuum, C. frutes-cens, C. chinense*	Floral characters Karyological studies	Jha and Saha (2016)
Korea	1	12	*Capsicum* sp.	Corolla color, white/ purple	Lu et al. (2012)
				Stem diameter (cm), 0.53–1.7	
				Leaf length (cm)- 5.17–18.83	
				Leaf width (cm), 2–8	
				Fruit length (cm), 3.5–14.43	
				Fruit width (cm), 1.43–4.53	
				Fruit wall thickness (cm), 1.53–4.8	
				Mean fruit weight (g), 4.31–40.92	
Brazil	347	50	*Capsicum* sp.	Stem color, shape, pubescence, length, and diameter; nodal anthocyanin (the whole plant); plant height, growth habit, and canopy width; branching habit; tillering; leaf density, color, shape, and pubescence; lamina margin; mature leaf length and width; number of flowers per axil; flower position; corolla color, spot color, shape, and length; anther color and length; filament color and length; Stigma exsertion; male sterility; calyx pigmentation, margin, and annular constriction; anthocyanin spots or stripes; fruit color at intermediate stage and mature stage; fruit shape, length, width, weight, wall thickness and surface; fruit shape at pedicel attachment; neck at base of	Barbieri et al. (2007)

TABLE 16.1 *(Continued)*

Region of study	No. of accessions	No. of characters studied	*Capsicum* species	Major findings	References
				fruit; fruit shape at blossom end and blossom end appendage; fruit cross-section corrugation; number of locules; ripe fruit persistence; seed color and surface; number of seeds per fruit.	
Brazil	49	13	*C. chinense*	Fruit length (mm), 14.15–76.22 Fruit width (mm), 8.69–42.89 Fruit fresh weight(g), 0.99–19.15 Extractable color (ASTA units), 30.35–595.84	Finger et al. (2010)
World wide	39	20	*C. annuum*	Corolla color, white, purple Flower position, pendant, intermediate, erect Fruit color at intermediate stage, light yellow/light green/ green/ deep green Mature fruit color, light red, red, dark red, brown Leaf color, green, dark green, dark purple Fruit shape, elongate, almost round, blocky Days to maturity, days to flowering, fruit maturation period, fruit length, fruit width, fruit weight, pericarp thickness, pedicel length, plant height, canopy width, arial fresh biomass, fruit number, fruit yield, harvest index	Geleta et al. (2005)
Italy	19		*C. annuum*	Plant height (cm), 57.3–125.8 Fruit length (cm), 2.6–12.5 Fruit width (cm), 1.14–2.61 Fruit weight (g), 3.1–14.5 Pericarp thickness (mm), 1.40–3.01	De Masi et al. (2007)

TABLE 16.1 (Continued)

Region of study	No. of accessions	No. of characters studied	Capsicum species	Major findings	References
India	139	8	C. annuum, C. frutescens, C. chinense	Fruit length (cm), 0.7–10.22	Sarpras et al. (2016)
				Fruit weight (g), 0.05–10.58	
				Seeds/fruit, 3–100	
				Seed weight, 0.035–0.071	
				Fruiting habit, pendant/erect	
				Fruit shape, elongated/almost round/block shaped/triangular/ovate/short slender	
				Fruit color at maturity, light red/yellow/dark red/red/orange/chocolate	
				Fruit shape at blossom end, pointed/ blunt/sunken	
India	56		C. annuum, C. frutescens, C. chinense	Plant growth habit, erect/intermediate/prostrate	Yumnam et al. (2012)
				Plant height (cm), 36–111	
				Corolla color, white/light yellow/yellow/yellow-green/ purple with white base/white with purple base/white with purple margin/purple	
				Fruit color at intermediate stage, white/yellow/green/yellow green/purple/deep purple	
				Fruit color at the mature stage, white/ lemon-yellow/pale orange-yellow/orange yellow/pale orange/orange/light red/red/dark red/purple/brown/black	
				Fruit shape, elongate/almost round/triangular/ campanulate/blocky (oblong)/star-shaped	
				Fruiting behavior, pendant/erect	
				Fruit width (cm), 0.6–4.54	
				Fruit surface, smooth/semi wrinkled/wrinkled	

TABLE 16.1 *(Continued)*

Region of study	No. of accessions	No. of characters studied	*Capsicum* species	Major findings	References
Turkey	6	10	*Capsicum* spp.	Fruit width (cm), 0.51–2.03	Yaldiz and
				Fruit length (cm), 2.91–6.12	Ozguven
				Plant height (cm), 51.02–94.98	(2011)
				Fruit/plant, 175.4–460.4	
				Yield/plant (g), 253.9–675.5	
				Yield (kg Ha^{-1}), 9412–24418	
Asia, America, Africa, and Europe	32		*Capsicum* spp.	Unripe fruit color, white/light green/green/dark green	Wahyuni et al. 2011
				Ripe fruit color, red/dark red/brown/dark brown/salmon/yellow/orange	
				Fruit shape, elongate/roundish/triangular/blocky (oblong)	
				Fruit size, very small/small/medium/large	
Brazil and Mexico	56	25	*Capsicum* spp.	Fruit length (cm), 2.7–10.3	Sudré et al. 2010
				Fruit diameter (cm), 1.0–3.5	
				Seed number per fruit, 26.2–155.5	
				Plant height (cm), 38.3–92.7	
				Canopy diameter (cm), 45.5–114.4	
				Weight of 1000 seeds (g), 3.3–5.7	
				Days to flowering, 36.6–71.3	
				Days to fruiting, 118.8–160.7	
				Fruit number per plant, 39.8–381.5	
				Fruit weight per plant (g), 238.2–1063.0	
				Fruit mean weight (g), 0.6–29.2	

TABLE 16.1 *(Continued)*

Region of study	No. of accessions	No. of characters studied	*Capsicum* species	Major findings	References
				Stem color, green/ green with purple stripes/ purple	
				Anther color, yellow/ pale blue/ blue/ purple	
				Corolla color, white/ purple/white with yellow-green spots/white-green/yellow with purple base/ purple with yellow base	
				Flower position, pendant/intermediate/erect	
				Immature fruit color, yellow/green/orange/purple	
				Mature fruit color, white/pale orange-yellow/ orange-yellow/pale orange/orange/light red/red/ dark red/purple	
				Fruit shape, elongate/almost round/triangular/ campanulate/blocky/ellipse/star shaped	
				Fruit surface, smooth/semiwrinkled/wrinkled	
				Number of locules, two/three/four	

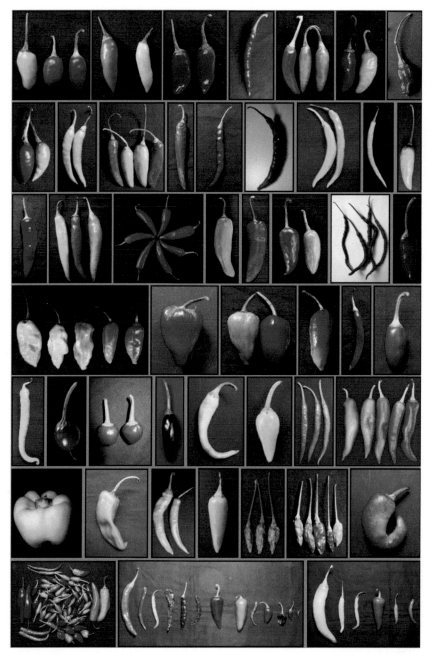

FIGURE 16.1 The wide range of variation in fruit morphology cultivated in different geographical regions.

Source: Paul et al. (2013).

C, vitamin E, and provitamin A are most abundant in chili fruits. Though their quantities showed wide variations, ripened fruits usually contained the maximum amounts (Wahyuni et al., 2011; Topuz and Ozdemir, 2007; Marín et al., 2004). The aforesaid parameters greatly influence the antioxidant activities of *Capsicum* fruits and, thereby, variations in these parameters lead to variable antioxidant activities (Dutta et al., 2016; Conforti et al.; 2007; Dubey et al., 2015). Nevertheless, sterols, triterpenes, organic acids, fatty acids, amino acids, oils, and volatile compounds are also reported to vary greatly in different accessions of chili fruits (Azabou et al., 2017; Gurnani et al. 2016). Variations in chili fruits often lead to qualitative variations in the products prepared and can lead to critical losses (Reilly et al., 2001). The major variations in chemical compounds including capsaicin, carotenoids, and vitamins among different accessions of capsicum are represented in Table 16.2. The identification of a suitable environment is prerequisite to cultivate specific pepper genotype with the highest quality of bioactive compounds. Since pungency is the key trait in capsicum, screening of variability of capsaicinoids content in different accessions would be not only helpful for researchers but to the pharmaceutical industries for commercial utilization.

16.4 ASSESSMENT OF MOLECULAR MARKER BASED GENETIC DIVERSITY

The characterization of genetically diverse germplasm is prerequisite in breeding programs for crop improvement strategies. This study will also be helpful to screen the elite clone for collection, maintenance, preservation, and utilization adequately. The characterization of germplasm serves essential link between the conservation and appropriate utilization of genetic resource (Paterson et al., 1991). Genetic diversity is usually analyzed by measurement of genetic distance, through which differences or similarities at the genetic level can be calculated efficiently. The analysis of molecular markers could be explored for genetic diversity analysis. The molecular marker-based genetic diversity analysis (MMGDA) play a pivotal role to identify different accessions of plants at the taxonomic level and evaluate diversity among species over different time point and geographic locations (Duwick 1984). The MMGDA including restriction fragment length polymorphism, random amplified polymorphic DNA (RAPD), simple sequence repeats (SSR), and amplified fragment length polymorphism (AFLP) are regularly being executed in analysis of genetic resources in different plant species

TABLE 16.2 The Wide Range of Variations of Different Chemical Constituents in Chili Fruits Cultivated in Different Geographical Locations.

Region of study	No. of accessions	Capsicum species	Parameters	Range	References
Mexico	13	*C. annuum*	Capsaicinoids ($\mu g \cdot g^{-1}$ DW)	250–1750	Rodriguez-Uribe et al. (2014)
			Dihydrocapsaicin ($\mu g \cdot g^{-1}$ DW)	146.7–1024.9	
			Capsaicin ($\mu g \cdot g^{-1}$ DW)	103.1–719.5	
			β-carotene ($\mu g \cdot g^{-1}$ DW)	5.0–22.0	
			β-cryptoxanthin ($\mu g \cdot g^{-1}$ DW)	29.9–87.8	
			Zeaxanthin ($\mu g \cdot g^{-1}$ DW)	73.8–169.0	
			Violaxanthin ($\mu g \cdot g^{-1}$ DW)	61.8–125.8	
			Capsanthin ($\mu g \cdot g^{-1}$ DW)	465.2–1006.8	
			Total carotenoids ($\mu g \cdot g^{-1}$ DW)	1697.7–3481.6	
Brazil	8	*C. annuum, C. chinense, C. baccatum*	Total carotenoids ($\mu g/g$)	59.86–1349.97	Carvalho et al. (2015)
			Vitamin C (mg/100 g)	82.55–264.13	
			Total phenolics (mg/100 g)	215.73–1103.20	
			Total anthocyanins (mg/100 g)	5.99–18.30	
			DPPH• (g/g DPPH)	1745.18–4905.06	
			ABTS+ (μM trolox/g)	46.79–113.08	
World-wide	101	*Capsicum* sp.	Chile pepper pungency (SHU)	1053.5–852404.6	Kantar et al. (2016)
			Vitamin A (IU/100 g pepper)	302.5–20840.0	
			Vitamin C (mg/100 g pepper)	11.85–195.75	
			Folate ($\mu g/100$ g pepper)	9.95–265.24	
India	139	*Capsicum* sp.	Total capsaicinoid (mg/g)	0.02–72.05	Islam et al. (2015)
			Pungency (SHU)	317–1,152,832	
			Capsaicin content (%)	25.52–83.10	
			Dihydrocapsaicin content (%)	16.9–74.48	
			Mean ratio of (Cap/Dhc)	0.33–4.92	

TABLE 16.2 *(Continued)*

Region of study	No. of accessions	Capsicum species	Parameters	Range	References
Spain	2	*Capsicum frutescens*	Betulin (mg/kg)	138.2–161.9	Silva et al. (2013)
			Campesterol (mg/kg)	42.3–54.1	
			Stigmasterol (mg/kg)	6.3–9.3	
			β-Sitosterol (mg/kg)	46.1–67.4	
			Organic acid (mg/kg)	8218.2–8527.4	
			Ascorbic acid (mg/kg)	66.6–230.4	
			Total fatty acid (mg/kg)	59104.9–59803.7	
			SFA (mg/kg)	30077.2–28140.3	
			MUFA (mg/kg)	6381.7–9200.2	
			PUFA (mg/kg)	22646.0–22463.2	
Peru and Bolivia	186	*Capsicum* sp.	Antioxidant capacity (mmol/100 g)	2.1–9.2	Zonneveld et al. (2015)
			Extractable color (ASTA)	1–146	
			Capsaicinoids (mg/100 g)	0.3–1244.3	
			Fat (g/100 g)	2.2–32.8	
			Flavonoids (mg/100 g)	0.4–46.8	
			Polyphenols (g/100 g)	1.09–3.69	
			Quercetin (mg/100 g)	0.4–42.6	
Peru, Guatemala, and Ecuador	5	*C. baccatum, C. pubescens, C. chinense*	Total capsaicinoid (mg/kg)	13–1605	Kollmannsberger et al. 2011
			Pungency (SHU)	200–23500	
			Capsaicin content (%)	33.6–83.0	
			Dihydrocapsaicin content (%)	13.9–43.3	
South Asia	6	*C. annuum, C. chinense*	Total capsaicinoid (SHU)	20867.4–187100.7	Gurung et al. (2012)
			Capsaicin content (SHU)	14047.3–115532.8	
			Dihydrocapsaicin content (SHU)	6820.0–74212.1	

TABLE 16.2 *(Continued)*

Region of study	No. of accessions	Capsicum species	Parameters	Range	References
Texas	7	*C. annuum, C. chinense, C. frutescens*	β-cryptoxanthin (µg/100 g)	131–973	Howard et al. (2000)
			α-carotene (µg/100 g)	222–2127	
			β-carotene (µg/100 g)	2–1187	
			Retinol equiv (RE/100 g)	0.33–336	
			Provitamin A (% RDA)	0.03–33.7	
			Capsanthin (µg/100 g)	984–20861	
			Lutein (µg/100 g)	61–955	
			Zeaxanthin (µg/100 g)	15–1958	
			Quercetin (mg/g)	0.88–64.47	
			Luteolin (mg/g)	1.75–81.30	
			Ascorbic Acid (mg/100 g)	74.55–202.40	
Peru	147	*Capsicum* spp.	Capsaicinoids (mg/100 g)	0.4–1560.1	Meckelmann et al. (2013)
			Nordihydrocapsaicin (mg/100 g)	0–81.5	
			Capsaicin (mg/100 g)	0.3–1074.3	
			Dihydrocapsaicin (mg/100 g)	0.2–459.8	
			Total Polyphenols (g GAE/100 g)	1.22–3.69	
			TEAC (mmol/100 g)	1.8–9.2	
			Ascorbic acid (mg/100 g)	0–295	
			Total Flavonoids (mg/100 g)	0.5–29.5	
			Quercetin (mg/100 g)	0.5–26.6	
			Luteolin (mg/100 g)	0.4–5.2	
			Extractable color (ASTA)	1–146	
			Fat (g/100 g)	2.2–19.6	
			Moisture (g/100 g)	0.4–6.6	

TABLE 16.2 *(Continued)*

Region of study	No. of accessions	Capsicum species	Parameters	Range	References
Mexico	4	*C. annuum*	Total protein (g/100 g DW)	13.4–15.5	Hervert-Hernández et al. (2010)
			Total fat (g/100 g DW)	7.4–13.2	
			Total dietary fiber (g/100 g DW)	27.9–41.7	
			Total polyphenols (mg/100 g DW)	2325.4–2843.5	
			Total carotenoids (mg/100 g DW)	87.6–373.3	
			FRAP (μmol TE/g DW)	37.5–66.5	
			ABTS (μmol TE/g DW)	18.6–36.4	
			β-carotene (mg/100 g DW)	7.3–85.7	
			β-cryptoxanthin (mg/100 g DW)	2.0–10.6	
			Zeaxanthin (mg/100 g DW)	0.9–10.3	
Peru	50	*Capsicum* sp.	Total terpenoids (%)	4.3–47.6	Patel et al. (2016)
			Copaene (%)	0.2–13.8	
			Limonene (%)	0.3–17.4	
			O-cymene (%)	0.3–7.9	
			Total esters (%)	1.6–72.0	
			n-hexyl hexanoate (%)	0.5–29.4	
			Total hydrocarbons (%)	1.9–71.8	
			2-methyl tridecane (%)	0.2–9.7	
			Pentadecane (%)	0.4–37.0	
			n-tetradecane (%)	0.2–5.3	
			Total aldehydes (%)	0.1–12.9	
			Cumaldehyde (%)	0.5–5.6	
			2-hexenal (%)	0.2–5.8	
			Total ketones	0.7–34.2	
			2-nonanone	0.4–23.8	

TABLE 16.2 *(Continued)*

Region of study	No. of accessions	Capsicum species	Parameters	Range	References
Peru	23	*Capsicum* sp.	Capsaicinoids (mg/100 g)	0.99–1515.53	Meckelmann et al. (2015a)
			Capsaicin (mg/100 g)	0.71–1199.10	
			Dihydrocapsaicin (mg/100 g)	0.29–307.89	
			Nordihydrocapsaicin (mg/100 g)	0.55–159.96	
			Total Polyphenols (g GAE /100 g)	1.34–2.77	
			TEAC (mmol/100 g)	2.0–7.0	
			Total Flavonoids (mg/100 g)	1.27–13.77	
			Quercetin (mg/100 g)	1.27–13.77	
			Luteolin (mg/100 g)	0.57–3.33	
			Tocopherols (mg/100 g)	0.23–29.09	
			α-Tocopherol (mg/100 g)	1.09–26.36	
			γ-Tocopherol (mg/100 g)	0.23–5.29	
			β-Tocopherol (mg/100 g)	0.03–0.78	
			Extractable color (ASTA)	3.50–94.23	
			Moisture (g/100 g)	0.43–2.60	
USA	90	*Capsicum* spp.	Capsaicin (mg/g)	0.00–2.89	Antonious and Jarret (2006)
			Dihydrocapsaicin (mg/g)	0.00–1.71	
Peru	32	*C. pubescens*	Capsaicinoids (mg/100 g)	55–410	Meckelmann et al. (2015b)
			Capsaicin (mg/100 g)	13–128	
			Dihydrocapsaicin (mg/100 g)	25–207	
			Nordihydrocapsaicin (mg/100 g)	9–122	
			Total Polyphenols (g GAE/100 g)	0.7–1.5	
			TEAC (mmol/100 g)	1.8–2.4	

TABLE 16.2 *(Continued)*

Region of study	No. of accessions	Capsicum species	Parameters	Range	References
			Total Flavonoids (mg/100 g)	2.4–4.6	
			Quercetin (mg/100 g)	6.8–16.9	
			Tocopherols (mg/100 g)	5.9–18.2	
			α-Tocopherol (mg/100 g)	0.1–1.8	
			γ-Tocopherol (mg/100 g)	0.0–0.2	
			β-Tocopherol (mg/100 g)	2.8–9.3	
			Extractable color (ASTA)	2–66	
			Moisture (g/100 g)	1.4–3.4	
India	136	*C. annuum, C. frutescens, C. chinense*	Capsaicinoids (µg/g DW)	168.5–64333.0	Sarpras et al. (2016)
			SHU	3188.4–1037305.0	
			Capsaicin (µg/g DW)	101.18–54543.0	
			Dihydrocapsaicin (µg/g DW)	5011.66–26455.189	
			Nordihydrocapsaicin (µg/g DW)	0.035–914.1	
			Nonivamide (µg/g DW)	0.006–816.7	
			Antioxdant activity (%)	3.52–81.78	
Netherlands	24	*C. annuum*	Glucose (g/100 g fw)	1.79–3.81	Eggink et al. (2012)
			Fructose (g/100 g fw)	1.89–3.75	
			Malic acid (mg/100 g fw)	11.71–159.27	
			Citric acid (mg/100 g fw)	185.7–609.7	
			Ascorbic acid (mg/100 g fw)	137.9–247.1	
India	30	*C. annuum*	Capsaicin content (%)	0.42–2.06	Yatung et al. (2014)
			Ascorbic acid (mg/100g)	175.23–328.26	
			Chlorophyll content (mg/g)	0.16–0.59	

TABLE 16.2 *(Continued)*

Region of study	No. of accessions	Capsicum species	Parameters	Range	References
Texas	12	*C. annuum*	Total Flavonoids (mg/100 g)	27.37–851.53	Lee et al. (1995)
			Quercetin (mg/100 g)	17.60–783.83	
			Luteolin (mg/100 g)	6.07–103.50	
			Ascorbic acid (mg/100g)	48.9–168.4	
			Total Polyphenols (mg/100 g)	178.2–384.9	
			Antioxidant activity (%)	50.1–81.5	
			Heat index	1–8	
Poland	4	*C. annuum*	Vitamin C (mg/100 g)	101.19–167.54	Perucka and Materska (2007)
			β-carotene (mg/100 g)	0.058–0.460	
			Xanthophylls (mg/100 g)	0.500–4.658	
			Phenolic compounds (mg/100 g)	37.54–67.35	
World-wide		*Capsicum* sp.	Vitamin C (mg/100 g)	76.1–243.1	Palevitch and Craker (1996)
			Vitamin E (μg/ g)	322–883	
Poland	4	*C. annuum*	Capsaicin (mg/g)	0.035–0.530	Materska and Perucka (2005)
			Dihydrocapsaicin (mg/g)	0.350–0.015	
Alabama	19	*C. annuum*	Ascorbic acid (mg/ 100g FW)	62–124	Simonne et al. (1997)
			Provitamin A (RE/ 100g FW)	29–127	
			Sodium (mg/ 100g DW)	7–12	
			Potassium (mg/ 100g DW)	80–139	
			Calcium (mg/ 100g DW)	3–6	
			Phosphorus (mg/ 100g DW)	9–18	
			Nitrogen (mg/ 100g DW)	335–743	
Côte d'Ivoire	5	*Capsicum* sp.	Beta carotene (μg/100 g FW)	68.47–535.98	Kouassi et al. (2012)
			Ascorbic acid (mg/100 g FW)	86.38–96.62	

(Williams et al., 1990; Vos et al., 1995; Meudt and Clarke, 2007; Agarwal et al., 2008). The studies of variation in phenotypic traits are essential for diversity analysis; they need to be corroborated with molecular markers to provide robust genetic diversity evaluations. A plethora of DNA markers has been developed and utilized for diversity analysis in capsicum germplasm from different geographic locations. Among the molecular markers, AFLP was first executed among 25 accessions in pepper from different locations of Mexico (Prince et al., 1992). In this pioneer work, principal component analysis combined with cluster analysis have revealed the significant correlation between genetic distance calculated through AFLP and distance measured through isozyme analysis. Subsequent to the above analysis, AFLP markers have been used in different chili germplasm for genetic diversity analysis (Aktas et al. 2009; Thul et al., 2006; Krishnamurthy et al., 2015; Islam et al., 2016; Prince et al. 1995; Wahyuni et al., 2013). The morphological classification of different *Capsicum* species was validated with germplasm analysis using RAPD and AFLP markers and these markers were also found to be helpful in identifications of different species of an accession. A comparative PCR-based molecular marker analysis was executed between 34 pepper cultivars of different geographic origin to assess the effectiveness between RAPD and AFLP markers (Paran et al., 1998). They have reported the higher efficiency of AFLP marker over RAPD and highlighted the divergence between the large-fruited sweet cultivars from the small-fruited pungent peppers using dendrogram based study. The AFLP markers combined with morphological traits were utilized to cluster different genotypes of *Capsicum* (Geleta et al., 2005). In another study, 134 accessions from six *Capsicum* species were genetically characterized using >100 RAPD markers at the Asian Vegetable Research and Development Center (Rodriguez et al., 1999). Due to the difficulty in scoring of major morphological traits used in the identification, they have deployed the diagnostic markers for better taxonomic characterization of *Capsicum* accessions. Lately, several studies have been executed by researchers throughout the world to assess genetic homology or diversity along with phylogenetic analysis using RAPD markers (Adetula 2006; Costa et al., 2006; Finger et al., 2010; Bhadragoudar and Patil 2011; Sitthiwong et al., 2005; Rad et al., 2009; Sanatombi et al., 2010; Thul et al., 2012). Among these different types of molecular markers, sequence-tagged microsatellite sites (STMS) based on microsatellite DNA loci have emerged as an important tool in molecular marker analysis. The variation in these microsatellite loci, termed as SSRs, have been comprehensively employed in plant genetics over the years due to their stability, codominance, multiallele genetic markers detection, as well as for better sensitivity (Mason 2015). However, single nucleotide polymorphisms (SNPs) analysis is an additional attractive molecular marker in breeding program. The SNPs are enormously abundant, mostly biallelic, easily scored and can be coupled with differences in phenotypic traits. The genetic diversity, along with structure of population of different accessions, was examined through a transcriptome-based SNPs marker and it was observed that *C. annuum* exhibited maximum diversity (Lee et al., 2016). The establishment of SNPs for genetic mapping, as well as for diversity analysis, were also executed by another group of researchers (Cheng et al., 2016). They have recognized SNP markers, constructed high-density genetic map, explored the genetic diversity of different capsicum species for the study of pepper molecular genetics and advanced breeding program. The pioneer work to develop polymorphic microsatellite markers of *Capsicum,* as well as molecular map, were executed in 2004 by a group of researchers (Lee et al., 2004). The investigators were able to successfully identify 32 microsatellite markers through screening of entire capsicum genome. Through EST-microsatellites analysis, polymorphism was detected between *C. annuum* cv TF68 and *C. chinense* cv Habanero. Consequently, SSR-based libraries were constructed from the *C. annum* genome and over six hundred unique SSR were detected (Minamiyama et al., 2006). Efficient breeding, as well as marker-assisted selection, could be executed through the construction of linkage map. In subsequent years, several groups of researchers have worked on pepper microsatellites markers to explore high-density linkage map in intra- and interspecific populations of *Capsicum* collected from different geographic locations (Ince et al., 2010; Mimura et al., 2012; Nagy et al., 2007; Patel et al., 2011; Rodrigues and Tam, 2010; Sugita et al., 2013; Huang et al. 2000; Yumnam et al., 2012; Ahn et al., 2013; Rana et al., 2014; Rivera et al., 2016). The genetic characterization along with interactions among different capsicum germplasm was analyzed through high-throughput genome-wide markers. Pepper GeneChip® array (Affymetrix) for analysis of genome-wide transcript-based markers was developed to evaluate capsicum's genetic polymorphism (Hill et al., 2013). The designed array offered maximum redundancy to detect single position polymorphism and more than 33,000 SSP markers were detected from 40 diverse *C. annuum* lines. The 'state-of-the-art' technology including next-generation sequencing was successfully deployed to the three pepper genotypes to identify SNPs and SSRs (Ashrafi et al., 2012). A large collection of transcriptomic data were analyzed through bioinformatics tools and thousands of SSRs and SNPs were detected among 65 *Capsicum* genotypes (Cheng et al., 2015). In order to explore genetic diversity among different pepper genotypes, SSRs combined with random amplified microsatellite polymorphism (RAMPO) markers were successfully deployed (Rai et al., 2013). Among them, 25 polymorphic SSR markers and seventeen RAMPO markers with better polymorphic information content were detected. The PCR-based molecular markers corroborated with EST-based markers has explored the genetic diversity in *Capsicum* germplasm and exposed the avenue towards mapping the populations. The comprehensive research work on the development of different types of molecular markers in *Capsicum* and their applications in genetic diversity analysis is represented in Table 16.3.

16.5   VARIATION IN DISEASE ETIOLOGY

Peppers fruits are susceptible to several pathogens including bacteria, fungi, mycoplasmas, viruses, insects, and nematodes that are major obstructive in yield of capsicum. On an average of about 40–60% yield losses can occur in chili worldwide due to various diseases (Ali, 2006; Mekonen and Chala, 2014). The intensity of disease etiology and types greatly vary on environmental condition as well as on geographic locations. *Colletotrichum* spp. causes chili anthracnose disease leading to degradation in quality and quantity of yield. *C. capsici* is the major pathogen causing this disease (Susheela, 2012; Chaisemsaeng et al., 2013; Than et al., 2008; Rao and Nandineni, 2017). The pathogenic bacteria *Xanthomonas campestris* produce the disease 'bacterial spot' and profusely affects the yield of peppers in high humid areas (Stall et al., 2009). It has been reported that 'scabby canker spots' was found in the pods of pepper due to the infection of the bacterium *Corynebacterium michiganense* (Volcani et al., 1970). The node of the pepper plants is susceptible to *Fusarium solani* (Fletcher, 1994). A devastating form of infection was recorded in pepper at higher humidity and temperature by the water mold *Phytophthora capsici* and *P. nicotianae* (Bosland and Lindsey, 1991; Alcantara and Bosland, 1994; Sy et al., 2005). It has been reported that *P. capsici* Leonian greatly induced wilting in different *Capsicum* sp. and it was rated as one of the most destructive diseases worldwide (Richins et al., 2010; García-Rodríguez et al., 2010; Gómez-Rodríguez et al., 2017). *Verticillium dahliae* is responsible for *Verticillium* wilt that possesses a serious threat to worldwide pepper production (Goicoechea, 2006; Gurung et al., 2015). Root rot of chili is instigated by *Rhizoctonia solani* Kuhn (Muhyi and Bosland, 1995). Among different types of the pathogen, the virus was found to be most serious disease problem in the tropic area (Green and Kim 1991; Naresh et al. 2017). Considerable economic losses are caused by pepper yellow

TABLE 16.3 The Wide Range of Variations of Different Chemical Constituents in chili Fruits Cultivated in Different Geographical Locations.

Region of study	No of accessions	Capsicum species	Parameters	Range	References
Mexico	13	*C. annuum*	Capsaicinoids (µg·g⁻¹ DW)	250– 1750	Rodriguez-Uribe et al. (2014)
			Dihydrocapsaicin (µg·g⁻¹ DW)	146.7–1024.9	
			Capsaicin (µg·g⁻¹ DW)	103.1–719.5	
			β-carotene (µg·g⁻¹ DW)	5.0–22.0	
			β-cryptoxanthin (µg·g⁻¹ DW)	29.9–87.8	
			Zeaxanthin (µg·g⁻¹ DW)	73.8–169.0	
			Violaxanthin (µg·g⁻¹ DW)	61.8– 125.8	
			Capsanthin (µg·g⁻¹ DW)	465.2– 1006.8	
			Total carotenoids (µg·g⁻¹ DW)	1697.7–3481.6	
Brazil	8	*C. annuum, C. chinense, C. baccatum*	Total carotenoids (µg/g)	59.86–1349.97	Carvalho et al. (2015)
			Vitamin C (mg/100 g)	82.55–264.13	
			Total phenolics (mg/100 g)	215.73–1103.20	
			Total anthocyanins (mg/100 g)	5.99–18.30	
			DPPH• (g/g DPPH)	1745.18–4905.06	
			ABTS+ (µM trolox/g)	46.79–113.08	
World-wide	101	*Capsicum* sp.	Chile Pepper Pungency (SHU)	1053.5– 852404.6	Kantar et al. (2016)
			Vitamin A (IU/100g pepper)	302.5–20840.0	
			Vitamin C (mg/100g pepper)	11.85– 195.75	
			Folate (µg/100g pepper)	9.95– 265.24	
India	139	*Capsicum* sp	Total capsaicinoid (mg/g)	0.02– 72.05	Islam et al. (2015)
			Pungency (SHU)	317– 1,152,832	
			Capsaicin content (%)	25.52– 83.10	
			Dihydrocapsaicin content (%)	16.9– 74.48	
			Mean ratio of (Cap/Dhc)	0.33– 4.92	

TABLE 16.3 *(Continued)*

Region of study	No of accessions	Capsicum species	Parameters	Range	References
Spain	2	*Capsicum frutescens*	Betulin (mg/kg)	138.2–161.9	Silva et al. (2013)
			Campesterol (mg/kg)	42.3–54.1	
			Stigmasterol (mg/kg)	6.3–9.3	
			β-Sitosterol (mg/kg)	46.1–67.4	
			Organic acid (mg/kg)	8218.2–8527.4	
			Ascorbic acid (mg/kg)	66.6–230.4	
			Total fatty acid (mg/kg)	59104.9–59803.7	
			SFA (mg/kg)	30077.2–28140.3	
			MUFA (mg/kg)	6381.7–9200.2	
			PUFA (mg/kg)	22646.0–22463.2	
Peru and Bolivia	186	*Capsicum* spp.	Antioxidant capacity (mmol/100g)	2.1–9.2	Zonneveld et al. (2015)
			Extractable color (ASTA)	1–146	
			Capsaicinoids (mg/100g)	0.3–1244.3	
			Fat (g/100g)	2.2–32.8	
			Flavonoids (mg/100g)	0.4–46.8	
			Polyphenols (g/100g)	1.09–3.69	
			Quercetin (mg/100g)	0.4–42.6	
Peru, Guatemala, and Ecuador	5	*C. baccatum, C. pubescens, C. chinense*	Total capsaicinoid (mg/kg)	13–1605	Kollmannsberget al. (2011)
			Pungency (SHU)	200–23500	
			Capsaicin content (%)	33.6–83.0	
			Dihydrocapsaicin content (%)	13.9–43.3	

TABLE 16.3 *(Continued)*

Region of study	No of accessions	Capsicum species	Parameters	Range	References
South Asia	6	*C. annuum, C. chinense*	Total capsaicinoid (SHU)	20867.4– 187100.7	Gurung et al. (2012)
			Capsaicin content (SHU)	14047.3– 115532.8	
			Dihydrocapsaicin content (SHU)	6820.0 – 74212.1	
Texas	7	*C. annuum, C. chinense, C. frutescens*	β-cryptoxanthin (μg/100 g)	131– 973	Howard et al. (2000)
			α-carotene (μg/100 g)	222– 2127	
			β-carotene (μg/100 g)	2–1187	
			Retinol equiv (RE/100 g)	0.33– 336	
			Provitamin A (% RDA)	0.03– 33.7	
			Capsanthin (μg/100 g)	984– 20861	
			Lutein (μg/100 g)	61–955	
			Zeaxanthin (μg/100 g)	15– 1958	
			Quercetin (mg/g)	0.88– 64.47	
			Luteolin (mg/g)	1.75– 81.30	
			Ascorbic Acid (mg/100 g)	74.55– 202.40	
Peru	147	*Capsicum* spp.	Capsaicinoids (mg/100 g)	0.4– 1560.1	Meckelmann et al. (2013)
			Nordihydrocapsaicin (mg/100 g)	0–81.5	
			Capsaicin (mg/100 g)	0.3– 1074.3	
			Dihydrocapsaicin (mg/100 g)	0.2– 459.8	
			Total Polyphenols (g GAE/100 g)	1.22– 3.69	
			TEAC (mmol/100 g)	1.8–9.2	
			Ascorbic acid (mg/100 g)	0–295	
			Total Flavonoids (mg/100 g)	0.5–29.5	
			Quercetin (mg/100 g)	0.5–26.6	

TABLE 16.3 *(Continued)*

Region of study	No of accessions	Capsicum species	Parameters	Range	References
Mexico	4	C. annuum	Luteolin (mg/100 g)	0.4–5.2	Hervert-Hernández et al. (2010)
			Extractable color (ASTA)	1–146	
			Fat (g/100 g)	2.2–19.6	
			Moisture (g/100 g)	0.4–6.6	
			Total protein (g/100 g DW)	13.4–15.5	
			Total fat (g/100 g DW)	7.4–13.2	
			Total dietary fiber (g/100 g DW)	27.9–41.7	
			Total polyphenols (mg/100 g DW)	2325.4–2843.5	
			Total carotenoids (mg/100 g DW)	87.6–373.3	
			FRAP (μmol TE/g DW)	37.5–66.5	
			ABTS (μmol TE/g DW)	18.6–36.4	
			β-Carotene (mg/100 g DW)	7.3–85.7	
			β-cryptoxanthin (mg/100 g DW)	2.0–10.6	
			Zeaxanthin (mg/100 g DW)	0.9–10.3	
Peru	50	Capsicum sp.	Total terpenoids (%)	4.3–47.6	Patel et al. (2016)
			Copaene (%)	0.2–13.8	
			Limonene (%)	0.3–17.4	
			O-cymene (%)	0.3–7.9	
			Total esters (%)	1.6–72.0	
			n-hexyl hexanoate (%)	0.5–29.4	
			Total hydrocarbons (%)	1.9–71.8	
			2-methyl tridecane (%)	0.2–9.7	

TABLE 16.3 *(Continued)*

Region of study	No of accessions	Capsicum species	Parameters	Range	References
			Pentadecane (%)	0.4–37.0	
			n-tetradecane (%)	0.2–5.3	
			Total aldehydes (%)	0.1–12.9	
			Cumaldehyde (%)	0.5–5.6	
			2-hexenal (%)	0.2–5.8	
			Total ketones	0.7–34.2	
			2-nonanone	0.4–23.8	
Peru	23	*Capsicum* sp.	Capsaicinoids (mg/100 g)	0.99–1515.53	Meckelmann et al. (2015a)
			Capsaicin (mg/100 g)	0.71– 1199.10	
			Dihydrocapsaicin (mg/100 g)	0.29–307.89	
			Nordihydrocapsaicin (mg/100 g)	0.55–159.96	
			Total Polyphenols (g GAE /100 g)	1.34– 2.77	
			TEAC (mmol/100 g)	2.0–7.0	
			Total Flavonoids (mg/100 g)	1.27–13.77	
			Quercetin (mg/100 g)	1.27–13.77	
			Luteolin (mg/100 g)	0.57–3.33	
			Tocopherols (mg/100 g)	0.23–29.09	
			α-Tocopherol (mg/100 g)	1.09–26.36	
			γ-Tocopherol (mg/100 g)	0.23– 5.29	
			β-Tocopherol (mg/100 g)	0.03– 0.78	
			Extractable color (ASTA)	3.50– 94.23	
			Moisture (g/100 g)	0.43– 2.60	

TABLE 16.3 *(Continued)*

Region of study	No of accessions	Capsicum species	Parameters	Range	References
USA	90	*Capsicum* spp.	Capsaicin (mg/g)	0.00– 2.89	Antonious and Jarret (2006)
			Dihydrocapsaicin (mg/g)	0.00– 1.71	
Peru	32	*C. pubescens*	Capsaicinoids (mg/100 g)	55–410	Meckelmann et al. (2015b)
			Capsaicin (mg/100 g)	13–128	
			Dihydrocapsaicin (mg/100 g)	25–207	
			Nordihydrocapsaicin (mg/100 g)	9–122	
			Total polyphenols (g GAE /100 g)	0.7–1.5	
			TEAC (mmol/100 g)	1.8–2.4	
			Total Flavonoids (mg/100 g)	2.4–4.6	
			Quercetin (mg/100 g)	6.8–16.9	
			Tocopherols (mg/100 g)	5.9–18.2	
			α-Tocopherol (mg/100 g)	0.1–1.8	
			γ-Tocopherol (mg/100 g)	0.0–0.2	
			β-Tocopherol (mg/100 g)	2.8–9.3	
			Extractable color (ASTA)	2–66	
			Moisture (g/100 g)	1.4–3.4	
India	136	*C. annuum, C. frutescens, C. chinense*	Capsaicinoids (µg/g DW)	168.5–64333.0	Sarpras et al. (2016)
			SHU	3188.4–1037305.0	
			Capsaicin (µg/g DW)	101.18–54543.0	
			Dihydrocapsaicin (µg/g DW)	5011.66–26455.189	
			Nordihydrocapsaicin (µg/g DW)	0.035– 914.1	
			Nonivamide (µg/g DW)	0.006–816.7	
			Antioxdant activity (%)	3.52– 81.78	

TABLE 16.3 *(Continued)*

Region of study	No of accessions	Capsicum species	Parameters	Range	References
Netherlands	24	*C. annuum*	Glucose (g/100 g fw)	1.79– 3.81	Eggink et al. (2012)
			Fructose (g/100 g fw)	1.89– 3.75	
			Malic acid (mg/100 g fw)	11.71– 159.27	
			Citric acid (mg/100 g fw)	185.7– 609.7	
			Ascorbic acid (mg/100 g fw)	137.9– 247.1	
India	30	*C. annuum*	Capsaicin content (%)	0.42– 2.06	Yatung et al. (2014)
			Ascorbic acid (mg/100g)	175.23– 328.26	
			Chlorophyll content (mg/g)	0.16– 0.59	
Texas	12	*C. annuum*	Total Flavonoids (mg/100 g)	27.37– 851.53	Lee et al. (1995)
			Quercetin (mg/100 g)	17.60– 783.83	
			Luteolin (mg/100 g)	6.07– 103.50	
			Ascorbic acid (mg/100g)	48.9– 168.4	
			Total Polyphenols (mg/100 g)	178.2– 384.9	
			Antioxidant activity (%)	50.1– 81.5	
			Heat index	1– 8	
Poland	4	*C. annuum*	Vitamin C (mg/100 g)	101.19–167.54	Perucka and Materska (2007)
			β-carotene (mg/100 g)	0.058– 0.460	
			Xanthophylls (mg/100 g)	0.500– 4.658	
			Phenolic compounds (mg/100 g)	37.54– 67.35	
World-wide		*Capsicum* sp.	Vitamin C (mg/100 g)	76.1– 243.1	Palevitch and Craker (1996)
			Vitamin E (µg/ g)	322–883	
Poland	4	*C. annuum*	Capsaicin (mg/g)	0.035– 0.530	Materska and Perucka (2005)
			Dihydrocapsaicin (mg/g)	0.350– 0.015	

TABLE 16.3 *(Continued)*

Region of study	No of accessions	Capsicum species	Parameters	Range	References
Alabama	19	*C. annuum*	Ascorbic acid (mg/ 100 g FW)	62–124	Simonne et al. (1997)
			Provitamin A (RE/ 100g FW)	29–127	
			Sodium (mg/ 100 g DW)	7–12	
			Potassium (mg/ 100 g DW)	80–139	
			Calcium (mg/ 100 g DW)	3–6	
			Phosphorus (mg/100 g DW)	9–18	
			Nitrogen (mg/100g DW)	335–743	
Côte d'Ivoire	5	*Capsicum* sp.	Beta carotene (µg/100 g FW)	68.47–535.98	Kouassi et al. (2012)
			Ascorbic acid (mg/100 g FW)	86.38–96.62	

mosaic virus, tobacco engraving virus, peppermint virus, tobacco mosaic virus, papaya leaf curl virus, cucumber mosaic virus, chili leaf curl virus, potato virus Y, and tomato leaf curl virus (Carvalho et al., 2017; Lucinda et al., 2012; Kumar et al., 2015; Senanayake et al., 2007; Srivastava et al., 2017). It has been reported that root-knot nematodes including *Meloidogyne* spp. and *Nacobbus aberrans* adversely affect the yield (Djian-Caporalino, 2012; Jones et al., 2013; Carvalho et al., 2017). Several accessions of *Capsicum* have been reported to be resistant to various pathogens including fungi (Kim, 2014), viruses (Naresh et al., 2017) and nematodes (Table 16.4). The extent of economic damages in pepper due to different biotic factors greatly vary with geographic locations along with type of pathogen. The use of fungicides or pesticides in field unable to decrease disease symptoms significantly. Therefore, the implementation of disease-resistant cultivars of pepper in very much essential to retain the quality of fruits.

16.6 CONCLUSIONS

The analysis of genetic resources of crop plants is vital for screening beneficial traits present within the enormous size of germplasm as well as for improvement in yield and stress resistance. The pepper is an important crop with versatile applications from vegetables to medicine. Therefore, we have explored the enormous variation in different *Capsicum* species grown in diverse agroclimatic environment for important traits including pungency, fruit size, and shape, resistance or susceptible to diseases. Nevertheless, due to the discrepancy in the major bioactive compounds including capsaicin, flavonoids, and vitamins among different accessions, it is pivotal to screen the potential genotypes with better phytochemical constituents toward improving the utilization of *Capsicum* species in pharmaceutical industries.

ACKNOWLEDGMENTS

The authors are thankful to Swami Kamalasthananda, Principal, Ramakrishna Mission Vivekananda Centenary College, Rahara, Kolkata (India), for the facilities provided as well as his continuous enthusiastic encouragement for the present study. The authors thank the Department of Biotechnology, Govt. of West Bengal for the financial assistance and research fellowships to AD. We are also thankful to DST-FIST for infrastructural support.

TABLE 16.4 List of Resistant Accessions of *Capsicum* sp. Against Different Pathogenic Organisms.

Accessions	Resistant against micro-organism	References
PI 439410, PI 555611	*Rhizoctonia solani*	Muhyi and Bosland (1995)
PI 201231, PI 201239, PI 593485, PI 439273 (top 5 of 37 resistant accessions)	*Phytophthora capsici*	Candole et al. (2010)
PI 187331, PI 123469, PI 201232, PI 188476, PI 201234	*Phytophthora capsici*	Kimble and Grogan (1960)
RTx638, RTxLB, 638xRT, RTx625, RTx625a, 638xNv;	*Phytophthora capsici*	Rodríguez Llanes et al. (2014)
PI 640833, PI 566811	*Phytophthora capsici*	Naegele et al. (2015)
CNPH-148, CM-334	*Phytophthora capsici*	Costa Ribeiro et al. (2012)
KC00807-1, KC01744, KC00937, PI201237-3, PI201237-4, PI566811-1, PI566811-2, PI593573-1, PI593573-3, PI640532-1, KC01322	*Phytophthora capsici*	Mo et al. (2014)
Italico II	*Phytophthora capsici*	Messaouda et al. (2015)
41-1, 41-2, 35-3	*Phytophthora capsici, Meloidogyne incognita, Nacobbus aberrans*	Gómez-Rodríguez et al. (2017)
PI 163192, PI 224451, PI 241670, PI 244670, PI 271322, PI 308787, PI 369994, PI 377688	*Xanthomonas campestris*	Kim (1988)
PI 123469, PI 201232, PI 201234, PI 224445, P 51, AC 2258, Riogrande, Gosung	*Phytophthora capsici*	Kim (1988)
DLS-Sel-10, WBC-Sel-5 and PBC-142	*Leaf curl virus*	Srivastava et al. (2017)
Paladin, Archimedes, AP4839	*Phytophthora capsici*	Krasnow et al. (2017)
Grif 9073, PI 281396, PI 281397, PI 438666, PI 439292, PI 439297, PI 555616, PI 594125	*Verticillium dahliae*	Gurung et al. (2015)
EC-631751, ACC-16, EC-631750	*Colletotrichum truncatum*	Katoch et al. (2017)
Chawa, Blanco, Maax, 'X'catic'	*Bemisia tabaci–Begomovirus complex*	Ballina-Gómez et al. (2013)

TABLE 16.4 *(Continued)*

Accessions	Resistant against micro-organism	References
5 lines (1; 6; 8; 11, 13) out of 18 hybrids between UENF 1381 and UENF 1421	*Xanthomonas euvesicatoria*	Moreira et al. (2015)
YG4, YG5, GMS x YG5, CMS x YG3	*Ralstonia solanacearum, Phytophthora capsici*	Abebe et al. (2016)
UENF 1718, UENF 1797	*Colletotricum gloeosporioides*	Silva et al. (2014)
Gola peshawari, Talhari, Harmal, Neelum, Burewala, Sanam, FSD-1	*Fusarium oxysporum f.sp. capsici*	Murtza et al. (2017)
PBC 80, PBC 81	*Colletotrichum gloeosporioides, C. acutatum*	Yoon et al. (2004)
P.I. 152225 from Peru, South Carolina No. 46252	*Tobacco-etch virus (TEV)*	Greenleaf (1953)
PBC 81,	*Colletotrichum capsici*	Prasath and Ponnuswami (2008)
BG2814-6	*Cucumber mosaic virus (CMV)*	Grube et al. (2000)
F1(PIX-044B-01-01 x Carolina Wonder, F1(PIX-044B-13-01 x Carolina Wonder), F1(PIM-013 x MYR-29-09-05), F1(PIX-045B-32-03 x MYR- 29-09-05), F1(PIX-052B-06-01 x MYR-29-09-05)	*Phytophthora capsici, Pepper yellow mosaic virus (PepYMV), Meloidogyne incognita*	Carvalho et al. (2017)
F1 (IHR 2451 x IHR 500), F1 (IHR 4503 x IHR 2451), F1 (IHR 4503 x IHR 500), F1 (IHR 2451 x IHR 500), F1 (IHR 3849 x IHR 2451), F1 (IHR 3849 x IHR 500)	*Cucumber mosaic virus (CMV), Chilli veinal mottle virus (ChiVMV)*	Naresh et al. (2016)

KEYWORDS

- **genetic resources**
- **chili, germplasm**
- **morphological diversity**
- **chemical diversity**
- **genetic diversity**
- **disease etiology**

REFERENCES

Abebe, A. M.; Wai, K. P. P.; Siddique, M. I.; Mo, H. S.; Yoo, H. J.; Jegal, Y.; Byeon, S. E.; Jang, K. S.; Jeon, S. G.; Hwang, J. E.; Kim, B. S. Evaluation of *Phytophthora* Root Rot and Bacterial Wilt-resistant Inbred Lines and Their Crosses for Use as Rootstocks in Pepper (*Capsicum annuum* L.). *Hortic. Environ. Biotechnol.* **2016,** *57,* 598–605.

Adetula, O. Genetic Diversity of Capsicum Using Random Amplified Polymorphic DNAs. *Afr. J. Biotech.* **2006,** *5,* 120–122.

Agarwal, M.; Shrivastava, N.; Padh, H.; Advances in Molecular Marker Techniques and Their Applications in Plant Sciences. *Plant Cell Rep.* **2008,** *27,* 617–631.

Ahn, Y.; Tripathi, S.; Cho, Y.; Kim, J.; Lee, H.; Kim, D.; Woo, J.; Cho, M. De novo Transcriptome Assembly and Novel Microsatellite Marker Information in *Capsicum annuum* Varieties Saengryeg 211 and Saengryeg 213. *Bot Stud.* **2013,** *54,* 58.

Aktas, H.; Abak, K.; Sensoy, S. Genetic Diversity in Some Turkish Pepper (*Capsicum annuum* L.) Genotypes Revealed by AFLP Analyses. *Afr. J. Biotech.* **2009,** *8,* 4378–4386.

Alcantara, T. P.; Bosland, P. W. An Inexpensive Disease Screening Technique for Foliar Blight of Chile Pepper Seedlings. *HortScience* **1994,** *29,* 1182−1183.

Ali, M. Chili (Capsicum spp.) Food Chain Analysis: Setting Research Priorities in Asia. Shanhua, Taiwan: AVRDC-The World Vegetable Center, Technical Bulletin. 2006, 38, 253.

Andrews, J. *Peppers: The Domesticated Capsicums*; University of Texas Press: Austin, TX, USA, 1995; p 274.

Antonious, G. F.; Jarret, R. L. Screening *Capsicum* Accessions for Capsaicinoids Content. *J. Environ. Sci. Health B.* **2006,** *41,* 717–729.

Ashrafi, H.; Hill, T.; Stoffel, K.; Kozik, A.; Yao, J.; Chin, W. S. R.; Deynze, A. V. *De novo* Assembly of the Pepper Transcriptome (*Capsicum annuum*): A Benchmark for in Silico Discovery of SNPs, SSRs and Candidate Genes. *BMC Genomics* **2012,** *13,* 571.

Azabou, S.; Taheur, F. B.; Jridi, M.; Bouaziz, M.; Nasri, M. Discarded Seeds from Red Pepper (*Capsicum annum*) Processing Industry as a Sustainable Source of High Added-value Compounds and Edible Oil. *Environ. Sci. Pollut. Res.* **2017,** *24,* 22196−22203.

Aziagba, B. O. Macro Morphological Observations in *Capsicum* Varieties Cultivated in Awka Anambre State South Eastern Nigeria. *Am. J. Life. Sci. Res.* **2015,** *3,* 30–34.

Baba, V. Y.; Rocha, K. R.; Gomes, G. P.; Ruas, C. F.; Ruas, P. M.; Rodrigues, R.; Gonçalves, L. S. A. Genetic Diversity of *Capsicum chinense* Accessions Based on Fruit Morphological Characterization and AFLP Markers. Genet. *Res. Crop Evol.* **2015**, *63*, 1371−1381.

Ballina, G. H.; Latournerie, M. L.; Ruíz, S. E.; Pérez, G. A.; Rosado, L. G. Morphological Characterization of *Capsicum annuum* L. Accessions from Southern Mexico and their Response to the *Bemisia tabaci-Begomovirus* Complex. *Chilean. J. Agric. Res.* **2013**, *73*, 329−338.

Barbieri, R. L.; Heiden, G.; Neitzke, R. S.; Choer, E.; Leite, D. L.; Garrastazu, M. C. *Capsicum* Gene Bank of Southern Brazil. *Acta Hortic.* **2007**, *745*, 319–322.

Bernal, M. A.; Calderon, A. A.; Pedreno, M. A.; Muñoz, R.; Ros, B. A. Capsaicin Oxidation by Peroxidase from *Capsicum annuum* (variety *annuum*) Fruits. *J. Agric. Food Chem.* **1993**, *41*, 1041−1044.

Bhadragoudar, M. R.; Patil, C. G. Assessment of Genetic Diversity Among *Capsicum annuum* L. genotypes Using RAPD Markers. *Afr. J. Biotechnol.* **2011**, *10*, 17477–17483.

Bharath, S. M.; Cilas, C.; Umaharan, P. Fruit Trait Variation in a Caribbean Germplasm Collection of Aromatic Hot Peppers (*Capsicum chinense* Jacq.). *Hort. Sci.* **2013**, *48*, 531–538.

Bianchi, P. A.; Dutra, I. P.; Moulin, M. M.; Santos, J. O.; Santos, J. A. C. Morphological Characterization and Analysis of Genetic Variability Among Pepper Accessions. *Ciência Rural.* **2016**, *46*, 1151−1157.

Bosland P. W. Capsicums: Innovative Uses of an Ancient Crop. Progress in New Crops. ASHS Press: Arlington, VA, 1996; pp 479–487.

Bosland, P. W.; Baral, J. B. 'Bhut Jolokia'—The world's Hottest Known Chile Pepper is a Putative Naturally Occurring Interspecific Hybrid. *HortScience* **2007**, *42*, 222−224.

Bosland, P. W., Lindsey, D. L. A Seedling Screen for *Phytophthora* Root Rot of Pepper, *Capsicum annuum. Plant Dis.* **1991**, *75*, 1048−1050.

Bosland, P. W.; Votava E. J. Peppers: Vegetable and spice Capsicums. *Crops Prod. Sci. Hortic.* **2012**, *12*, 1–11.

Butcher, J. D.; Crosby, K. M.; Yoo, K. S.; Patil, B. S.; Ibrahim, A. M. H.; Leskovar D. I.; Jifon, J. L. Environmental and Genotypic Variation of Capsaicinoid and Flavonoid Concentrations in Habanero (*Capsicum chinense*) Peppers. *HortScience* **2012**, *47*, 574–579.

Candole, B. L.; Conner P. J.; Ji P. Screening *Capsicum annuum* Accessions for Resistance to Six Isolates of Phytophthora capsici. *HortScience* **2010**, *45*, 254–259.

Careaga, M.; Fernández, E.; Dorantes, L.; Mota, L.; Jaramillo, M. E.; Hernandez, S. H. Antibacterial Activity of *Capsicum* Extract Against *Salmonella typhimurium* and *Pseudomonas aeruginosa* Inoculated in Raw Beef Meat. *Int. J. Food Microbiol.* **2003**, *83*, 331–335.

Carvalho, A. V.; Mattietto, R. A.; Rios, A. O.; Maciel, R. A.; Moresco, K. S.; Oliveira, T. C. S. Bioactive Compounds and Antioxidant Activity of Pepper (*Capsicum* sp.) Genotypes. *J. Food Sci. Technol.* **2015**, *52*, 7457–7464.

Carvalho, R. C.; Nogueira, D. W.; Ticona, B. C. A.; Nogueira, D. G.; Maluf, W. R.; Gonçalves, R. J. S.; Silva L. F. L. Assessment of Resistances to Multiple Pathogens in Experimental Sweet Pepper Hybrids. *Hortic. Bras.* **2017**, *35*, 048–056.

Caterina, M. J.; Leffler, A.; Malberg, A. B.; Martin, W. J.; Trafton, J.; Petersen, Z. K. R.; Koltzenburg, M.; Basbaum, A. I.; Julius, D. Impaired Nociception and Pain Sensation in Mice Lacking the Capsaicin Receptor. *Science* **2000**, *288*, 306−313.

Chaisemsaeng, P.; Mongkolthanaruk, W.; Bunyatratchata, W. Screening and Potential for Biological Control of Anthracnose Disease (*Colletotrichum capsici*) on Chili Fruits by Yeast Isolates. *J. Life Sci. Technol.* 2013, *1*, 201–204.

Cheng, J.; Qin, C.; Tang, X.; Zhou, H.; Hu, Y.; Zhao, Z.; Cui, J.; Li, B.; Wu, Z.; Yu, J., Hu, K. Development of a SNP Array and its Application to Genetic Mapping and Diversity Assessment in Pepper (*Capsicum* spp.). Sci. Rep. **2016**, *6*.

Cheng, J.; Zhao, Z.; Li, B., Qin, C.; Wu, Z.; Trejo, S. D. L.; Luo, X.; Cui, J.; Rivera, B. R. F.; Li, S.; Hu, K. A Comprehensive Characterization of Simple Sequence Repeats in Pepper Genomes Provides Valuable Resources for Marker Development in *Capsicum*. *Sci. Rep.* **2015**, *6*.

Cichewicz, R. H. The Antimicrobial Properties of Chile Peppers (*Capsicum* species) and Their Uses in Mayan Medicine. *J. Ethnopharmacol.* **1996**, *52*, 61–70.

Conforti, F., Statti, G. A., Menichini, F. Chemical and Biological Variability of hot Pepper Fruits (*Capsicum annuum* var. *acuminatum* L.) in Relation to Maturity Stage. *Food Chem.* **2007**, *102*, 1096–1104.

Cooke, R. J.; Bredemeijer, G. M. M.; Ganal, M. W.; Peeters, R.; Isaac, P.; Rendell, S.; Jackson, J.; Röder M. S.; Korzun V.; Wendehake K.; Areshchenkova T. Assessment of the Uniformity of Wheat and Tomato Varieties at DNA Microsatellite Loci. *Euphytica* **2003**, *132*, 331–342.

da Costa, F. R.; Pereira, T. N. S.; Vitória, A. P.; de Campos, K. P.; Rodrigues, R, da Silva, D. H.; Pereira, M. G. Genetic Diversity Among *Capsicum* Accessions Using RAPD Markers. *Crop Breed. Appl. Biotechnol.* **2006**, *6*, 18–23.

da Costa Ribeiro, C. S.; Bosland, P. W. Physiological Race Characterization of *Phytophthora capsici* Isolates from Several Host Plant Species in Brazil Using New Mexico Recombinant Inbred Lines of *Capsicum annuum* at Two Inoculum Levels. *J. Amer. Soc. Hort. Sci.* **2012**, *137*, 421–426.

Davis C. B.; Markey C. E.; Busch M. A.; Busch K. W. Determination of Capsaicinoids in Habanero Peppers by Chemometric Analysis of UV Spectral Data. *J. Agric. Food Chem.* **2007**, *55*, 5925–5933.

De Masi, L.; Siviero, P.; Castaldo, D.; Cautela, D.; Esposito, C.; Laratta, B. Agronomic, Chemical and Genetic Profiles of Hot Peppers (*Capsicum annuum* ssp.). *Mol. Nutr. Food Res.* **2007**, *51*, 1053–1062.

Demirbilek, S.; Ersoy M. O.; Demirbilek, S.; Karaman, A.; Gurbuz, N.; Bayraktar, N.; Bayraktar, M. Small-dose Capsaicin Reduces Systemic Inflammatory Responses in Septic Rats. *Anesth. Analog.* **2004**, *99*, 1501–1507.

Djian, C. C. Root-knot Nematodes (*Meloidogyne* spp.), A Growing Problem in French Vegetable Crops, *EPPO Bulletin* **2012**, *42*, 127–137.

Dubey, R. K.; Singh, V.; Upadhyay, G.; Pandey, A. K.; Prakash, D. Assessment of Phytochemical Composition and Antioxidant Potential in Some Indigenous Chilli Genotypes from North East India. *Food Chem.* **2015**, *188*, 119–125.

Dutta, S. K.; Singh, S. B.; Saha, S.; Akoijam, R. S.; Boopathi, T.; Banerjee, A.; Roy, S. Diversity in Bird's Eye Chilli (*Capsicum frutescens* L.) landraces of North-East India in Terms of Antioxidant Activities. *Proc. Nat. Acad. Sci. India* Sect B 1–10. **2016**.

Duwick, D. N. Genetic Diversity in Major Farm Crops on the Farm and Reserve. *Econ. Bot.* **1984**, *32*, 161–178.

Eggink, P. M.; Maliepaard, C.; Tikunov, Y.; Haanstra, J. P. W.; Bovy, A. G.; Visser, R. G. F. A Taste of Sweet Pepper: Volatile and Non-volatile Chemical Composition of Fresh Sweet Pepper (*Capsicum annuum*) in Relation to Sensory Evaluation of *Taste. Food Chem.* **2012**, *132*, 301–310.

Esquinas-Alcázar, J. Science and Society: Protecting Crop Genetic Diversity for Food Security: Political, Ethical and Technical Challenges. *Nat. Rev. Genet.* **2005**, *6*, 946–953.

FAOSTAT. (2013). www.fao.org

Finger, F. L.; Lannes, S. D.; Schuelter, A. R.; Doege, J.; Comerlato, A. P.; Gonçalves, L. S. A.; Ferreira,, F. R. A.; Clovis L. R.; Scapim, C. A. Genetic Diversity of *Capsicum chinensis* (Solanaceae) Accessions Based on Molecular Markers and Morphological and Agronomic Traits. *Genet. Mol. Res.* **2010,** 9, 1852–1864.

Fletcher, J. T. *Fusarium* Stem and Fruit Rot of Sweet Peppers in the Glasshouse. *Plant Pathol.* **1994,** *43,* 225–227.

Ganguly, R. P.; Bhat, K. V. Analysis of Economically Important Morphological Traits Diversity in *Vigna radiata*. National Research Centre on DNA Fingerprinting, Agricultural Research Institute, New Delhi, 2012.

García, R. M.; Chiquito, A. E.; Loeza, L. P. D.; Godoy, H. H.; Villordo, P. E.; Pons, H. J. L.; Anaya, L. J. L. Producción de chile ancho injertado sobre criollo de Morelos 334 para el control de *Phytophthora capsici*. *Agrociencia* **2010,** *44,* 701–709.

Geleta, L. F.; Labuschagne, M. T.; Viljoen, C. D. Genetic Variability in Pepper (*Capsicum annuum* L.) Estimated by Morphological Data and Amplified Fragment Length Polymorphism Markers. *Biodivers. Conserv.* **2005,** *14,* 2361–2375.

Goicoechea, N. *Verticillium*-induced Wilt in Pepper: Physiological Disorders and Perspectives for Controlling the Disease. *Plant Pathol. J.* **2006,** *5,* 258–265.

Gómez, R. O.; Corona, T. T.; Heber Aguilar, R. V. Differential Response of Pepper (*Capsicum annuum* L.) Lines to *Phytophthora capsici* and Root-knot Nematodes. *Crop Prot.* **2017,** *92,* 148–152.

Green, S. K.; Kim, J. S. Characteristics and Control of Viruses Infecting Peppers: A Literature Review. Asian Vegetable Development Center Technical Bulletin, 1991, 18, 60.

Greenleaf, W. H. Effects of Tobacco-etch Virus on Peppers (*Capsicum* sp.). *Phytopathology* **1953,** *43,* 564–570.

Grube, R. C.; Zhang, Y.; Murphy, J. F.; Loaiza, F. F.; Lackney, V. K.; Provvidenti, R.; Jahn, M. K. New Source of Resistance to *Cucumber mosaic virus* in *Capsicum frutescens*. *Plant Dis.* **2000,** *84,* 885–891.

Gurnani, N.; Gupta, M.; Mehta, D.; Mehta, B. K. Chemical Composition, Total Phenolic and Flavonoid Contents, and In Vitro Antimicrobial and Antioxidant Activities of Crude Extracts from Red Chilli Seeds (*Capsicum frutescens* L.). *J. Taibah. Univ. Sci.* **2016,** *10,* 462–470.

Gurung, S.; Short, D. P. G.; Hu. X.; Sandoya, G. V.; Hayes, R. J.; Subbarao K. V.; Screening of Wild and Cultivated *Capsicum* Germplasm Reveals New Sources of *Verticillium* Wilt Resistance. *Plant Dis.* **2015,** *99,* 1404–1409.

Gurung, T.; Techawongstien, S.; Suriharn, B.; Techawongstien, S. Stability Analysis of Yield and Capsaicinoids Content in Chili (*Capsicum* spp.) Grown Across Six Environments. *Euphytica* **2012,** *187,* 11–18.

Guzman, I.; Hamby, S.; Romero, J.; Bosland, P. W.; O'Connell, M. A. Variability of Carotenoid Biosynthesis in Orange Colored *Capsicum* spp. *Plant Sci.* **2010,** *179,* 49–59.

Hageman, C.; Fahselt, D. Enzyme Electromorph Variation in the Lichen Family Umbilicariaceae: Within Stand Polymorphism in Umbilicate Lichens of Eastern Canada. *Can. J. Bot.* **1990,** *68,* 2636–2643.

Hammer, K.; Arrowsmith, N.; Gladis, T. Agrobiodiversity with Emphasis on Plant Genetic Resources. *Naturwissenschaften* **2003,** *90,* 241–250.

Henderson, D. E.; Slickman, A. M.; Henderson, S. K. Quantitative HPLC Determination of the Antioxidant Activity of Capsaicin on the Formation of Lipid Hydroperoxides of

Linoleic Acid: A Comparative Study Against BHT and Melatonin. *J. Agric. Food Chem.* **1999**, *47*, 2563–2570.

Hervert, H. D.; Sáyago, A. S. G.; Goñi, I. Bioactive Compounds of Four Hot Pepper Varieties (*Capsicum annuum* L.), Antioxidant Capacity, and Intestinal Bioaccessibility. *J. Agric. Food. Chem.* **2010**, *58*, 3399–3406.

Hill, T. A.; Ashrafi, H.; Reyes, C. W. S.; Yao, J.; Stoffel, K.; Truco, M. J.; Kozik, A.; Michelmore, R. W.; Van Deynze, A. Characterization of *Capsicum annuum* Genetic Diversity and Population Structure Based on Parallel Polymorphism Discovery with a 30K Unigene Pepper Gene Chip. *PLoS One* **2013**, *8*.

Hogaboam, C. M.; Wallace, J. L. Inhibition of Platelet Aggregation by Capsaicin. An Effect Unrelated to Actions on Sensory Afferent Neurons. *Eur. J. Pharmacol.* **1991**, *202*, 129–131.

Howard, L. R.; Talcott, S. T.; Brenes, C. H.; Villalon, B. Changes in Phytochemical and Antioxidant Activity of Selected Pepper Cultivars (*Capsicum* species) as Influenced by Maturity. *J. Agric. Food Chem.* **2000**, *48*, 1713–1720.

Huang, S.; Zhang, B.; Milbourne, D.; Cardle, L.; Yang, G.; Guo, J. Development of Pepper SSR Markers from Sequence Databases. *Euphytica* **2000**, *117*, 163–167.

Ince, A. G.; Karaca, M.; Onus, A. N. Polymorphic Microsatellite Markers Transferable Across *Capsicum* Species. *Plant Mol. Biol. Rep.* **2010**, *28*, 285–291.

Islam, M. A.; Sharma, S. S.; Sinha, P.; Negi, M. S.; Neog, B.; Tripathi, S. B. Variability in Capsaicinoid Content in Different Landraces of *Capsicum* Cultivated in North-eastern India. *Sci Hort.* **2015**, *183*, 66–71.

Islam, M. A.; Sinha, P.; Sharma, S. S.; Negi, M. S.; Neog B.; Tripathi S. B. Analysis of Genetic Diversity and Population Structure in *Capsicum* Landraces from North Eastern India Using TE-AFLP Markers. *Plant Mol. Biol. Rep.* **2016**, *34*, 869–875.

Jarret, R. L.; Bolton, J.; Perkins, B. A *Capsicum annuum* Pepper Germplasm Containing High Concentrations of Capsinoids. *Hortscience* **2014**, *49*, 107–108.

Jha, T. B.; Saha, P. S. Characterization of Some Indian Himalayan Capsicums Through Floral Morphology and EMA-based Chromosome Analysis. *Protoplasma* **2017**, *254*, 921–933.

Jones, J. T.; Haegeman, A.; Danchin, E. G.; Gaur, H. S.; Helder, J.; Jones, M. G.; Kikuchi, T.; Manzanilla, L. R.; Palomares, R. J. E.; Wesemael, W. M.; Perry, R. N. Top 10 Plant Parasitic Nematodes in Molecular Plant Pathology. *Mol. Plant Pathol.* **2013**, *14*, 946–961.

Kaale, E.; Van Schepdael, A.; Roets, E.; Hoogmartens, J. Determination of Capsaicinoids in Topical Cream by Liquid–liquid Extraction and Liquid Chromatography. *J. Pharm. Biomed. Anal.* **2002**, *30*, 1331–1337.

Kantar, M. B.; Anderson, J. E.; Lucht, S. A.; Mercer, K.; Bernau, V.; Case, K. A.; Le, N. C.; Frederiksen, M. K.; De Keyser, H. C.; Wong, Z. Z.; Hastings, J. C. Vitamin Variation in *Capsicum* spp. Provides Opportunities to Improve Nutritional Value of Human Diets. *PloS One* **2016**, *11* (8), e0161464. doi: 10.1371/journal.pone.0161464.

Katoch, A.; Sharma, P.; Padder, B. A.; Sharma, P. N. Population Structure of *Colletotrichum truncatum* in Himachal Pradesh and Identification of broad-Spectrum Resistant Sources in *Capsicum*. *Agric. Res.* **2017**, *6* (3), 296–303.

Kehie, M.; Kumaria, S.; Tandon, P. *In vitro* Plantlet Regeneration from Nodal Segments and Shoot Tips of *Capsicum chinense* jacq. *cv*. Naga King chili. *3 Biotech.* **2012**, *2*, 31–35.

Khan, F. A.; Mahmood, T.; Ali, M.; Saeed, A.; Maalik A. Pharmacological Importance of an Ethnobotanical Plant: *Capsicum annuum* L. *Nat. Prod. Res.* **2014**, *28*, 1267–1274.

Kim, B. S. Characteristics of Bacterial Spot Resistant Lines and Phytophthora Blight Resistant Line of Capsicum Pepper. *J. Korean. Soc. Hort. Sci.* **1988**, *29*, 247–252.

Kim, B. S. Phytophthora Blight of Pepper and Genetic Control of the Disease. *Curr. Res. Agric. Life Sci.* **2014**, *32*, 111–117.

Kimble, K. A.; Grogan, R. G. Resistance to *Phytophthora* Root Rot in Pepper. *Phytopathology* **1960**, 50.

Kobata, K.; Kawamura, M.; Toyoshima, M.; Tamura, Y.; Ogawa, S.; Watanabe, T. Lipase Catalyzed Synthesis of Capsaicin Analogs by Amidation of Vanillylamine with Fatty Acid Derivatives. *Biotechnol. Lett.* **1998**, *20*, 451⁻454.

Kollmannsberger, H.; Rodríguez, B. A.; Nitz, S.; Nuez, F. Volatile and Capsaicinoid Composition of ají (*Capsicum baccatum*) and Rocoto (*Capsicum pubescens*), Two Andean Species of Chile Peppers. *J. Sci. Food Agr.* **2011**, *91*, 1598–1611.

Kothari, S. L.; Joshi, A.; Kachhwaha, S.; Ochoa, A. N. Chilli Peppers: A Review on Tissue Culture and Transgenesis. *Biotechnol. Adv.* **2010**, *28*, 35–48.

Kouassi, C. K.; Nanga, Z. Y.; Lathro, S. J.; Aka, S.; Koffi Nevry, R. Bioactive Compounds and Some Vitamins from Varieties of Pepper (*Capsicum*) Grown in Côte d'Ivoire. *Pure Appl. Biol.* **2012**, *1*, 40.

Kozukue, N.; Han, J. S.; Kozukue, E.; Lee, S. J.; Kim, J. A.; Lee, K. R.; Levin, C. E.; Friedman, M. Analysis of Eight Capsaicinoids in Peppers and Pepper-Containing Foods by High-performance Liquid Chromatography and Liquid Chromatography⁻mass Spectrometry. *J. Agric. Food Chem.* **2005**, *53*, 9172–9181.

Krasnow. C. S.; Wyenandt. A. A.; Kline. W. L.; Carey. J. B.; Hausbeck. M. K. Evaluation of Pepper Root Rot Resistance in an Integrated *Phytophthora* Blight Management Program. *HortTechnology* **2017**, *27*, 408–415.

Krishnamurthy, S. L.; Prashanth, Y.; Rao, A. M.; Reddy, K. M.; Ramachandra, R. Assessment of AFLP Marker Based Genetic Diversity in Chilli (*Capsicum annum* L. & *C. baccatum* L.). *Indian J. Biotechnol.* **2015**, *14*, 49–54.

Kumar, R. V.; Singh, A. K.; Singh, A. K.; Yadav, T.; Basu, S.; Kushwaha, N.; Chattopadhyay, B.; Chakraborty, S. Complexity of Begomovirus and Betasatellite Populations Associated with Chilli Leaf Curl Disease in India. *J. Gen. Virol.* **2015**, 96.

Kundu, S.; Das, A.; Ghosh B. Modulation of Pungency and Major Bioactive Compounds in Pepper Due to Agro-climatic Discrepancy: A Case Study with *Capsicum chinense* Bhut Jolokia Fruit. *Int. J. Pharm. Sci.* **2015**, *7*, 294⁻298.

Lanteri, S.; Acquadro, A.; Quagliotti, L.; Portis, E. RAPD and AFLP Assessment of Variation in a Landrace of Pepper (*Capsicum annuum* L.) Grown in North-West Italy. *Genet Res. Crop Evol.* **2003**, *50*, 723–735.

Lee, H.; Ro, N.; Jeong, H.; Kwon, J.; Jo, J.; Ha, Y.; Jung, A.; Han, J.; Venkatesh, J.; Kang, B. Genetic Diversity and Population Structure Analysis to Construct a Core Collection from a Large *Capsicum* Germplasm. *BMC Genetics* **2016**, *17*, 142.

Lee, J. J.; Crosby, K. M.; Pike, L. M.; Yoo, K. S.; Leskovar, D. I. Impact of Genetic and Environmental Variation on Development of Flavonoids and Carotenoids in Pepper (*Capsicum* spp.). *Sci. Hort.* **2005**, *106*, 341–352.

Lee, J. M.; Nahm, S. H.; Kim, Y. M.; Kim, B. D. Characterization and molecular Genetic Mapping of Microsatellite Loci in Pepper. *Theor. Appl. Genet.* **2004**, *108*, 619–627.

Lee, Y.; Howard, L. R.; Villalon, B. Flavonoids and Antioxidant Activity of Fresh Pepper (*Capsicum annuum*) Cultivars. *J. Food Sci.* **1995**, *60*, 1–4.

Lijun, O.; Xuexiao, Z. Inter Simple Sequence Repeat Analysis of Genetic Diversity of Five Cultivated Pepper Species. *Afr. J. Biotechnol.* **2012**, *11*, 752–757.

López, E. R. G.; Hernández, V. S.; Parra, T. S.; Porras, F.; Pacheco, O. A.; Valdez O. A.; Osuna E. T.; Muy Rangel M. D. Geographical Differentiation of Wild Pepper (*Capsicum annuum* L.

var. *glabriusculum*) Populations from North-western Mexico. Phyton (Buenos Aires) **2016,** *85,* 131–141.

Lu, F. H.; Kwon, S. W.; Yoon, M. Y.; Kim, K. T.; Cho, M. C.; Yoon, M. K.; Park, Y. J. SNP Marker Integration and QTL Analysis of 12 Agronomic and Morphological Traits in F8 RILs of Pepper (*Capsicum annuum* L.). *Mol. Cells* **2012,** *34,* 25–34.

Lucinda, N.; Rocha, W. B.; Inoue, N. A. K.; Nagata, T. Complete Genome Sequence of Pepper Yellow Mosaic Virus, A Potyvirus, Occurring in Brazil. *Arch. Virol.* **2012,** *157,* 1397−1401.

Luo, X. J.; Peng, J.; Li, Y. J. Recent Advances in the Study on Capsaicinoids and Capsinoids. *Eur. J. Pharm.* **2011,** *650,* 1–7.

Luqman, S.; Rizvi, S. I. Protection of Lipid Peroxidation and Carbonyl Formation in Proteins by Capsaicin in Human Erythrocytes Subjected to Oxidative Stress. *Phytother Res.* **2006,** *20,* 303−306.

Marín, A.; Ferreres, F.; Tomás, B. F. A.; Gil M. I. Characterization and Quantitation of Antioxidant Constituents of Sweet Pepper (*Capsicum annuum* L.). *J. Agr. Food Chem.* **2004,** *52,* 3861–3869.

Martinez, A. L. A.; Araújo, J. S. P.; Ragassi, C. F.; Buso, G. S. C.; Reifschneider, F. J. B. Variability Among *Capsicum baccatum* Accessions from Goiás, Brazil, Assessed by Morphological Traits and Molecular Markers. *Genet. Mol. Res.* **2017,**16.

Mason, A. S. *SSR Genotyping; In Batley, J. ed. Plant Gen.* Springer: New York, NY, 2015; pp 77–89.

Materska, M.; Perucka I. Antioxidant Activity of the Main Phenolic Compounds Isolated from Hot Pepper Fruit (*Capsicum annuum* L.). *J. Agric. Food Chem.* **2005,** *53,* 1750–1756.

Meckelmann, S. W.; Jansen, C.; Riegel, D. W.; van Zonneveld, M.; Ríos, L.; Peña, K.; Mueller, S. E.; Petz, M. Phytochemicals in Native Peruvian *Capsicum pubescens* (rocoto). *Eur. Food Res. Technol.* **2015,** *241,* 817–825.

Meckelmann, S. W.; Riegel, D. W.; van Zonneveld, M.; Ríos, L.; Peña, K., Mueller, S. E.; Petz, M. Capsaicinoids, Flavonoids, Tocopherols, Antioxidant Capacity and Color Attributes in 23 Native Peruvian Chili Peppers (*Capsicum* spp.) Grown in Three Different Locations. *Eur. Food Res. Technol.* **2015,** *240,* 273–283.

Meckelmann, S. W.; Riegel, D. W.; van Zonneveld, M. J., Ríos L.; Peña, K.; Ugas, R.; Quinonez, L.; Mueller, S. E.; Petz, M. Compositional Characterization of Native Peruvian Chili Peppers (*Capsicum* spp.). *J. Agric. Food Chem.* **2013,** *61,* 2530–2537.

Mehmood, S.; Bashir, A.; Akram A. A. Z.; Jabeen N.; Gulfraz M. Molecular Characterization of Regional *Sorghum bicolor* Varieties from Pakistan. *Pak. J. Bot.* **2008,** *40,* 2015–2021.

Mekonen. S., Chala. A. Assessment of Hot Pepper (*Capsicum* species) Diseases in Southern Ethiopia. *Int. J. Sci. Res.* **2014,** *3,* 91–95.

Messaouda, B.; Abdelhadi, G.; Samia, M. A. Susceptibility of Algerian Pepper Cultivars (*Capsicum annuum* L) to *Phytophthora capsici* Strains from Different Geographic Areas. *Afr. J. Biotechnol.* **2015,** *14,* 3011–3018.

Meudt, H. M.; Clarke, A. C. Almost Forgotten or Latest Practice? AFLP Applications, Analyses and Advances. *Trends Plant Sci.* **2007,** *12,* 106–117.

Mimura, Y.; Inoue, T.; Minamiyama Y.; Kubo, N. An SSR Based Genetic Map of Pepper (*Capsicum annuum* L.) Serves as an Anchor for the Alignment of Major Pepper Maps. *Breed Sci.* **2012,** *62,* 93–98.

Min, J. K.; Han, K. Y.; Kim, E. C.; Kim, Y. M.; Lee, S. W.; Kim, O. H.; Kim, K. W.; Gho, Y. S.; Kwon, Y. G. Capsaicin Inhibits *In Vitro* and *In Vivo* Angiogenesis. *Can. Res.* **2004,** *64,* 644−651.

Minamiyama, Y.; Tsuro, M.; Hirai, M. An SSR-based Linkage Map of *Capsicum annuum*. *Mol. Breed*. **2006**, *18*, 157–169.

Mo, H.; Kim, S.; Wai, K. P. P.; Siddique, M. I.; Yoo, H.; Kim, B. S. New Sources of Resistance to *Phytophthora capsici* in *Capsicum* spp. *Hortic. Environ. Biotechnol*. **2014**, *55*, 50–55.

Moreira, S. O.; Rodrigues, R.; Sudré, C. P.; Riva, S. E. M. Bacterial Spot Resistance and Agronomic Characteristic in *Capsicum annuum* Recombinant Inbred Lines. *Braz. J. Agric. Sci*. **2015**, *10*, 198-204.

Morrison, D. A.; Weston, P. H. Analysis of Morphological Variation in a Field Sample of *Caladenia catenata* (Smith) Druce (Orchidaceae). *Aust. J. Bot*. **1985**, *33*, 185–195.

Muhyi, R.; Bosland, P. W. Evaluation of *Capsicum* Germplasm for Sources of Resistance to *Rhizoctonia solani*. *Hortscience*. **1995**, *30*, 341–342.

Murtza, A.; Bokhari, S. A.; Ali, Y.; Ahmad, T.; Habib, A.; Mazhar, K.; Hussain, M.; Randhawa, S. Anti-fungal Potential of Chilli Germplasm Against *Fusarium* Wilt. *Pak. J. Phytopathol*. **2017**, *29*, 57–61.

Naegele, R. P.; Tomlinson, A. J.; Hausbeck, M. K. Evaluation of a Diverse, Worldwide Collection of Wild, Cultivated, and Landrace Pepper (*Capsicum annuum*) for Resistance to *Phytophthora* Fruit Rot, Genetic Diversity, and Population Structure. *Phytopathology* **2015**, *105*, 110–118.

Nagy, I.; Stagel, A.; Sasvari, Z.; Roder, M.; Ganal, M. Development, Characterization, and Transferability to Other Solanaceae of Microsatellite Markers in Pepper (*Capsicum annuum* L.). *Genome* **2007**, *50*, 668–688.

Naresh, P.; Reddy, M. K.; Reddy, A. C.; Lavanya, B.; Reddy, D. C. L.; Reddy, K. M. Isolation, Characterization and Genetic Diversity of NBS-LRR Class Disease-Resistant Gene Analogs in Multiple Virus Resistant Line of Chili (*Capsicum annuum* L.). *3 Biotech*. **2017**, *7*, 114.

Naresh, P.; Reddy, M. K.; Reddy, P. H. C.; Reddy, K. M. Screening Chilli (*Capsicum* spp.) Germplasm Against *Cucumber mosaic virus* and *Chilli veinal mottle virus* and Inheritance of Resistance. *Eur. J. Plant Pathol*. **2016**, *146*, 451–464.

Nsabiyera, V.; Logose, M.; Ochwo, S. M.; Sseruwagi, P.; Gibson, P.; Ojiewo, C. Morphological Characterization of Local and Exotic Hot Pepper (*Capsicum annuum* L.) Collections in Uganda. *Biorem. Biodiv. Bioavail*. **2013**, *7*, 22–32.

Ogundiwin. E. A.; Berke. T. F.; Massoudi. M.; Black. L. L.; Huestis, G.; Choi, D.; Lee, S.; Prince, J. P. Construction of 2 Intraspecific Linkage Maps and Identification of Resistance QTLs for *Phytophthora capsici* Root-rot and Foliar-blight Diseases of Pepper (*Capsicum annuum* L.). *Genome* **2005**, *48*, 698–711.

Olmstead, R. G.; Bohs, L.; Migid, H. A.; Santiago, V. E.; Garcia, V. F.; Collier, S. M. A Molecular Phylogeny of the Solanaceae. *Taxon* **2008**, *57*, 1159–1181.

Onus, A. N.; Pickersgill, B. Unilateral Incompatibility in *Capsicum* (Solanaceae): Occurrence and Taxonomic Distribution. *Ann. Bot*. **2004**, *94*, 289–295.

Ortiz, R.; Flora, F.; Alvarado, G.; Crossa J. Classifying Vegetable Genetic Resources—A Case Study with Domesticated *Capsicum* spp. *Sci Hort*. **2010**, *126*, 186–191.

Padilha, H. K. M.; Sigales, C. V.; Villela, J. C. B.; Valgas R. A.; Barbieri, R. L. Agronomic Evaluation and Morphological Characterization of Chili Peppers (*Capsicum annuum*, Solanaceae) from Brazil. *Aust. J. Basic. Appl. Sci*. **2016**, *10*, 63–70.

Palevitch, D.; Craker, L. E. Nutritional and Medical Importance of Red Pepper (*Capsicum* spp.). *J. Herbs Spices Med. Plants* **1996**, *3*, 55–83.

Paran, I.; Knaap, E. Genetic and Molecular Regulation of Fruit and Plant Domestication Traits in Tomato and Pepper. *J. Exp. Bot*. **2007**, *58*, 3841–3852.

Paran, I.; Aftergoot, E.; Shifriss, C. Variation in *Capsicum annuum* Revealed by RAPD and AFLP Markers. *Euphytica* **1998**, 99, 167–174.

Patel, A. S.; Sasidharan, N.; Vala, A. G. Genetic Relation in *Capsicum annum* L. Cultivars Through Microsatellite Markers: SSR and ISSR. *Electr. J. Plant Breed.* **2011**, *2*, 67–76.

Patel, K.; Ruiz, C.; Calderon, R.; Marcelo, M.; Rojas, R. Characterisation of Volatile Profiles in 50 Native Peruvian Chili Pepper Using Solid Phase Microextraction–Gas Chromatography Mass Spectrometry (SPME–GCMS). *Food Res. Int.* **2016**, *89*, 471–475.

Paterson, A. H.; Tanksley, S. D.; Sorrells, M. E. DNA Markers in Plant Improvement. *Adv. Agron.* **1991**, *46*, 39–90.

Paul, S.; Das, A.; Sarkar, N. C.; Ghosh, B. Collection of Chilli Genetic Resources from Different Geographical Regions of West Bengal, India. *Int. J. Biores. Stress Manag.* **2013**, *4*, 147–153.

Perucka, I.; Materska, M. Antioxidant Vitamin Contents of *Capsicum annuum* Fruit Extracts as Affected by Processing and Varietal Factors. *Acta Sci. Pol. Technol. Aliment.* **2007**, *6*, 67–73.

Prasath, D.; Ponnuswami, V. Screening of Chilli (*Capsicum annuum* L.) Genotypes Against *Colletotrichum capsici* and Analysis of Biochemical and Enzymatic Activities in Inducing Resistance. *Indian J. Genet.* **2008**, *68*, 344–346.

Prince, J. P.; Lackney, V. K.; Angeles, C.; Blauth J. R.; Kyle, M. M. A Survey of DNA Polymorphism Within the Genus *Capsicum* and the Fingerprinting of Pepper Cultivars. *Genome* **1995**, *38*, 224–231.

Prince, J. P.; Loaiza, F. F.; Tanksley, S. D. Restriction Fragment Length Polymorphism and Genetic Distance Among Mexican Accessions of *Capsicum*. *Genome* **1992**, *35*, 726–732.

Rad, M. B.; Hassani, M. E.; Mohammadi, A.; Lessan, S.; Zade, S. G. Evaluation of Genetic Diversity in *Capsicum* spp. as Revealed by RAPD Markers. *Acta Hortic.* **2009**, *829*, 275–278.

Rahman, S.; Hossain, M. A.; Afroz, R. Morphological Characterization of Chilli Germplasm in Bangladesh. *Bang. J. Agril. Res.* **2017**, *42*, 207–219.

Rai, V. P.; Kumar, R.; Kumar, S.; Rai, A.; Kumar, S.; Singh, M.; Singh, S. P.; Rai, A. B.; Paliwal, R. Genetic Diversity in *Capsicum* Germplasm Based on Microsatellite and Random Amplified Microsatellite Polymorphism Markers. *Physiol. Mol. Biol. Plants* **2013**, *19*, 575–586.

Ramanna, A. India's Plant Variety and Farmers' Rights Legislation: Potential Impact on Stakeholder Access to Genetic Resources, Environment and Production Technology Division, International Food Policy Research Institute, Washington, 2003, 96.

Rana, M.; Sharma, R.; Sharma, P.; Bhardwaj, S. V.; Sharma M. Estimation of Genetic Diversity in *Capsicum annuum* L. Germplasm Using PCR-based Molecular Markers. *Natl. Acad. Sci. Lett.* **2014**, *37*, 295–301.

Rao, S.; Nandineni, M. R. Genome Sequencing and Comparative Genomics Reveal a Repertoire of Putative Pathogenicity Genes in Chilli Anthracnose Fungus *Colletotrichum truncatum*. *PloS One* **2017**, 12.

Reilly, C. A.; Crouch, D. J.; Yost, G. S. Quantitative Analysis of Capsaicinoids in Fresh Peppers, Oleoresin Capsicum and Pepper Spray Products. *J. Forensic. Sci.* **2001**, *46*, 502–509.

Richins, R. D.; Micheletto, S.; O'Connell M. A. Gene Expression Profiles Unique to Chile (*Capsicum annuum* L.) Resistant to *Phytophthora* Root Rot. *Plant Sci.* **2010**, *178*, 192–201.

Rivera, A.; Monteagudo, A. B.; Igartua, E.; Taboada, A.; García, U. A.; Pomar, F.; Riveiro, L. M.; Silvar C. Assessing Genetic and Phenotypic Diversity in Pepper (*Capsicum annuum* L.) Landraces from North-West Spain. *Sci. Hort.* **2016**, *203*, 1–11.

Rodrigues, K. F.; Tam, H. K. Molecular Markers for *Capsicum frutescens* Varieties Cultivated in Borneo. *J. Plant Breed Crop Sci.* **2010**, *2*, 165–167.

Rodriguez, J. M.; Berke, T.; Engle, L.; Nienhuis, J. Variation Among and Within *Capsicum* Species Revealed by RAPD Markers. *Theor. Appl. Genet.* **1999**, *99*, 147–156.

Rodríguez, L.; Depestre, M.; Palloix, A. Behavior of New Pepper (*Capsicum annuum* L.) F1 Hybrid and Varieties with Multiresistance to Virus in Open Field Conditions. *Cult. Trop.* **2014**, *35*, 51–59.

Rodriguez, U. L.; Hernandez, L.; Kilcrease, J. P.; Walker, S.; O'Connell, M. A. Capsaicinoid and Carotenoid Composition and Genetic Diversity of Kas I and Ccs in New Mexican *Capsicum annuum* L. Landraces. *HortScience* **2014**, *49*, 1370–1375.

Saidu, A. N.; Garba, R. Antioxidant Activity and Phytochemical Screening of Five Species of *Capsicum* Fruits. *Int. Res. J. Biochem. Bioinformat.* **2011**, *1*, 237–241.

Sanatombi, K.; Sen, M. S.; Sharma, G. J. DNA Profiling of *Capsicum* Landraces of Manipur. *Sci. Hortic.* **2010**, *124*, 405–408.

Sanchez, A. M.; Malagarie, C. S.; Olea, N.; Vara, D.; Chiloeches, A.; Diaz, L. I. Apoptosis Induced by Capsaicin in Prostate PC-3 Cells Involves Ceramide Accumulation, Neutral Sphingomyelinase, and JNK Activation. *Apoptosis* **2007**, *12*, 2013–2024.

Sarpras, M.; Gaur, R.; Sharma, V.; Chhapekar, S. S.; Das J., Kumar, A.; Yadava, S. K.; Nitin, M.; Brahma, V.; Abraham, S. K.; Ramchiary, N. Comparative Analysis of Fruit Metabolites and Pungency Candidate Genes Expression Between Bhut Jolokia and Other *Capsicum* Species. *PloS One* **2016**, 11.

Senanayake, D. M. J. B.; Mandal, B., Lodha, S.; Varma, A. First Report of Chilli leaf Curl Virus Affecting Chilli in India. *Plant Pathol.* **2007**, *56*, 343.

Silva, L. R.; Azevedo, J.; Pereira, M. J.; Valentão, P.; Andrade, P. B. Chemical Assessment and Antioxidant Capacity of Pepper (*Capsicum annuum* L.) Seeds. *Food Chem. Toxicol.* **2013**, *53*, 240–248.

Silva, S. A.; Rodrigues, R.; Gonçalves, L. S.; Sudré, C. P.; Bento, C. S.; Carmo, M. G.; Medeiros, A. M. Resistance in *Capsicum* spp. to Anthracnose Affected by Different Stages of Fruit Development During Pre-and Post-harvest. *Trop. Plant Pathol.* **2014**, *39*, 335–341.

Simonne, A. H.; Simonne, E. H.; Eitenmiller, R. R.; Mills, H. A.; Green, N. R. Ascorbic Acid and Provitamin A Contents in Unusually Colored Bell Peppers (*Capsicum annuum* L.). *J. Food. Comp. Anal.* **1997**, *10*, 299–311.

Sitthiwong, K.; Matsui, T.; Sukprakarn, S.; Okuda, N.; Kosugi, Y. Classification of Pepper (*Capsicum annuum* L.) Accessions by RAPD Analysis. *Biotechnology* **2005**, *4*, 305–309.

Smith, J. S. C.; Smith, O. S. The Description and Assessment of Distances Between Inbred Lines of Maize: The Utility of Morphological, Biochemical and genetic Descriptors and a Scheme for the Testing of Distinctiveness Between Inbred Lines. *Maydica.* **1989**, *34*, 151–161.

Srivastava, A.; Mangal, M.; Saritha, R. K.; Kalia, P. Screening of Chilli Pepper (*Capsicum* spp.) Lines for Resistance to the Begomoviruses Causing Chilli Leaf Curl Disease in India. *Crop Prot.* **2017**, *100*, 177–185.

Stall, R. E.; Jones, J. B.; Minsavage, G. V. Durability of Resistance in Tomato and Pepper to Xanthomonads Causing Bacterial Spot. *Annu. Rev. Phytopathol.* **2009**, *47*, 265–284.

Sudré, C. P.; Gonçalves, L. S. A.; Rodrigues, R.; Amaral Júnior, A. D.; Riva, S. E. M.; Bento, C. D. S. Genetic Variability in Domesticated *Capsicum* spp. as Assessed by Morphological and Agronomic Data in Mixed Statistical Analysis. *Genet. Mol. Res.* **2010**, *9*, 283–294.

Sugita, T.; Semi, Y.; Sawada, H.; Utoyama, Y.; Hosomi, Y.; Yoshimoto, E.; Maehata Y.; Fukuoka H.; Nagata R.; Ohyama A. Development of Simple Sequence Repeat Markers and Construction of a High-density Linkage Map of *Capsicum annuum*. *Mol. Breed.* **2013**, *31*, 909–920.

Susheela, K. Evaluation of Screening Methods for Anthracnose Disease in Chilli. *Pest Manag. Hort. Ecosyst.* **2012**, *18*, 188–193.

Sy, O.; Bosland, P. W.; Steiner, R. Inheritance of *Phytophthora* Stem Blight Resistance as Compared to *Phytophthora* Root Rot and *Phytophthora* Foliar Blight Resistance in *Capsicum annuum* L. J. *Am. Soc. Hort. Sci.* **2005**, *130*, 75–78.

Szolcsányi, J. Forty Years in Capsaicin Research for Sensory Pharmacology and Physiology. *Neuropeptides* **2004**, *38*, 377–84.

Taranto, F.; D'Agostino, N.; Greco, B.; Cardi, T.; Tripodi, P. Genome-wide SNP Discovery and Population Structure Analysis in Pepper (*Capsicum annuum*) Using Genotyping by Sequencing. *BMC Genom.* **2016**, *17*, 943.

Than, P. P.; Jeewon, R.; Hyde, K. D.; Pongsupasamit, S.; Mongkolporn, O.; Taylor P. W. J. Characterization and Pathogenicity of *Colletotrichum* Species Associated with Anthracnose on Chilli (*Capsicum* spp.) in Thailand. *Plant Pathol.* **2008**, *57*, 562–572.

Thul, S. T.; Darokar, M. P.; Shasany, A. K.; Khanuja, S. P. Molecular Profiling for Genetic Variability in *Capsicum* Species Based on ISSR and RAPD Markers. *Mol. Biotechnol.* **2012**, *51*, 137–147.

Thul, S. T.; Shasany, A. K.; Darokar, M. P.; Khanuja, S. P. AFLP Analysis for Genetic Diversity in *Capsicum annuum* and Related Species. *Nat. Prod. Commun.* **2006**, *3*, 223–228.

Topuz, A.; Ozdemir, F. Assessment of Carotenoids, Capsaicinoids and Ascorbic Acid Composition of Some Selected Pepper Cultivars (*Capsicum annuum* L.) Grown in Turkey. *J. Food. Compost. Anal.* **2007**, *20*, 596–602.

van Zonneveld, M.; Ramirez, M.; Williams, D. E.; Petz, M.; Meckelmann, S.; Avila, T.; Bejarano, C.; Ríos, L.; Peña, K.; Jäger, M.; Libreros, D. Screening Genetic Resources of *Capsicum* Peppers in Their Primary Center of Diversity in Bolivia and Peru. *PloS One* **2015**, *10* (9), e0134663. doi: 10.1371/journal.pone.0134663

Volcani, Z.; Zootra, D.; Cohen, R. Bacterial Canker Disease of Tomatoes and Capsicums. *Hassadeh* **1970**, *50*, 1028–1032.

Vos, P.; Hogers, R.; Bleeker, M.; Reijans, M.; Van der Lee, T.; Hornes, M.; Frijters, A.; Pot, J.; Peleman, J.; Kuiper, M.; Zabeau, M. AFLP: A New Technique for DNA Fingerprinting. *Nucleic Acids Res.* **1995**, *23*, 4407–4414.

Votava, E. J.; Baral, J. B.; Bosland, P. W. Genetic Diversity of Chile (*Capsicum annuum* var. *annuum* L.) Landraces from Northern New Mexico, Colorado, and Mexico. *Econ. Bot.* **2005**, *59*, 8–17.

Wahyuni, Y.; Ballester, A. R.; Sudarmonowati, E.; Bino, R. J.; Bovy A. G. Metabolite Biodiversity in Pepper (*Capsicum*) Fruits of Thirty-two Diverse Accessions: Variation in Health-related Compounds and Implications for Breeding. *Phytochemistry* **2011**, *72*, 1358–1370.

Wahyuni, Y.; Ballester, A. R.; Tikunov, Y.; de Vos, R. C.; Pelgrom, K. T.; Maharijaya, A.; Sudarmonowati, E.; Bino, R. J.; Bovy, A. G. Metabolomics and Molecular Marker Analysis to Explore Pepper (*Capsicum* sp.) Biodiversity. *Metabolomics* **2013**, *9*, 130–144.

Wall, M. M.; Waddell, C. A.; Bosland, P. W. Variation in β-carotene and Total Carotenoid Content in Fruits of *Capsicum*. *HortScience*. **2001**, *36*, 746–749.

Walpole, C. S.; Bevan, S.; Bloomfield, G.; Breckenridge, R.; James, I. F.; Ritchie, T.; Szallasi, A.; Winter, J.; Wrigglesworth, R. Similarities, and Differences, in the Structure-activity Relationships of Capsaicin and Resiniferatoxin Analogues. *J. Med. Chem.* **1996**, *39*, 2939–2952.

Weir, B. S. *Genetic Data Analysis. Methods for Discrete Population Genetic Data*. Sinauer Associates, Inc. Publishers: USA, 1990.

Williams, J. G. K.; Kubelik, A. R.; Livak, K. J.; Rafalski, J. A.; Tingey, S. V. DNA Polymorphisms Amplified by Arbitrary Primers are Useful as Genetic Markers. *Nucleic Acids Res.* **1990,** *18*, 6531–6535.

Yaldiz, G.; Ozguven, M. A Study of Yield and Yield Components of Different Ornamental Pepper (*Capsicum* sp.) Species and Lines in Cukurova Ecological Conditions. *Pak. J. Biol. Sci.* **2011,** *14*, 273–281.

Yatung, T.; Dubey, R. K.; Singh, V.; Upadhyay, G. Genetic Diversity of Chilli (*Capsicum annuum* L.) Genotypes of India Based on Morpho-chemical Traits. *Aust. J. Crop. Sci.* **2014,** *8*, 97–102.

Yoon. J. B.; Yang. D. C.; Lee. W. P.; Ahn. S. Y.; Park, H. G. Genetic Resources Resistant to Anthracnose in the Genus *Capsicum. Hort. Environ. Biotechnol.* **2004,** *45*, 318–323.

Yoshitani, S. I.; Tanaka, T.; Kohno, H.; Takashima, S. Chemoprevention of Azoxymethane-Induced rat Colon Carcinogenesis by Dietary Capsaicin and Rotenone. *Int. J. Oncol.* **2001,** *19*, 929–939.

Yumnam, J. S.; Tyagi, W.; Pandey, A.; Meetei, N. T.; Rai, M. Evaluation of Genetic Diversity of Chilli Landraces from North Eastern India Based on Morphology, SSR Markers and the Pun1 Locus. *Plant Mol. Biol. Rep.* **2012,** *30*, 1470–1479.

Zewdie, Y.; Bosland P. W. Evaluation of Genotype, Environment, and Genotype-by-Environment Interaction for Capsaicinoids in *Capsicum annuum* L. *Euphytica* **2000,** *111*, 185–190.

Zhang, R.; Humphreys, I.; Sahu, R. P.; Shi, Y.; Srivastava, S. K. *In Vitro* and *In Vivo* Induction of Apoptosis by Capsaicin in Pancreatic Cancer Cells is Mediated Through ROS Generation and Mitochondrial Death Pathway. *Apoptosis* **2008,** *13*, 1465−1478.

Zhigila, D. A.; Rahaman, A. A. A.; Kolawole, O. S.; Oladele, F. A. Fruit Morphology as Taxonomic Features in five Varieties of *Capsicum annuum* L. Solanaceae. *J. Bot.* 2014.

Zunun, P. A. Y.; Guevara, F. T.; Jimenez, G. S. N.; Feregrino, P. A. A.; Gautier, F.; Guevara, G. R. G. Effect of Foliar Application of Salicylic Acid, Hydrogen Peroxide and a Xyloglucan Oligosaccharide on Capsiate Content and Gene Expression Associated with Capsinoids Synthesis in *Capsicum annuum* L. *J. Biosci.* **2017,** *42*, 245–250.

CHAPTER 17

Ex Situ Conservation of Chili (*Capsicum* spp.)

TARUN HALDER and BISWAJIT GHOSH*

Plant Biotechnology Laboratory, Department of Botany, Ramakrishna Mission Vivekananda Centenary College, Rahara, Kolkata, India

Corresponding author. E-mail: ghosh_b2000@yahoo.co.in

ABSTRACT

Plant genetic resources are essential to check the diminishing of genetic erosion and for development of improved high-yielding commercial varieties that are a better response against biotic and abiotic stresses as well as combat new climatic conditions. Chili is an important vegetable and cash crop around the world. The genus Capsicum is mainly cultivated for its nonpungent (sweet pepper), pungent, and ornamental values. It is rich in bioactive compounds, which contribute to the improvement of human health. For future agricultural development and improvement of the food security program, plant genetic resources must be conserved in the form of seeds, plants, tissues, etc. Biotechnology approach involving plant tissue culture is a powerful technique that can be an alternative to conventional breeding and advance germplasm improvement. Several techniques are applied for conservation of Capsicum that are more effective, like seed bank, greenhouse, tissue culture, in vitro conservation, cryopreservation, etc. For long-term ex situ conservation of disease-free materials, the only in vitro conservation method can be adopted, it reducing the growth rate of plant material and increasing subculture intervals. For prolonged conservation, ultralow temperature (cryopreservation) can be used in the contamination-free state of chili materials.

Some useful germplasm for continuous agricultural methods and diversity of breeding lines are lost due to the constant refinement activities, which are only focused on elite genotypes or germplasms and their proper conservation. This conservation method avoids the conservation of wild genotypes and wild crop-relatives that are very important for further improvement of crop cultivar. An effective and well-organized conservation system is required to support from different nations and a true continuation of this program needs an effective initiative for regular collection of plant genetic resource from wild and their good conservation management.

17.1   INTRODUCTION

Preservation of genetic diversity of a specific plant species or genetic stock is primarily required for germplasm conservation. Ex situ conservation is now an important mode for conservation of crop varieties and wild genetic resources because of its utility in future crop improvement. The words chili and chile basically come from people of Nahuatl, the Uto-Aztecan language family of central Mexico. Since 7500 BCE, the red peppers have been common in a part of the world populations' diet. It is now assumed that chili was domesticated in Mexico more than 6000 years ago.

Bosland (1996) reported that chili was the first self-pollinating crop cultivated in Mexico and South America. Even at that time, the people of Central and South American countries believed the myth that capsicum plants acted as the god of war, used to counter magic and protection rituals. Sprinkled around the house, they were expected to clean the area of illegal demons and vampires; however, burning them laterally with garlic and other pungent spices were anticipated to fumigate and purify the house. Parenthetically this practice is also reputed to disperse vermin and insects.

The world center creates improved inbred and its germplasm accession lines resulting from its improvement breeding programs available for international use as global public crop materials (Keatinge et al., 2012). Globally, in most developing countries, chili researchers, in both public and private sectors, now use germplasms for better crop products. In Capsicum, a total of 8235 accessions have collected under AVRDC, which is the world's largest accession center comprising about 11% of all crops and vegetable accessions maintained globally (Reddy et al., 2015). Out of the total collected accessions are 66% (*C. annuum*), 8% (*C. frutescens*), 6% (*C. chinense*), 5% (*C. baccatum*), and others (Lin et al., 2013).

BOX 17.1 Capsicum Genebank, Country and Collection

Genebank Institute code	Genebank Acronym	Country	Accessions No.
TWN001	AVRDC	Taiwan	7914
USA016	S9	USA	4698
MEX008	INIFAP	Mexico	4661
IND001	NBPGR	India	3835
BRA006	IAC	Brazil	2321
JPN003	NIAS	Japan	2271
PHL130	IPB-UPLB	Philippines	1880
TWN005	TSS-PDAF	Taiwan	1800
DEU146	IPK	Germany	1526
CHN004	BVRC	China	1394
	Others (176)	Others	41,272
		World	73,572

[a]Actual data (May 2011) from Asian Vegetable Genetic Resources Information System.

Capsicum is an important commercial vegetable and spice crop all over the world. Generally, 400 different capsicum varieties are found, but there are thought to be 38 species of Capsicum (Table 17.1), of which only 5–6 species are cultivated, major one is *C. annuum, C. frutescens, C. baccatum*, and *C. baccatum*, etc. (Kothari et al., 2010; Ramchiary et al., 2014; Reddy et al., 2015; Haque et al., 2016; Hegde et al., 2017). Capsicum is rich in pharmaceutically high-valued bioactive compounds that contribute to the betterment of human health (McCormack, 2010) (Fig. 17.1).

Other than medicinal and nutritional reputation, breeders have improved agricultural practices of pepper, such as pungency, fruit shape, disease resistance, that is, biotic stress and abiotic stress tolerance, etc. (Lee et al., 2016). For food security and sustainable agricultural development of the plant, genetic resources of wild genotypes and commercially less important cultivars are conserved in the form of plants, seeds, tissues, etc. (Babu et al., 2012).

Due to the pressure of more and more production, all agricultural policy-makers and scientists are concerned only on superior varieties that create a homogeneity, on the other hand, wild genotypes are gradually eroded due to lack of our interest but, at present, due to environmental problems, we try to collect genetically variant genotypes that are already missing. This standing action for the conservation of germplasm is essential at species, gene pool, or ecosystem level for successors (Frankel, 1975). It is a fact that a lot of useful genes in the landraces and genetic diversity of breeding lines have been lost due to the continuous breeding among high-yielding cultivars (Tang et al., 2010; Lee et al., 2016; Hedge et al., 2017). Ex- situ conservation is a safe and efficient approach to conserve chili genetic resources and to make the germplasm readily available to breeders, plant biotechnologists, and other researchers. The duty of the plant breeder or genetic engineer is to create an improved variety with respect to their nutritional value, stress tolerance, as well as high-yielding cultivars. For ex situ conservation, different modes of preservation are adopted for chili from a traditional approach to modern methods (Fig. 17.2).

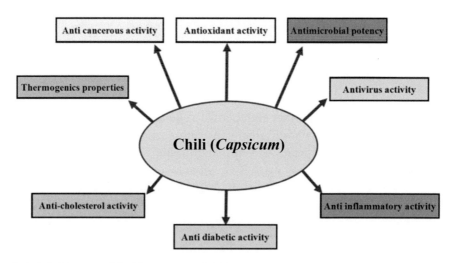

FIGURE 17.1   Medicinal importance of chili.

17.2   FIELD GENE BANK

Physical facilities for maintaining collections of live plant materials under field conditions are called field gene bank. According to Plant Genetic Resources for Food and Agriculture, gene banks are assured in two activities (1) germplasm secure in the long term and (2) are made available for use by farmers, plant breeders, and researchers. Among all areas of plant genetic resources (PGR) activities, exchange of germplasm has become crucial for the formation of a legal framework to protect their biodiversity

TABLE 17.1 Different *Capsicum* spp. with Their Geographical Distribution.

S. No.	Species	Locality
1.	*Capsicum. annuum* L.	Southern USA, Mexico, Antilles, Belize, Panama, Costa Rica, Guatemala, Surinam, Venezuela, Colombia, Ecuador, Peru, northern and northeastern Brazil
2.	*C. baccatum* L.	Colombia, Peru, Bolivia, Paraguay, southern and southeastern Brazil, northern Argentina, Chile, Argentina, India
3.	*C. buforum* Hunz.	Brazil
4.	*C. caballeroi* M. Nee	Bolivia
5.	*C. campylopodium* Sendtn.	Brazil
6.	*C. cardenasii* Heiser & P. G. Sm.	Bolivia
7.	*C. ceratocalyx* M. Nee	Bolivia
8.	*C. chacoense* Hunz.	Southern Bolivia, Paraguay, northern and central Argentina
9.	*C. chinense* Jacq.	Cultivated in USA, Mexico, Central America, Ecuador, Peru, Bolivia, Brazil, Argentina, China, Japan, Thailand
10.	*C. coccineum* (Rusby) Hunz.	Peru, Bolivia
11.	*C. cornutum* (Hiern) Hunz.	Brazil
12.	*C. dimorphum* (Miers) Kuntze	Colombia, Ecuador
13.	*C. dusenii* Bitter	South-East Brazil
14.	*C. eximium* Hunz.	Southern Bolivia, northern Argentina
15.	*C. flexuosum* Sendtn.	Paraguay, southern and southeastern Brazil, northeastern Argentina
16.	*C. friburgense* Bianch. & Barboza	Brazil
17.	*C. frutescens* L.	USA, Mexico, Central and South America, Africa, India, China, Japan, Thailand
18.	*C. galapagoense* Hunz.	Ecuador
19.	*C. geminifolium* (Dammer) Hunz.	Colombia, Ecuador, Peru

TABLE 17.1 *(Continued)*

S. No.	Species	Locality
20.	*C. havanense* Kunth	Colombia
21.	*C. hookerianum* (Miers) Kuntze	Southern Ecuador, northern Peru
22.	*C. hunzikerianum* Barboza & Bianch	Brazil
23.	*C. lanceolatum* (Greenm.) C. V. Morton & Standl	Mexico, Guatemala
24.	*C. leptopodum* (Dunal) Kuntze	Brazil
25.	*C. lycianthoides* Bitter	Peru
26.	*C. minutiflorum* (Rusby) Hunz.	South America, Northern and Central America
27.	*C. mirabile* Mart. ex Sendtn.	Brazil
28.	*C. parvifolium* Sendtn.	Colombia, Venezuela, northeastern Brazil
29.	*C. pereirae* Barboza & Bianch.	Brazil
30.	*C. pubescens* Ruiz & Pav.	Mexico, Central and South America
31.	*C. ramosissimum* Witasek	Africa, Madagascar, South Africa, Afghanistan
32.	*C. recurvatur* Witasek	Brazil
33.	*C. rhomboideum* (Dunal) Kuntze	Mexico, Guatemala, Honduras, Colombia, Venezuela, Ecuador, Peru
34.	*C. schottianum* Sendtn.	Brazil
35.	*C. scolnikianum* Hunz.	Ecuador
36.	*C. spina-albc* (Dunal) Kuntze	Africa
37,	*C. stramoniifolium* (Kunth) Standl.	Peru
38.	*C. villosum* Sendtn.	Brazil

and interest of future needs for conservation of particular crop diversity and crop improvement (Nair et al., 2017).

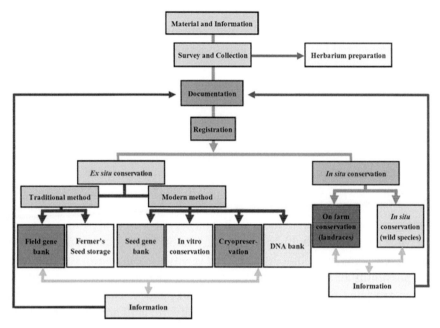

FIGURE 17.2   Flowchart for documentation and conservation.

Diversity or variation of all biological species are essential and this biological diversity could be at three levels: Variation in genes and genotypes (genetic diversity), species richness (species diversity), and ecological diversity for communities of species. It must be recognized that only diversity can allow sustainability and can lead to development in several human activities, like social and economic systems to flourish, which can ensure to meet food security and avoiding the malnutritional problem in poorest communities of different countries (Shiva, 1994).

For more than two decades, there has been a growing awareness of the wholesome view of biodiversity, particularly agrodiversity, and conservation for sustainable use and development (Jacobsen et al., 2013). A very common but serious loss of plant genetic resources from natural disasters, such as floods, fires, snow, volcanoes, earthquakes, and hurricanes, is another important criterion for ensuring the physical safety of collections. Furthermore, physical security and potential of anthropogenic extortion, such as theft and vandalism, should be taken into consideration. The designing and location of a field gene bank should be considered to retain the characteristic feature of a particular genotype. Though conservation and utilization of genetic resources are well recognized, during the last decade, their importance has been further highlighted in two global conventions. The first CBD held at Rio (1992), Brazil, and second, at the International Technical Conference on the Conservation and Use of Plant Genetic Resources for Food and Agriculture (Iwanaga, 1994; FAO, 1996).

The 1992 and 1996 resolutions equally have recognized the authority of countries where the PGR accessible surrounded by their borders but the problem to conserve and use PGR rests with developing countries and stresses on the significance of impartial sharing of these resources and knowledge related to their proper exploitation. Among the 20 priority activities of the Global Plan of Action, network of PGR for food and agriculture is also included. Due to the highly specific nature of different environments, such domestication has resulted in many 'ecospecific' adaptations, which resulted in the formation of landraces, well-matched to local environments (Bennett et al., 1987).

Most of the chili cultivars grown are known to be susceptible to pest, insect, and some microbial disease. That is why there is a necessity to explore the possibility of relative tolerance and resistance of the cultivar's cultures under restricted field conditions (Singh and Pandey, 2015, Samanta et al., 2017). In a few cases, insect resistance and hybrid chili are also conserved in separate field places (Samanta et al., 2017).

17.3   GREENHOUSE

A good technology involved for the conservation of plants, popularly known as "greenhouse," is now adopted to provide favorable environment condition to the plants. During the unfavorable environmental conditions, to some extent, it is used to save the plants from abiotic and biotic stresses like wind, cold, precipitation, extreme temperature, excessive radiation, insects, and diseases (Yadav et al., 2014). Under greenhouse or playhouse, where the environmental conditions are changed manually, one can grow any plant in any place at any time by providing suitable environmental conditions. During the winter season, changing the climatic temperature at that conditions cold air does not enter inside the playhouse and inside environment becomes favorable for rapid germination of seed and growth of seedlings. Several times farmers produce an increase in fruit yield of capsicum (Singh et al., 2011).

It is difficult to grow some important vegetables like capsicum, tomato, etc., in the open field condition due to abiotic cold stress. Therefore, greenhouse technology was introduced for off-season production of vegetable nurseries as well as conservation of high-value selected germplasm.

Capsicum field trial was conducted in the playhouse to assess the yield performance (Singh and Naik, 1990; Singh et al., 2010). Fruit yield of capsicum differed significantly with open and control environment also reported (Shahak et al., 2007; Khan et al., 2010; Patel and Rajput, 2010; Roy et al., 2011). Sometimes, significantly, higher plant height, number of branches, and the total number of fruits in capsicum were noted under the playhouse condition (Jovicich et al., 2005). Sweet peppers germplasm conserved under greenhouse is worldwide also reported by Lin and Saltveit (2012).

17.4   SEED BANK

Seed banks are an important effective way of ex situ conservation where a huge number of genetic diversities is maintained in very small places. The advantages of seed bank are that about 90% of seed plants have orthodox seeds, multiple collections be able to conserve in a small space and database systems empower the recording of multiple ecogeographic details on each seed population (Babu et al., 2014; Ruiz-González et al., 2017; Lei and Middleton, 2017).

Requirement of seeds from seed banks can be used both for conservation or preservation and restoration (Fig. 17.3) of plant populations (Rodríguez-Arévalo et al., 2017). Classically, ex situ conservation arrangement works only as back-ups to in situ conservation systems. In the past few years, many collections were maintained without the help of storage facilities, which would extend the viability of seeds. It is a fact that about 1750 gene banks are now involved worldwide for conservation of more than 7 million plant germplasm accessions and nearly 2 million accessions are estimated to be unique (Fu, 2017).

Sometimes conserved accessions had to be regenerated very frequently leading to loss of genetic diversity in gene banks (Frankel and Hawkes, 1975; Nair et al., 2017). For the maintenance of genetic pureness of the conserved germplasm accessions, troubles arise primarily due to the selection during regeneration, outcrossing with other access and genetic drift, differential survival in storage (Allard, 1970; Lawan et al., 2016). Appropriate storage conditions related to understanding the genetic control of best discriminating among the studied traits would bring a significant contribution to the genetic improvement and proper grow-outs are expected to reduce the effects of such problems (Rao, 1980; Garba et al., 2015).

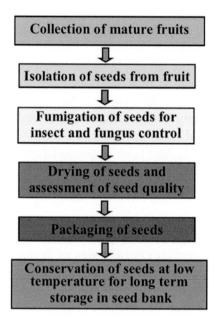

FIGURE 17.3   Steps involved for seed's conservation.

The genetic resources of wild chili pepper or *Capsicum* in the population are valuable assets and the information of the germination ability is of great priority for its management and conservation (España et al., 2017). A total of 372 accessions were conserved that is collected from 31 provinces in China (Zhang Xiao-min et al., 2016). Conservation and collection of some wild and domesticated species of *Capsicum* from Bolivia contains 487 accessions and Peruvian capsicum contains 712 accessions (Zonnevel et al., 2015).

17.5   BIOTECHNOLOGICAL APPROACH FOR CONSERVATION

The biotechnological methods are used to select genotypes with desirable traits, to identify and insert the important desirable genes that induce resistance and tolerance to biotic and abiotic stress. Plant tissue culture method particularly micropropagation techniques are now used to multiply and preserve plant genetic biodiversity outside its natural habitat. Furthermore, plant tissue culture methods offer a safe means for the international exchange of germplasm, which allow the establishment of extensive collections with minimal space requirements.

Biotechnological approaches also allow a valuable supply of in vitro regenerated plant materials for recovery of wild population, they promise the repository of pathogen-free material and elite plants and assist the progress of the performance of molecular investigations and ecological studies (Tandon and Kumaria, 2005). Some biotechnological techniques, such as in vitro culture, are very helpful in keeping up ex situ germplasm collections of plant species that have asexual mode of propagation than the species that are impossible to maintain as seeds or in field gene banks (Chatterjee and Ghosh, 2015, 2016; Haque and Ghosh, 2013a, 2013b, 2016, 2017; Kundu et al., 2015).

Totipotency is a unique inherent character of all plant cells that are now been exploited through in vitro techniques, this concept was basically proposed by Haberlandt (1902) and initially, it was clearly demonstrated by Steward et al. (1958). In vitro plant regeneration via callus culture, multiplication, and clonal propagation of the plant are essential for improvement of disease-free plant and it is a compulsory application of biotechnology branch to plant genetic improvement. It is also important for the conservation of genetically pure planting materials.

Micropropagation is now widely used for large scale propagation of novel plants as an alternative of conventional propagation methods, even genetically modified as well as hybrid cultivars are also multiplied in this biotechnological technique. This method is also used for mass-propagation of new genotypes. Meristem culture also adopted for generation of large-scale virus-free and other pathogen-free plant material that trigger the impressive improvement the yield of established cultivars.

17.5.1 IN VITRO CULTURE AND MICROPROPAGATION

Plant tissue culture is an ideal procedure that is now widely used in academic as well as commercial purposes. Several aseptic in vitro culture procedures are now adopted especially in as in vitro seed germination, micropropagation, callus and cell suspension culture (Wilson and Roberts, 2012).

In contrast to any other plant propagation system, the in vitro aseptic micropropagation method gain highest appreciation for large-scale multiplication of any elite clone without natural climatic influences like temperature, light, humidity, any seasonal variation, etc. (Costa et al., 2013). Even micropropagation method generated genetically stable can also be used for the purpose of conservation of recalcitrant and endanger species. In vitro culture and micropropagation form the base for establishing tissue cultures and developing in vitro and cryo-conservation technology.

Plant tissue-cultured should be maintained for their genetic stability as well as morphological nature. Micropropagation provides continuous stable supply of any plant genetic resources that can serve in two way firstly it involved in different crop improvement program and secondly, for germplasm conservation purpose. A huge number of plant species are now enlisted in successfully in vitro micropropagation system including horticultural species. Among the most important in vitro technique applications, is the micropropagation of vegetable plants, medicinal and aromatic threatened plant species (Matkowski, 2008; Purohit, 2013).

In current scenario, conservation of a particular plant species and plant biodiversity of a population conservation is an important issue and this problem can be satisfied by in vitro micropropagation that can provide huge number of propagules from a cross-section of the genetic diversity of a region (Rogers, 2003) it also provides additional backup collections and provides alternative propagation and conservation of *Capsicum* species (Fig. 17.4) (Haque et al., 2016; Haque and Ghosh, 2017). Recent reports on in vitro multiplication of Capsicum (Fig. 17.5) and conservation (Haque et al., 2016, Haque and Ghosh, 2017).

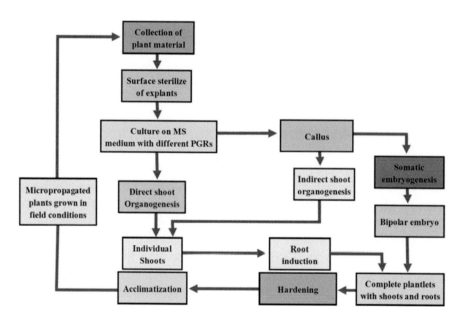

FIGURE 17.4   Flow diagram of plant tissue culture for mass propagation and conservation.

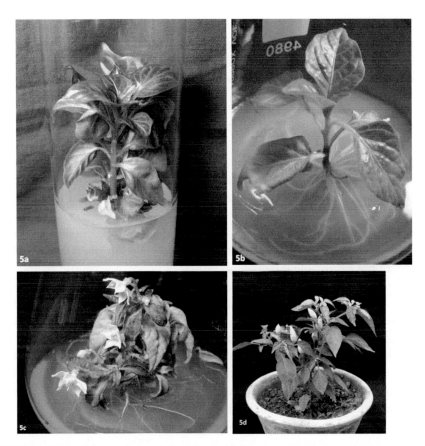

FIGURE 17.5 Tissue culture of Capsicum. (a) Shoot multiplication and (b) complete regenerated plant with shoot and roots. (c) In vitro flowering and (d) ex vitro condition after hardening.

The in vitro plant cell culture of *Capsicum* is an important system for understanding the mechanism of synthesis of capsaicin and other commercially viable secondary metabolites both at cellular and molecular level (Kumari et al., 2015). In spite of this, a collection of research work has been directed to explore the morphogenic potential and to attain the successful repeatable protocol for regeneration of whole plantlets of chili and constant efforts are still in progress to achieve more improvement in the arena of pepper biotechnology.

The maximum success of in vitro regeneration of chili has been attained through organogenesis process, but the other methods of regeneration through tissue culture, like somatic embryogenesis and anther of pollen culture for androgenic haploid production, have also been explored. A summary list of in vitro morphogenic response of different explants, composition of culture media in approach toward the micropropagation of different species of *Capsicum* is given below (Table 17.2).

17.5.1.1 EFFECT OF DIFFERENT CULTIVARS ON IN VITRO RESPONSE

The genotype is one of the main factors that influence the organogenic response of cultures in different plant species. Cultivar specific regeneration protocol is now essential because cultivar, as well as specific genotype or chemotype, also plays an important differential role for regeneration purposes due to cultivars specific differential gene expression and culture media response. So, in this context, recommendation of single standard protocol not acceptable it demands cultivar or genotype-specific protocol.

Various factors like explant type, composition of nutrient media, different physical conditions (light, temperature, humidity, volume of the culture vessels, etc.) highly influenced the regeneration efficacy of the plant species *Capsicum*. It is reported by Ochoa-Alejo and Ireta-Moreno (1990) that the same explant type ware used from different sources of cultivars showed clear differential response when cultured in same PGRs supplemented MS media. The differential shoot bud morphogenic response was observed in different cultivars when culture was maintained with same condition.

Differential response in organogenic potentiality of chili have also been observed in different genotypes (Rodeva et al., 2006; Valadez-Bustos et al., 2009; Manzur et al., 2013; Mythili et al., 2017), different cultivars (Ezura et al., 1993; Szász et al., 1995; Sanatombi and Sharma, 2008; Orlinska and Nowaczyk, 2015; Hegde et al., 2017), various species (Christopher and Rajam, 1996; Rodeva et al., 2006; Joshi and Kothari, 2007; Kehie et al., 2013; Maligeppagol et al., 2016), and different culture media (Ochoa-Alejo and Ireta-Moreno, 1990; Ezura et al., 1993; Rodeva et al., 2006; Bonilla and Chen, 2015; Ashwani et al., 2017; Mythili et al., 2017).

17.5.1.2 CHOICE OF THE EXPLANTS

The selection of right explant is very important aspect in plant tissue culture practices, particularly growth and morphogenesis, including the different genotypes of chili. The regeneration process of chili is also controlled by the selection of appropriate explant. Various types of explants including cotyledons,

TABLE 17.2 In Vitro Shoot Bud Proliferation in Different *Capsicum* spp.

S. No.	Species	Explants/tissues	PGR's+medium	References
1	*Capsicum annuum*	Zygotic embryo	BAP (5.0 mgL^{-1})	Agrawal and Chandra (1983)
2	*C. annuum*	Hypocotyl, cotyledon, stem, leaf, root, shoot-tip, embryo	BAP (5.0 mgL^{-1})	Agrawal et al. (1989)
3	*C. annuum*	shoot-tip and hypocotyl	BAP (5.0 mgL^{-1})+NAA (0.1 mgL^{-1})	Ebida and Hu (1993)
4	*C. annuum*	Shoot tip, seedlings	BAP (2.0 mgL^{-1})	Madhuri and Rajam (1993)
5	*C. praetermissum*	Shoot tip	BAP (2.0 mgL^{-1})	Christopher and Rajam (1994)
6	*C. annuum*	Cotyledon	BAP (8.88 μM)+IAA (2.85 μM)+AgNO$_3$ (5.85 μM)	Hyde and Phillips (1996)
7	*C. annuum*	Hypocotyl, cotyledon, leaf	BAP (13.3 μM)+IAA (5.71 μM), BAP (44.4 μM), BAP (22.2 μM)	Christopher and Rajam (1996)
8	*C. praetermissum*	Hypocotyl, cotyledon, leaf	BAP (13.3 μM)+IAA (5.71 μM), BAP (44.4 μM), BAP (22.2 μM)	Christopher and Rajam (1996)
9	*C. baccatum*	Hypocotyl, cotyledon, leaf	BAP (13.3 μM)+IAA (5.71 μM), BAP (44.4 μM), BAP (22.2 μM)	Christopher and Rajam (1996)
10	*C. annuum*	Cotyledon	BAP (13.35 μM)+IAA (3.4–5.9 μM)+EBR (0.1 μM)	Franck-Duchenne et al. (1998)
11	*C. annuum*	Cotyledon	BAP (5.0 mgL^{-1})+PAA (2.0 mgl^{-1})	Husain et al. (1999)
12	*C. annuum*	Zygotic embryos	BAP (5.0 mg L^{-1})+NAA (1.0 mgL^{-1})	Arous et al. (2001)
13	*C. annuum*	Seedling explants, embryonal explants	TDZ (1.0–2.0 mgL^{-1})	Dabauza and Pena (2001)
14	*C. annuum*	Leaf, cotyledon	TDZ (1.0–3.0 mgL^{-1})	Venkataiah et al. (2003)
15	*C. annuum*	Cotyledon	TDZ (1.5 μM) + IAA (0.5 μM)	Siddique and Anis, (2006)

TABLE 17.2 *(Continued)*

S. No.	Species	Explants/tissues	PGR's+medium	References
16	C. frutescens	Shoot tip	Zeatin (10.0 mgL^{-1}), BAP (5.0 mgl^{-1})+IAA (1.0 mgl^{-1})	Sanatombi and Sharma (2007)
17	C. annuum	Cotyledon	BAP (22.2 µM)+PAA (14.7 µM)	Joshi and Kothari (2007)
18	C. annuum	Leaf, cotyledon, hypocotyl	BAP (8.8 µM)+IAA (11.4 µM)	Sanatombi and Sharma (2008)
19	C. frutescens	Leaf, cotyledon, hypocotyl	BAP (8.8 µM)+IAA (11.4 µM)	Sanatombi and Sharma (2008)
20	C. chinense	Leaf, cotyledon, hypocotyl	BAP (8.8 µM)+IAA (11.4 µM)	Sanatombi and Sharma (2008)
21	C. annuum	Cotyledons	BAP (6.0 mgL^{-1})+IBA (1.0 mgl^{-1})	Otroshy et al. (2011)
22	C. chinense	Nodal segments and shoot tips	BAP (35.52 µM)+TDZ (18.16 µM)	Kehei et al. (2012)
23	C. annuum	Cotyledon	BAP (6.0 mgL^{-1})+IAA (0.3 mgl^{-1})	Verma et al., (2013)
24	C. annuum	Cotyledonary leaves and hypocotyls	BAP (10.0 mgL$^{-1)}$+IAA (1.0 mgL^{-1})	Rizwan et al. (2013)
25	C. annuum	Shoot	BAP (2.0 mgL$^{-1)}$+IAA (0.5 mgL^{-1})	Swamy et al. (2014)
26	C. chinense	Leaf	Kin (45.0 µM)+2,4-D (3.5µM) + AgNO$_3$ (35.0 µM)	Bora et al. (2014)
27	C. annuum	Nodal segments and shoot tips	IBA (1.0 mgL^{-1})+NAA (1.0 mgL^{-1})+Spermidin (1.5 mM)	Haque and Ghosh (2017)
28	C. annuum	Cotyledons	BAP (44.44 µM)+IAA (5.71 µM) AgNO$_3$ (10.0 µM)+n-morpholine (1.98 mgL^{-1})	Ashwani et al. (2017)
29	C. annuum	Cotyledons	BAP (44.38 µM)+TDZ (9.0 µM) GA$_3$ (5.77 µM)+PAA (14.7 µM)	Mythili et al. (2017)
30	C. annuum	Hypocotyl	Zeatin (7.55 mgL^{-1}) + GA$_3$ (2.0 mgL^{-1})	Hegde et al. (2017)

hypocotyls, leaves, shoot tips, zygotic embryos, embryonic leaves, stems, internodes, mature seeds, and roots have been employed for plant regeneration in capsicum (Agrawal, 1983; Agrawal et al., 1989; Ebida and Hu, 1993; Ezura et al., 1993; Gatz and Rogozinska, 1994; Ramirez-Malagon and Ochoa-Alejo, 1996; Berljak, 1999; do Rêgo et al., 2016; Ashwani et al., 2017; Mythili et al., 2017, Hedge et al., 2017).

17.5.2   CALLUS CULTURE

Developments in biotechnology, particularly methods for callus culture, should provide new means for the commercial handling of economically important plants for continuous production of different cell lines, regenerated plants for conservation, and the secondary metabolites they provide (Mula-bagal and Tsay, 2004). This method can be used for the quality improvement program of elite genotype of chili plants that will be utilized as renewable resources of capsaicin production. It can provide the system to produce and accumulate maximum amount of capsaicin by manipulating the parameters of the tissue culture environment and medium, selecting high-yielding cell clones, precursor feeding, and elicitation in different cultivars of chili (Table 17.3). The naturally grown medicinal plants are moreover different from before, they are facing more and more insecticide, herbicide, and heavy metals, which will cause contamination to the metabolites and finally generate side effects.

Moreover, due to the complex structures of secondary metabolites, chemical synthesis is not achieving maximum productivity in most cases. The huge demand for raw materials for photochemical production from various medicinal plant sources in pharmaceutical industry of the whole world can be satisfied by in vitro production of cell and tissue. Scientists are developed a different way to produce the conservation strategies and corresponding secondary metabolites from this way. A lot of effort is involved for the continuous round the year supply of pharmaceutically important bioactive compounds by manipulating the plant tissue culture system in different way.

This in vitro tissue culture methods are now involved for predictable production of raw materials that are independent of weather and season. In vitro plant callus and cell culture now involved for the production of different types of economically viable secondary metabolites. Synthesis of bioactive natural products from callus culture and plant cell cultures has been presently used for pharmaceutical industry. Production of flavor components and secondary metabolites in vitro using immobilized cells is a perfect method

TABLE 17.3   Callus Culture of Different *Capsicum* spp.

S. No.	Species	Explants/tissues	PGR's+MS medium	References
1	*Capsicum annuum*	Cotyledon, Hypocotyl	BAP (1.0–3.0 mgL^{-1})+IAA (1.0 mgL^{-1})+GA$_3$ (0.5mgL^{-1})	Rodeva et al. (2006)
2	*C. annuum*	Leaf, Shoot and nodal region	2,4-D (2.0 mgL^{-1})+Kin (0.5 mgl^{-1})	Umamaheswai and Lalitha (2007)
3	*C. annuum*	Cotyledon	Kin (0.5 mgL^{-1})+2,4-D (5.0 mgL^{-1})+NAA (2.0 mgL^{-1})	Rakshit et al. (2008)
4	*C. annuum*	Internode	BAP (2.0 µM)+2,4-D (10.0 µM)	Khan et al. (2011)
5	*C. annuum*	Hypocotyls	BAP (1.0 mgL^{-1})+IAA (0.8 mgL^{-1})+AgNO$_3$ (4.0 mgL^{-1})	Xie et al. (2013)
6	*C. chinense*	Immature green pods	2,4-D (2.0 mgL^{-1})+Kin (0.5 mgl^{-1})	Mangang (2014)
7	*C. annuum*	Seedlings	BAP (2.0 mgL^{-1})+NAA (0.1 mgL^{-1})	Swamy et al. (2014)
8	*C. chinense*	Stem	BAP (3.0 mgL^{-1})+NAA (1.0 mgL^{-1})	Raj et al. (2015)
9	*C. annuum*	Seedlings	BAP (0.1 µM)+2,4-D (0.1 µM)	Suthar and Shah (2015)
10	*C. chinense*	Leaf and internod	BAP (6.66 µM)+2,4-D (9.05 µM)	Gayathri et al. (2015)
11	*C. annuum*	Leaf and stem	BAP (1.0–5.0 mgL^{-1})+GA$_3$ (0.5–1.5 mgL^{-1})	Ikhajiagbe et al. (2016)
12	*C. annuum*	leaf, cotyledon, epycotyl and hypocotyl	BAP (4.0 mgL^{-1}) + IAA (0.5 mgL^{-1})+L2 vitamin.	Renfiyeni and Trisno (2016)
13	*C. annuum*	Leaf and Internode	BAP (2.2 µM)+2,4-D (18.10 µM)	Santos et al. (2017)

for spices crops like chili. Production of capsaicin was reported using such system (Johnson et al., 1996; Prasad et al., 2006; Umamaheswai and Lalitha, 2007; Kehie et al., 2014, 2016; Giri and Zaheer, 2016; Ferri et al., 2017).

17.5.3 SOMATIC EMBRYOGENESIS

Somatic embryogenesis is an unique in vitro method that can help to justify the totipotency concept in all plant cells. This potential character is now widely used in different aspects of plant biotechnology including ex situ conservation. It is also used to study the development of the embryo it can be used to produce plants commercially or to carry out basic studies including cell differentiation, gene expression, molecular genetics, and many others aspects also. The reports of somatic embryogenesis study are huge that cover different aspects of induction and subsequent development of various natures from the role of plant growth regulators, mainly auxins and cytokinin, to the function of the components of the media of culture (Loyola-Vargas, 2016).

Somatic embryogenesis can accelerate the steps of genetic improvement program of commercial crop species (Stasolla and Yeung, 2003). Somatic embryogenesis refers to the development of structures that resemble zygotic embryo from somatic cells through an orderly chain of characteristic morphological stages and is contemplated superior over other in vitro propagation systems as it reduces the propagation time and potentially offers an effective system for regenerating whole plants with high-genetic uniformity (Kothari et al., 2010).

Harini and Lakshmi Sita (1993) first time reported the somatic embryogenesis and regeneration in chili from immature zygotic embryos. Both direct or indirect mode of somatic embryogenesis and plant regeneration successfully achieved from various explants, like immature or mature zygotic embryos, seedlings, leaves, stem segments, etc. (Binzel et al., 1996; Buyukalaca and Mavituna, 1996; Kintzios et al., 2000; Kintzios et al., 2001; Kaparakis and Alderson, 2002; Steinitz et al., 2003; Khan et al., 2006; Santana-Buzzy et al., 2009; Avilés-Viñas et al., 2013; Venkataiah et al., 2016). MS medium supplemented with 2,4-D and different percentage of sucrose and sometimes undefined media has been observed to promote somatic embryos induction in chili explants (Binzel et al., 1996; Buyukalaca and Mavituna, 1996; Avilés-Viñas et al., 2013, Venkataiah et al., 2016), whereas cytokinins seem not to have significant role or even instead of induction they can inhibit somatic embryogenesis in chili pepper (Kaparakis and Alderson, 2008).

In few cases, cytokinin is involved in the regulation of plant cell cycling, division, and differentiation, playing key roles in somatic embryogenesis (Zapata-Castillo et al., 2007; Santana-Buzzy et al., 2009). Conversion of mature somatic embryos to complete plantlets has been induced by GA3 or TDZ, alone or in combination (Binzel et al., 1996; Venkataiah et al., 2016). Role of cytokinin on somatic embryos maturation and germination also reported by several groups (Harini and Lakshmi Sita, 1993; Binzel et al., 1996; Solís-Ramos et al., 2009), whereas abscisic acid (ABA) has also been used to promote maturation of somatic embryos (Buyukalaca and Mavituna, 1996). Plant regeneration and direct somatic embryogenesis from hypocotyl, stem segments, and shoot tips of *C. annuum* on TDZ supplemented medium has been studied by (Khan et al., 2006; Aboshama, 2011).

17.5.4 HAPLOID CULTURE

Haploid culture first reported from India, anther culture for the androgenic haploid plant was carried out on *Datura innox*ia by Guha and Maheshwari (1964). Haploid culture is one of the useful methods in plant breeding which may be utilized to facilitate the detection of mutations and the recovery of unique recombinants (Kothari et al., 2010; Roshany et al., 2013). Haploids may occur spontaneously in nature in some specific plant species or they may be induced experimentally to occur in *Capsicum* species (Pochard and Dumas de Vaulx, 1979; Ahmad et al., 2006). Several reports are available on anther culture and regeneration of haploid plants of *Capsicum* species and hybrids (Wang et al., 1973; Kuo et al., 1973; George and Narayanaswamy, 1973; Sibi et al., 1979; Silva Monteiro et al., 2011; Roshany et al., 2013; Barroso et al., 2015; Nowaczyk et al., 2015; Ari et al., 2016). Wang et al. (1973), Kuo et al. (1973), and others have discussed haploid production of chili through anther culture and haploid plant regeneration (Table 17.4).

Chili is now recognized to be the third Solanaceous crop that could be defined as recalcitrant in regard to the response to androgenesis induction (Segui-Simarro et al., 2011). Anthers with microspore at the uninucleate stage were cultured on MS medium modified in some micronutrients and vitamins and supplemented with either Kinetin, NAA, or 2,4-D. Several factors influence the haploid plant regeneration from microspore or anther culture of the *Capsicum* species, hybrid, cultivar, or even genotype (Munyon et al., 1989; Mityko et al., 1995; Nowaczyk and Kisiala, 2006; Koleva-Godeva et al., 2007; Lantos et al., 2009; Alremi et al., 2014; Barroso et al., 2015). Pretreatments of anther donor plants (Kristiansen and Andersen,

TABLE 17.4 Androgenic Culture of Chili.

S. No.	Species	Culture	Media supplement	References
1	*Capsicum annuum*	Anther	Kin (0.1 mgL^{-1})+2,4-D (0.001 mgL^{-1})+Vitamin B$_{12}$ (0.04 mgL^{-1})	Rodeva et al. (2006)
2	*C. annuum*	Microspore	Zeatin (2.5 μM)+IAA (5.0 μM)	Supena et al. (2006)
3	*C. annuum*	Flower bud, Anther	Kin (1.0 mgL^{-1})+IAA (0.001 mgl^{-1})+2,4-D (0.01 mgL^{-1})	Koleva-Godeva et al. (2007)
4	*C. annuum*	Anther	BAP (1.0 mgL^{-1})+NAA (4.0 mgL^{-1})+AgNO$_3$ (15.0 mgL^{-1})	Taskin et al. (2011)
5	*C. annuum*	microspore culture	Kin (0.2 mgL^{-1})+2,4-D (0.1 mgL^{-1})	Lantos et al. (2012)
6	*C. annuum*	Anther	BAP (0.5 mgL^{-1})+NAA (0.5 mgL^{-1})+2,4-D (0.1 mgL^{-1})	Roshany et al. (2013)
7	*C. annuum*	Anther	Kin (0.1 mgL^{-1})+2,4-D (0.01 mgL^{-1})	Nowaczyk et al. (2015)
8	*C. annuum*	Anther	BAP (6.0 mgL^{-1})+NAA (0.5 mgL^{-1})+AgNO$_3$ (6.0 mgL^{-1})	Taskin et al. (2013); Ari et al. (2016)
9	*C. annuum*	Anther	Kin (0.1 mgL^{-1})+2,4-D (0.1 mgL^{-1})	Akyol et al. (2016)
10	*C. annuum*	Anther	Zeatin (1.0 mgL^{-1})+2,4-D (0.2 mgL^{-1})+AgNO$_3$ (15.0 mgL^{-1})	Hegde et al. (2017)

1993) or floral buds before in vitro culture are very common for increasing the regeneration ability of haploids in chili pepper (Sibi et al., 1979; Barroso et al., 2015).

17.5.5   TRANSFORMED CULTURE OF CHILI

Orthodox plant breeding has paid meaningfully to crop upgrading over the past 50 years. However, there is intense pressure to produce further improvements in crop quality and quantity due to the result of population growth, social demands, health requirements, environmental stress, and ecological considerations. Traditional plant breeding is not able to withstand this increasing demand due to the limited gene pool, restricted range of organism between which genes can be moved in the species barriers. Genetic transformation holds countless ability for improving these major restrictions to crop productivity. Chili is second only to tomato in terms of vegetable production in advanced countries, and its breeding and production, as with other major crops, are constantly faced by plentiful pests, diseases, and abiotic stresses (Rizwan et al., 2013).

Genetic manipulation is an attractive proposition where it involves recombination of an efficient cell or tissue culture regeneration system with recombinant DNA technology, which would transfer specific genes from other taxa, or the modified expression of specific native genes (Kothari et al., 2010). It is very common, *Agrobacterium tumefaciens* and *A. rhizogenes* has been used as the vector for genetic transformation of diverse dicotyledonous species, In the case of chili pepper, genetic transformation via Agrobacterium is surely an important tool to help genetic improvement against many diseases caused by phytopathogenic fungi, bacteria, and viruses (Aarrouf et al., 2012; Rizwan et al., 2013). However, advances in this area have been limited because of low efficiency for in vitro plant regeneration of the reported systems. Liu et al. (1990) published the first report on chili pepper genetic transformation employing in vitro seedling explants (hypocotyls, cotyledons, and leaves) cocultured with the wild tumorigenic strains A281 and C58 of *A. tumefaciens* and with a disarmed strain bearing the plasmid pGV 3850.

Callus normally developed from cotyledon and leaf tissues leaf-like structures, and occasional shoot buds in the presence of kanamycin. Although a number of kanamycin-resistant shoot buds were obtained, no further elongation and plant formation occurred. Usually Agrobacterium has been the only used vector for chili pepper genetic transformation (Liu et al., 1990; Wang et al., 1991; Dong et al., 1992; Lee et al., 1993; Ye et al., 1993; Zhu et al., 1996; Kim et al., 1997; Christopher and Rajam, 1997; Subhash and Christopher, 1997; Lim et al., 1997; Mihalka et al., 2000; Aarrouf et al., 2012; Rizwan et al., 2013). Plant regeneration and transformation studies have been mainly focused on *C. annuum* (Liu et al., 1990; Dong et al., 1992; Christopher and Rajam, 1997; Lee et al., 1993; Ye et al., 1993; Zhu et al., 1996; Harpster et al., 2002; Kim et al., 2002; Shin et al., 2002; Dabauza and Pena, 2003; Li et al., 2003). Most transformation studies in chili pepper refer to the use of marker (npt II) or reporter genes (gus) in order to establish adequate protocols; however, some genes have also been utilized to generate transgenic plants with tolerance to Cucumber mosaic virus (Dong et al., 1992; Lee et al., 1993; Zhu et al., 1996; Kim et al., 1997; Chen et al., 2003; Lee et al., 2009) or tolerant to multiple pathogenic organisms (Shin et al., 2002), and drought-tolerant (Maligeppagol et al., 2016).

17.6   IN VITRO CONSERVATION

During the last four decades, in vitro techniques have been increasingly used throughout the world for plant conservation. They consist of growing and multiplying parts of plants in flask or tubes in arterial media under control environments and sterile conditions. Gradually, an increasing number of countries have invested in tissue culture facilities for the propagation of genetically suitable cloned plants. In vitro conservation techniques are the expertise and facilities are also present. They are more economical and less risky in a long-term perspective. The conservation of plant organs that are propagates vegetatively, instead of whole plant, helps to reduce the large space. Recently advanced biotechnological techniques are used that offer alternative strategies, including slow growth in vitro culture for short-, medium-, and long-term conservation. Due to edaphic factors, it has minimal possibilities of losses and ensures more secure conservation of germplasm for future generation. Cost of preservation is highly dependent on location and when in vitro conservation is taken into consideration.

The recent advances in vitro conservation technology encapsulation of in vitro plant propagules serve different potential attributes to be an effective alternative pathway for ex situ conservation. Synthetic seed production is a modern technique which induces regrowth, rooting and converts into a complete plantlets. Recently, there has been a much prominence use of synthetic seeds for the conservation programmed of different elite germplasm of chili (Sharma and Shahzad, 2012; Parveen and Shahzad, 2014; Kundu et al., 2015). For short-term storage using either somatic embryos or vegetative propagules that were mixed with sodium alginate containing MS liquid medium dropped individually into a complexing solution of calcium chloride in a beaker placed on a magnetic stirrer. The encapsulated explants and nonencapsulated explants cultures were stored for few months under 4–15°C. These positive attributes of synthetic seeds are well enough to be emphasized for the propagation economically important plant species as well as for short-term ex situ conservation under low temperature.

For the successful execution of these techniques, in vitro culture may be considered as prerequisite phenomena. Therefore, micropropagation or in vitro culture techniques are effective tools that could be exploited for mass propagation and may be further used for conservation and utilization of genetic resources. In vitro collection maintaining cannot be considered a perfect method of regular subcultivations. A large number of subcultures was required for maintaining germplasm and at every step risk of contamination that is increase and this may lead to loss of genetic uniformity. Therefore, for optimizing in vitro conservation protocol should provide maximum survival rate of plants with a minimum rate of relapse of subculture (Srivastava et al., 2013). On the one hand, the stable growth of aseptic culture is a necessary prerequisite and important indicator of the efficiency of conservation method. Wide range of species and culture systems was gain through in vitro conservation of cultures it is also give varying degrees of success and successful slow growth systems were developed for different plant species (Negri et al., 2000; Thomas and Jacob, 2004; Piovan et al., 2010; Engelmann, 2011; Phulwaria et al., 2012; Cheruvathur et al., 2013). Ozudogru et al. (2010) reported that slow-growth conservation and cryopreservation of ornamental species that refers to the in vitro conservation of shoot cultures by minimizing their periodic subcultures without affecting the viability and revival of shoot cultures. In vitro conservation, most importantly is used to conserve the stored genetic material with maximum vigor, disease-free, and without somaclonal variation (Lata et al., 2010). Generally, slow growth is succeeded by either adding osmotic agent in the form of variable concentrations of sucrose, mannitol, and sorbitol or by removing growth regulator with the medium (Gonçalves and Romano, 2007; Lata et al., 2010; Scherwinski-Pereira et al., 2010). Addition of osmotic agent in culture media there is a significant increase in the storage life of *in vitro* tissues (Sharaf et al., 2012). Slow growth *in vitro* may be obtained by low temperature (Janeiro et al., 1995; Negri et al., 2000), which is required for minimum growth of plantlets usually 4–8°C storage temperature is required for temperate crops and

10–15°C for tropical germplasm (Keller et al., 2006). Germplasm for in vitro conservation of *Capsicum* for long- and medium-term storage was performed through medium composition rearrangement or facilitate to genetic manipulation were performed different authors (Batau et al., 2005; Valera-Montero et al., 2005; Montalvo-Peniche et al., 2007; Vilma et al., 2014).

17.7 CRYOPRESERVATION

For long-term conservation of the problem species, cryopreservation is the only method currently available. Dramatic progress has been made in recent years in the development of new cryopreservation techniques and cryopreservation protocols have been established for over 100 different plant species. Cryopreservation is an attractive option for long-term storage. Liquid nitrogen (–196°C) is routinely used for cryogenic storage, since it is relatively cheap and safe, requires little maintenance, and is widely available. Preparation of plant material could be considered for cryopreservation as dictated by the actual needs of conservation. Conservation here includes cell, callus, meristems, and protoplast cultures, somatic and zygotic embryos, anthers, pollen and whole seeds (Withers, 1985; Kartha, 1985). Plant germplasm stored in liquid nitrogen (–196°C) does not undertake cellular divisions. In addition, metabolic and most physical processes are stopped at this low temperature. As such, plant cells and organs can be stored for very long time periods and both the problem of genetic instability and the risk of losing accessions due to contamination or human error during subculturing are overcome. Maximum activities of cryopreservation contract with recalcitrant or refractory seeds vegetatively propagated in vitro crop tissues, species with a particular gene combination (elite genotypes) and dedifferentiated plant cell, tissue, organ, and callus. Care must be taken to avoid ice crystallization during the freezing process, which otherwise would cause physical damage to the tissues. The existing cryogenic policies depend on air-drying, osmotic dehydration, freeze dehydration, the addition of penetrating, cryoprotective substances and adaptive metabolism, encapsulation combinations of these processes. Cryopreservation is one of the impotent technical methods that have been developed for more than 80 different plant species in various forms like cell suspensions, calluses, and apices, somatic and zygotic embryos (Kartha and Engelmann, 1994; Engelmann et al., 1995; Engelmann, 2000). However, their routine utilization is still restricted almost exclusively to the conservation of cell lines in research laboratories. For small volumes, long-term storage is practicable through storage of cultures or materials in cryopreservation at ultralow temperature, usually by using liquid nitrogen (–196°C). At this low temperature, all cellular divisions and metabolic activities are virtually halted and therefore, plant material can be indefinitely stored without alteration or modification. The normal approach of tissue culture is to find a medium and set of conditions that favor the most rapid rate of growth with a subculture interval of 20–30 days. For cryopreservation storage, biological materials are stored in liquid nitrogen for long-term preservation without any subculturing. Cryopreservation, that is, the storage of biological material at ultralow temperature usually that of liquid nitrogen (–196°C) can be achieved by different techniques like direct freezing, encapsulation dehydration, encapsulation, and vitrification. Cryopreservation of *Capsicum* is meager and limited for the status of chili conservation as reported by different authors (Alexander et al., 1991; Rajasekharan and Ganeshan, 2003).

17.8   DNA BANK

Concurrent with the advancements in gene cloning and transfer has been the development of technology for the removal and analysis of DNA. DNAs from the nucleus, mitochondrion, and chloroplast are now routinely extracted and immobilized onto nitrocellulose sheets where the DNA can be probed with numerous cloned genes. In addition, the rapid development of polymerase chain reaction (PCR) now means that one can routinely amplify specific oligonucleotides or genes from the entire mixture of genomic DNA. These advances, coupled with the prospect of the loss of significant plant genetic resources throughout the world, have led to the establishment of DNA bank for the storage of genomic DNA. The conserved DNA will have numerous uses viz, molecular phylogenetic and systematic analysis of extinct taxa, production of previously characterized secondary compounds in transgenic cell cultures, production of transgenic plants using genes from gene families, in vitro expression and study of enzyme structure and function and genomic probes for research laboratories. The vast resources of dried specimens in the world's herbaria may hold considerable DNA that would be suitable for PCR. It seems likely that the integrity of DNA would decrease with the age of specimens. Because there are many types of herbarium storage environments, preservation, and collections, there is a need for systematic investigations of the effect of modes of preparation, collection, and storage on the integrity of DNA in the world's major holdings. Storing DNA advantage is that it is very simple, efficient, and overcomes many physical limitations then constraints that characterize other forms of storage (Adams, 1994). The disadvantage lies in problems with subsequent gene isolation, cloning, and transfer and, most importantly, it does not allow the regeneration of live organisms (Maxted et al., 1997). The plant taxonomy and systematics community have responded to the biodiversity crisis by defining three major challenges summarized by Blackmore (2002): (1) completing the inventory of life, (2) discovering evolutionary relationships through phylogenetic, and (3) providing information via the Internet. DNA collections can help with all three of those activities. DNA sequence analysis is useful in the identification and delimitation of species and higher taxa and is also set to become increasingly important via DNA taxonomy and DNA barcoding (Tautz et al., 2003; Lipscomb et al., 2003; Kristiansen et al., 2005; Chase et al., 2005). It is a powerful resource for molecular phylogenetic and efforts to reconstruct the 'tree of life' (Palmer et al., 2004).

Capsicum GENE banks for collections of germplasm predominantly retain domesticated accessions, with emphasis on complex *C. annuum* species. This is also observed for the characterization and evaluation of germplasm. In studies involving multiple species, 89% of the accessions belong to the *C. annuum* complex, 9.5% correspond to *C. baccatum*, 0.61% to *C. pubescens*, and 0.78% to other species (Leite et al., 2016). Some authors are followed to store of chloroplast DNA (Buso et al., 2002; Albrecht et al., 2012; Raveendar et al., 2015).

17.9 CONCLUSIONS

Ex situ conservation of chili is essential for present and future utilization and exploration for both conventional breedings as well as modern biotechnological purposes. No one method is compulsory for ex situ conservation that can be done by any means as per their available facility and purposes.

ACKNOWLEDGMENTS

We acknowledge Swami Kamalasthananda, Principal, Ramakrishna Mission Vivekananda Centenary College, Rahara, Kolkata (India), for the facilities provided during the present study. Also, DST-FIST program for infrastructural facilities is acknowledged. BG thanks the Department of Science and Technology, West Bengal (DST-WB) for providing a research grant.

KEYWORDS

- **chili**
- **ex situ conservation**
- **conservation strategies**
- **germplasm conservation**

REFERENCES

Aarrouf, J.; Castro-Quezada, P.; Mallard, S.; Caromel, B.; Lizzi, Y.; Lefebvre, V. Agrobacterium Rhizogenes-dependent Production of Transformed Roots from Foliar Explants of Pepper (*Capsicum annuum*): A New and Efficient Tool for Functional Analysis of Genes. *Plant Cell. Rep.* **2012,** *31*, 391–401.

Aboshama, H. M. S. Direct Somatic Embryogenesis of Pepper *(Capsicum annuum* L.). *World J. Agric. Sci.* **2011,** *7*, 755–762.

Adams, R. P. Conservation of Plant Genes II. Missouri Botanical Garden, 1994.

Agrawal, S.; Chandra, N. Differentiation of Multiple Shoot Buds and Plantlets in Cultured Embryos of *Capsicum annuum* L. var Mathania. *Curr Sci.* **1983,** *52*, 645–6.

Agrawal, S.; Chandra, N.; Kothari, S. L. Plant Regeneration in Tissue Cultures of Pepper (*Capsicum annuum* L. cv. Mathania). *Plant Cell Tiss. Org. Cult.* **1989,** *16*, 47–55.

Ahmad, N.; Siddique, I.; Anis, M. Improved Plant Regeneration in *Capsicum annum* L from Nodal Segments. *Biol. Plantarum* **2006,** *50*, 701–704.

Akyol, B.; Işİk, D.; İlbİ, H.; Gürel, A. Effect of Plant Growth Regulators in Anther Cultures of Different Pepper (*Capsicum annuum* L.) Varieties. Radovi Poljoprivrednog Fakulteta Univerziteta u Sarajevu (Works of the Faculty of Agriculture University of Sarajevo) **2016,** *61*, 189–192.

Albrecht, E.; Zhang, D.; Saftner, R. A.; Stommel, J. R. Genetic Diversity and Population Structure of *Capsicum baccatum* Genetic Resources. *Genet. Resour. Crop. Evol.* **2012,** *59*, 517–538.

Alexander, M. P.; Ganeshan, S.; Rajasekharan, P. E. Freeze Preservation of *capsicum* Pollen in Liquid Nitrogen (−196 C) for 42 Months-effect on Pollen Viability and Fertility. *Plant Cell Incompat. Newsl.* **1991,** *23*, 1–4.

Allard, R. W. Population Structure and Sampling Methods. In *Genetic Resources in Plants–Their Exploration and Conservation*; Frankel, O. H., Bennett, E., Eds.; Blackwell Scientific Publications: USA, 1970; pp 97–107.

Alremi, F.; Taşkın, H.; Sönmez, K.; Büyükalaca, S.; Ellialtıoğlu, Ş. Effect of Genotype and Nutrient Medium on Anther Culture of Pepper (*Capsicum annuum* L.). *Turk. J. Agric. Nat. Sci.* **2014,** *1*, 108–116.

Ari, E.; Yildirim, T.; Mutlu, N.; Büyükalaca, S.; gökmen. Ü.; Akman, E Comparison of Different Androgenesis Protocols for Doubled Haploid Plant Production in Ornamental Pepper (*Capsicum annuum* L.). *Turkish J. Biol.* **2016,** *40*, 944–954.

Arous, S.; Boussaid, M.; Marrakchi, M. Plant Regeneration from Zygotic Embryo Hypocotyls of Tunisian chili (*Capsicum annuum* L.). *J. Appl. Hortic.* **2001,** *3*, 17–22.

Ashwani, S.; Ravishankar, G. A.; Giridhar, P. Silver Nitrate and 2-(N-morpholine) Ethane Sulphonic Acid in Culture Medium Promotes Rapid Shoot Regeneration from the Proximal Zone of the Leaf of *Capsicum frutescens* Mill. *Plant Cell Tiss. Org. Cult.* **2017**, *129*, 175–180.

Avilés–Viñas, S. A.; Lecona-Guzmán, C. A.; Canto-Flick, A.; López-Erosa, S.; Santana-Buzzy, N. Morpho-histological and Ultrastructural Study on Direct Somatic Embryogenesis of *Capsicum chinense* Jacq. in Liquid Medium. *Plant Biotechnol. Rep.* **2013**, *7*, 277–286.

Babu, B. K.; Agrawal, P. K.; Pandey, D.; Jaiswal, J. P.; Kumar, A. Association Mapping of Agro-morphological Characters Among the Global Collection of Finger Millet Genotypes Using Genomic SSR Markers. *Mol. Biol. Rep.* **2014**, *41*, 5287–5297.

Babu, K. N.; Yamuna, G.; Praveen, K.; Minoo, D.; Ravindran, P. N.; Peter, K. V. Cryopreservation of Spices Genetic Resources (Chapter 16). In *Current Frontiers in Cryobiology*; IntechOpen: 2012, pp 457–484.

Bennett, E., Sykes, T., Bunting, H., Eds. *Plant Genetic Resources: Historical Survey*; CGIAR/ IBPGR: Rome, 1987.

Blackmore, S. Biodiversity Update-Progress in Taxonomy. *Science* **2002**, *298*, 365–365.

Bosland, P. W. Capsicums: Innovative Uses of An Ancient Crop. In *Progress in New Crops*; Janick, J., Ed.; ASHS Press: Arlington, VA, 1996; pp 479–487.

Barroso, P. A.; Rêgo, M. M.; Rêgo, E. R.; Soares, W. S. Embryogenesis in the Anthers of Different Ornamental Pepper (*Capsicum annuum* L.) Genotypes. *Genet. Mol. Res.* **2015**, *14*, 13349–13363.

Binzel, M. L.; Sankhla, N.; Joshi, S.; Sankhla, D. Induction of Direct Somatic Embryogenesis and Plant Regeneration in Pepper (*Capsicum annuum* L.). *Plant Cell Rep.* **1996**, *15*, 536–540.

Berljak, J. *In Vitro* Plant Regeneration from Pepper (*Capsicum annuum* L. cv.Soroksari') Seedling Explants. *Phyton. Horn.* **1999**, 39, 289–292.

Bonilla, M. D. O.; Chen, F. C. Effect of 6-benzyladenine (BA) and Indole-3-acetic Acid (IAA) on the *In Vitro* Regeneration of Chili Pepper (*Capsicum annuum* L.). *J. Int. Coop.* **2015**, *10*, 109–120.

Bora, G.; Gogoi, H. K.; Handique, P. J. Effect of Silver Nitrate and Gibberellic Acid on *in Vitro* Regeneration, Flower Induction and Fruit Development in Naga Chilli. *As Pac. J. Mol. Bio. Biotech.* **2014**, *22*, 137–144.

Buso, G. S. C.; de Amaral, S. P.; Bianchetti, L. B.; Ferreira, M. E. Análise de seqüências de DNA chloroplástico de especies do gênero *Capsicum.* Boletim de Pesquisa e Desenvolvimento, **2002**, *37*, 1–21.

Buyukalaca, S. Mavituna, F. Somatic Embryogenesis and Plant Regeneration of Pepper in Liquid Media. *Plant Cell Tiss. Org. Cult.* **1996**, *46*, 227–235.

Campos, F. F.; Morgan, Jr. D. T. Haploid Pepper from A Sperm: An Androgenetic Haploid of *Capsicum frutescens.* [J. Hered. **1985**, *49*, 135–137.

Chase, M. W.; Salamin, N.; Wilkinson, M.; Dunwell, J. M.; Kesanakurthi RP, Haidar N Savolainen V Land plants and DNA Barcodes: Short-term and Long-term Goals. *Philos. Trans. R. Soc. Lond. B. Biol. Sci.* **2005**, *360*, 1889–1895.

Chatterjee, T.; Ghosh, B. Simple Protocol for Micropropagation and In Vitro Conservation of *Plumbago zeylanica* L: An Important Indigenous Medicinal Plant. *Int. J. Biores. Stress Manag.* **2015**, *6*, 068–075.

Chatterjee, T.; Ghosh, B. Efficient Stable *In Vitro* Micropropagation and Conservation of *Tinospora cordifolia* (Willd.) Miers: An Anti-diabetic Indigenous Medicinal. *Int. J. Bio-Res. Stress Manag.* **2016**, *7*, 814–822.

Chen, Z. L.; Gu, H.; Li, Y.; Su, Y.; Wu, P.; Jiang, Z.; Ming, X.; Tian, J.; Pan, N.; Qu, L. J. Safety Assessment for Genetically Modified Sweet Pepper and Tomato. *Toxicology* **2003**, *188*, 297–307.

Christopher, T.; Rajam, M. V. *In Vitro* Clonal Propagation of *Capsicum* spp. *Plant Cell Tiss. Org. Cult.* **1994**, *38*, 25–29.

Christopher, T.; Rajam, M. V. Effect of Genotype, Explant and Medium on *In Vitro* Regeneration of Red Pepper. *Plant Cell. Tiss. Org. Cult.* **1996**, *46*, 245–250.

Christopher, T. Rajam, M. V. *In Vitro* Plant Regeneration and *Agrobacterium* Mediated Transformation in Red Pepper. *In vitro* **1997**, *33*, 73.

Costa, P.; Gonçalves, S.; Valentão, P.; Andrade, P. B.; Romano, A. Accumulation of Phenolic Compounds in *In Vitro* Cultures and Wild Plants of Lavandula viridis L'Her and Their Antioxidant and Anti-cholinesterase Potential. *Food Chem. Toxicol.* **2013**, *57*, 69–74.

Dabauza, M.; Pena, L. High Efficiency Organogenesis in Sweet Pepper (*Capsicum annuum* L.) Tissues from Different Seedling Explants. *Plant Growth Regul.* **2001**, *33*, 221–229.

Dabauza, M.; Peña, L. Response of Sweet Pepper (*Capsicum annuum* L.) Genotypes to Agrobacterium Tumefaciens as a Means of Selecting Proper Vectors for Genetic Transformation. *J. Hortic. Sci. Biotechnol.* **2003**, *78*, 39–45.

Dong, C.; Chunxiao, J.; Lanxiang, F.; Jiazhen, G. Transgenic Pepper Plants (*Capsicum annuum* l.) Containing CMV Sat-RNA cDNA. *Acta Hortic. Sinica.* **1992**, *2*, 019.

do Rêgo, M. M.; do Rêgo, E. R.; Barroso, P. A. Tissue Culture of *Capsicum* spp. In Production and Breeding of Chilli Peppers (*Capsicum* spp.). Springer International Publishing: USA, 2016; pp 97–127.

Ebida, A. I.; Hu, C. Y. *In Vitro* Morphogenetic Responses and Plant Regeneration from Pepper (*Capsicum annuum* L. cv. Early California Wonder) Seedling Explants. *Plant Cell Rep.* **1993**, *13*, 107–110.

Engelmann, F.; Dumet, D.; Chabrillange. N.; Abdelnour-Esquivel. A.; Assy Bah, B.; Dereuddre, J.; Duval, Y. Cryopreservation of Zygotic and Somatic Embryos from Recalcitrant and Intermediate-seed Species. *Plant Genet. Res. Newsl.* **1995**, *103*, 27–31.

Engelmann, F. Importance of Cryopreservation for the Conservation of Plant Genetic Resources. In *Cryopreservation of Tropical Plant Germplasm: Current Research Progress and Application*. Proceedings of an International Workshop, International Plant Genetic Resources Institute, Tsukuba, Japan, October, 1998, pp 8–20.

Engelmann, F. Use of Biotechnologies for the Conservation of Plant Biodiversity in Vitro Cellular and Development Biology. *Plant.* **2011**, *47*, 5–16.

España, R. G. L.; López-Hernández, E. R.; Hernández-Morales, T.; Charrez-Cruz, A.; González-Guzmán, Y.; Muñoz-Jimarez, N. A.; Quintero, J. A. O. Effects of Temperature on Wild Chili Pepper (*Capsicum annuum* var. glabriusculum) Germination Grown Under Two Light Conditions. *Acta Agronómica* **2017**, *66*, 69–74.

Ezura, H.; Nishimiya, S.; Kasumi, M. Efficient Regeneration of Plants Independent of Exogeneous Growth Regulators in Bell Pepper (*Capsicum annuum* L.). *Plant Cell Rep.* **1993**, *12*, 676–680.

FAO Global Plan of Action for the Conservation and Sustainable Utilization of Plant Genetic Resources for Food and Agriculture. FAO, Rome, 1996.

Ferri, M.; Gruarin, N.; Barbieri, F.; Tassoni, A. *Capsicum spp* In Vitro Liquid Cell Suspensions: A Useful System for the Pr oduction of Capsaicinoids and Polyphenols. *Plant Biosyst.* **2017**, *152*, 1–9.

Franck-Duchenne, M.; Wang, Y.; Tahar, S. B.; Beachy, R. N. *In Vitro* Stem Elongation of Sweet Pepper in Media Containing 24-epi-Brassinolide. *Plant Cell Tiss. Org. Cult.* **1998**, *53*, 79–84.

Frankel, O. H., Hawkes, J. G., Eds. *Crop Genetic Resources for Today and Tomorrow*; Cambridge University Press: Cambridge, 1975; p 492.

Fu, Y. B. The Vulnerability of Plant Genetic Resources Conserved Ex Situ. *Crop Sci.* 2017. DOI: 10.2135/cropsci2017.01.001.

Gatz, A.; Rogozińska, J. *In Vitro* Organogenetic Potential of Cotyledon and Leaf Explants of *Capsicum annuum* L., cv. Bryza. *Acta Soc. Bot. Pol.* **1994**, *63*, 255–258.

Garba, N. M. I.; Bakasso, Y.; Zaman-Allah, M.; Atta, S.; Mamane, M. I.; Adamou, M.; ... Saadou, M. Evaluation of Agro-morphological Diversity of Groundnut (Arachis hypogaea L.) in Niger. *Afr. J. Agric. Res.* **2015**, *10*, 334–344.

Gayathri, N.; Gopalakrishnan, M.; Sekar, T. *In Vitro* Micropropagation of *Capsicum chinense* Jacq. (Naga King Chili). *Asian J. Plant. Sci. Res.* **2015**, *5,* 13–18.

George, L.; Narayanaswamy, S. Haploid *Capsicum* Through Experimental Androgenesis. *Protoplasma* **1973**, *78*, 467–470.

Giri, C. C. Zaheer, M. Chemical Elicitors Versus Secondary Metabolite Production In Vitro Using Plant Cell, Tissue and Organ Cultures: Recent Trends and a Sky Eye View Appraisal. *Plant Cell Tiss. Org. Cult.* **2016**, *126*, 1–18.

Gonçalves, S.; Romano, A. In Vitro Minimum Growth for Conservation of *Drosophyllum lusitanicum*. *Biol. Plantarum.* **2007**, *51*, 795–798.

Guha, S.; Maheshwari, S. C. *In Vitro* Production of Embryos from Anthers of Datura. *Nature* **1964**, *204*, 497–497.

Haberlandt, G. Culturversuche mit isolierten Pflanzenzellen. In Plant Tissue Culture. Springer: Vienna, 2003; pp 1–24.

Haque, S. M. Ghosh, B. High Frequency Microcloning of *Aloe Vera* and their True-to-type Conformity by Molecular Cytogenetic Assessment of Two Years Old Field Growing Regenerated Plants. *Bot. Stud.* **2013a**, *54*, 46.

Haque, S. M.; Ghosh, B. Field Evaluation and Genetic Stability Assessment of Regenerated Plants Produced Via Direct Shoot Organogenesis from Leaf Explant of an Endangered 'Asthma Plant' (*Tylophora indica*) Along with Their *In Vitro* Conservation. *Natl. Acad. Sci. Lett.* **2013b**, *36*, 551–562.

Haque, S. M.; Ghosh, B. An Improved Micropropagation Protocol for the Recalcitrant Plant *Capsicum*–a Study with Ten Cultivars of *Capsicum spp.* (*C. annuum, C. chinense, and C. frutescens*) Collected from Diverse Geographical Regions of India and Mexico. *J. Hortic. Sci. Biotechnol.* **2017**, 1–9.

Haque, S. M.; Paul, S.; Ghosh, B. High-frequency in Vitro Flowering, Hand-pollination and Fruit Setting in Ten Different Cultivars of *Capsicum* spp. (*C. annuum, C. chinense*, and *C. frutescens*): An Initial Step Towards In Vitro Hybrid Production. *Plant Cell, Tiss. Org. Cult.* **2016**, *127*, 161–173

Harini, I.; Sita, G. L. Direct Somatic Embryogenesis and Plant Regeneration from Immature Embryos of Chilli (*Capsicum annuum* L.). *Plant Sci.* **1993**, *89*, 107–112.

Harpster, M. H.; Brummell, D. A.; Dunsmuir, P. Suppression of a Ripening-related endo-1, 4–β-glucanase in Transgenic Pepper Fruit does not Prevent Depolymerization of Cell Wall Polysaccharides During Ripening. *Plant Mol. Biol.* **2002**, *50*, 345–355.

Hegde, V.; Partap, P. S.; Yadav, R. C. Plant Regeneration from Hypocotyl Explants in *Capsicum* (*Capsicum annuum* L.). *Int. J. Curr. Microbiol. App Sci.* **2017**, *6*, 545–557.

Hegde, V.; Partap, P. S.; Yadav, R. C.; Baswana, K. S. *In Vitro* Androgenesis in *Capsicum* (*Capsicum annuum* L.). *Int. J. Curr. Microbiol. App Sci*. 2017, 6, 925–933.

Husain, S.; Jain, A.; Kothari, S. L. Phenylacetic Acid Improves Bud Elongation and *In Vitro* Plant Regeneration Efficiency in *Capsicum annuum* L. *Plant Cell Rep.* **1999**, *19*, 64–68.

Hyde, C. L.; Phillips, G. C. Silver Nitrate Promotes Shoot Development and Plant Regeneration of Chile Pepper (*Capsicum annuum* L.) via Organogenesis. *In Vitro Cell Dev. Biol. Plant.* **1996,** *32,* 72–80.

Ikhajiagbe, B.; Eke, R. C.; Guobadia, B. O. Induction of Callus from Leaf and Stem Tissues Obtained from *Capsicum annuum* Explant Grown on Waste Engine Oil-polluted Soils. *J. Microbiol. Biotechnol. Food Sci.* **2016,** *6,* 966.

Iwanaga, M. Global Needs for Plant Genetic Resources Conservation. Presented at the Symposium on the Genetic Resources of Farm Animals and Plants, Norway, 1994.

Jacobsen, S. E.; Sørensen, M.; Pedersen, S. M.; Weiner, J. Feeding the World: Genetically Modified Crops Versus Agricultural Biodiversity. *Agron. Sustain. Dev.* **2013,** *33,* 651–662.

Janeiro, L. V.; Vieitez, A. M.; Ballester, A. Cold Storage of *In Vitro* Cultures of Wild Cherry, Chest Nut and Oak. *Ann. Sci.* **1995,** *52,* 287–93.

Johnson, T. S.; Ravishankar, G. A.; Venkataraman, L. V. Biotransformation of Ferulic Acid and Vanillylamine to Capsaicin and Vanillin in Immobilized Cell Cultures of *Capsicum frutescens. Plant Cell. Tiss. Org. Cult.* **1996,** *44,* 117–121.

Joshi, A. Micronutrient Optimization in Culture Media Improves Plant Regeneration in Regeneration in *Capsicum annuum Capsicum annuum Capsicum annuum* L. IISUniv. *J. Sc. Tech.* **2016,** *5,* 24–28.

Joshi, A.; Kothari, S. L. High Copper Levels in the Medium Improves Shoot Bud Differentiation and Elongation from the Cultured Cotyledons of *Capsicum annuum* L. *Plant Cell Tiss. Org. Cult.* **2007,** *88,* 127–133.

Jovicich, E.; Cantliffe, D. J.; Stoffella, P. J. Fruit Yield and Quality of Greenhouse-grown Bell Pepper as Influenced by Density, Container, and Trellis System. *Hort. Technol.* **2004,** *14,* 507–513.

Kaparakis, G.; Alderson, P. G. Influence of High Concentrations of Cytokinins on the Production of Somatic Embryos by Germinating Seeds of Tomato, Aubergine and Pepper. *J. Hortic. Sci. Biotechnol.* **2002,** *77,* 186–190.

Kaparakis, G.; Alderson, P. G. Role for Cytokinins in Somatic Embryogenesis of Pepper (*Capsicum annuum* L.)? *J. Plant Growth Regul.* **2008,** *27,* 110–114.

Kartha, K. K. *Meristem Culture and Germplasm Preservation. Cryopreservation of Plant Cells and Organs*; CRC Press: Boca Raton, FL, USA, 1985.

Kartha, K. K.; Engelmann, F. Cryopreservation and Germplasm Storage. In *Plant Cell and Tissue Culture*; Vasil, I. K., Thorpe T. A., eds.; Kluwer: Dordrecht, 1994; pp 195–230.

Keatinge, J. D.; Chadha, M. L.; Hughes, J. D. A.; Easdown, W. J.; Holmer, R. J.; Tenkouano, A.; … Luther, G. Vegetable Gardens and Their Impact on the Attainment of the Millennium Development Goals. *Biol. Agri. Horti.* **2012,** *28,* 71–85.

Kehie, M.; Kumaria, S.; Tandon, P. *In Vitro* Plantlet Regeneration from Nodal Segments and Shoot Tips of *Capsicum chinense* Jacq. cv. Naga King Chili. 3 *Biotech* **2012,** *2,* 31–35.

Keller, E. R. J.; Senula, A.; Leunufna, S.; Grübe, M. Slow Growth Storage and Cryopreservation Tools to Facilitate Germplasm Maintenance of Vegetatively Propagated Crops in Living Plant Collections. *Intl. J. Refrig.* **2006,** *29,* 411–417.

Khan, H.; Siddique, I.; Anis, M. Thidiazuron Induced Somatic Embryogenesis and Plant Regeneration in *Capsicum annuum. Biol Plant.* **2006,** *50,* 789–792.

Khan, M. S. I.; Roy, S. S.; Pall, K. K. Nitrogen and Phosphorus Efficiency on the Growth and Yield Attributes of *capsicum. Acad. J. Plant Sci.* **2010,** *3,* 71–78.

Khan, H.; Siddique, I.; Anis, M.; Khan, P. R. *In Vitro* Organogenesis from Internode Derived Callus Cultures of *Capsicum annuum* L. *J. Plant Biochem. Biot.* **2011,** *20,* 84–89.

Kim, S. J.; Lee, S. J.; Kim, B. D.; Paek, K. H. Satellite-RNA-mediated Resistance to Cucumber Mosaic Virus in Transgenic Plants of Hot Pepper (*Capsicum annuum* cv. Golden Tower). *Plant Cell Rep.* **1997**, *16*, 825–830.

Kim, J. Y.; Jung, M.; Kim, H. S.; Lee, Y. H.; Choi, S. H.; Lim, Y. P.; ... Harn, C. H.; A New Selection System for Pepper Regeneration by Mannose. *J. Plant Biotechnol.* **2002**, *4*, 129–134.

Kintzios, S.; Drossopoulos, J. B.; Shortsianitis, E.; Peppes, D. Induction of Somatic Embryogenesis from Young, Fully Expanded Leaves of Chilli Pepper (*Capsicum annuum* L.): Effect of Leaf Position, Illumination and Explant Pretreatment with High Cytokinin Concentrations. *Sci. Hort.* **2000**, *85*, 137–144.

Kintzios, S.; Drossopoulos, J. B.; Lymperopoulos, C. Effect of Vitamins and Inorganic Micronutrients on Callus Growth and Somatic Embryogenesis from Leaves of Chilli Pepper. *Plant Cell Tiss. Org. Cult.* **2001**, *67*, 55–62.

Koleva-Godeva, L. R.; Spasenoski, M.; Trajkova, F. Somatic Embryogenesis in Pepper Anther Culture: The Effect of Incubation Treatment and Different Media. *Sci. Hort.* **2007**, *111*, 114–119.

Kothari, S. L.; Joshi, A.; Kachhwaha, S.; Ochoa-Alejo, N. Chilli Peppers—A Review on Tissue Culture and Transgenesis. *Biotechnol. Adv.* **2010**, *28*, 35–48.

Kristiansen, K.; Andersen, S. B. Effects of Donor Plant Temperature, Photoperiod, and Age on Anther Culture Response of *Capsicum annuum* L. *Euphytica* **1993**, *67*, 105–109.

Kristiansen, K. A.; Cilieborg, M.; Drábková, L.; Jørgensen, T.; Petersen, G.; Seberg, O. DNA Taxonomy—The Riddle of Oxychloe (Juncaceae). *Syst Bot.* **2005**, *30*, 284–289.

Kumari, T.; Sharma, C.; Bajpai, V.; Kumar, B.; Srivastava, M.; Arya, K. R. Qualitative Determination of Bioactive Metabolites Through Q-TOF LC/MS in Different Parts and Undifferentiated Cultures of *Ulmus wallichiana* Planchon. *Plant Growth Regul.* **2015**, *75*, 331–340.

Kundu, S.; Das, A.; Haque, S. M.; Ghosh, B. Chemotypic Diversity in Different Bhut Jolokia Fruits: In Vitro Conservation and Mass Propagation of Superior Ecotype. *Int. J. Pharm. Sci. Rev. Res.* **2015**, *34*, 47–53.

Kuo, J. S.; Wang, Y. Y.; Chien, N. F.; Ku, S. J.; Kung, M. L. Hsu, H. C. Investigations on the Anther Culture *In Vitro* of *Nicotiana tabacum* L. and *Capsicum annuum* L. *Acta Bot. Sin.* **1973**, *15*, 47–52.

Lantos, C.; Juhasz, A. G.; Somogyi, G.; Otvos, K.; Vagi, P.; Mihaly, R.; Kristof, Z.; Somogyi, N.; Pauk, J. Improvement of Isolated Microspore Culture of Pepper (*Capsicum annuum* L.) via Co-culture with Ovary Tissues of Pepper or Wheat. *Plant Cell Tiss. Org. Cult.* **2009**, *97*, 285–293.

Lantos, C.; Juhász, A. G.; Vági, P.; Mihály, R.; Kristóf, Z.; Pauk, J. Androgenesis Induction in Microspore Culture of Sweet Pepper (*Capsicum annuum* L.). *Plant Biotechnol. Rep.* **2012**, *6*, 123–132.

Lata, H.; Moraes, R. M.; Bertoni, B.; Pereira, A. M. S. In Vitro Germplasm Conservation of Podophyllum peltatum L. Under Slow Growth Conditions. *In Vitro Cell. Dev. Biol. Plant* **2010**, *46*, 22–27.

Lee, S. J.; Paik, K. H.; Kim, B. D. *In vitro* plant regeneration and Agrobacterium-mediated Transformation from Cotyledon Explants of Hot Pepper (*Capsicum annuum* cv Golden Tower). *Korean J. Plant. Tiss. Cult.* **1993**, *20*, 289–294.

Lee, H. Y.; Ro, N. Y.; Jeong, H. J.; Kwon, J. K.; Jo, J.; Ha, Y.; ... Kang, B. C. Genetic Diversity and Population Structure Analysis to Construct a Core Collection from a Large *Capsicum* Germplasm. BMC Gen. **2016**, *17*, 142.

Lee, Y. H.; Jung, M.; Shin, S. H.; Lee, J. H.; Choi, S. H.; Her, N. H.; ... Harn, C. H. Transgenic Peppers that are Highly Tolerant to a New CMV Pathotype. *Plant Cell Rep.* **2009,** *28,* 223–232.

Lei, T.; Middleton, B. A. Repeated Drought Alters Resistance of Seed Bank Regeneration in Baldcypress Swamps of North America. *Ecosystems.* **2017,** *21,* 1–12.

Leite, P. S. S.; Rodrigues, R.; Silva, R. N. O.; Pimenta, S.; Medeiros, A. M.; Bento, C. S.; Gonçalves, L. S. A. Molecular and Agrono mic Analysis of Intraspecific Variability in *Capsicum baccatum* var. Pendulum Accessions. *Gen. Mol. Res.* **2016,** *15,* 1–16

Li, D.; Zhao, K.; Xie, B.; Zhang, B.; Luo, K. Establishment of a Highly Efficient Transformation System for Pepper (*Capsicum annuum* L.). *Plant Cell Rep.* **2003,** *21,* 785–788.

Lin, W. C.; Saltveit, M. Greenhouse Production. In *Peppers: Botany, Production and Uses*); Russo, V. M., Ed.; CABI Publishing: Wallingford, 2012; pp 57–71.

Lin, S. W.; Chou, Y. Y.; Shieh, H. C.; Ebert, A. W.; Kumar, S.; Mavlyanova, R.; ... Gniffke, P. A. Pepper (*Capsicum* spp.) Germplasm Dissemination by AVRDC–The World Vegetable Center: An Overview and Introspection. *Chron. Hort.* **2013,** *53,* 21–27.

Lipscomb, D.; Platnick, N.; Wheeler, Q. The Intellectual Content of Taxonomy: A Comment on DNA Taxonomy. *Trends Ecol. Evolut.* **2003,** *18,* 65–66.

Liu, W.; Parrott, W. A.; Hildebrand, D. F.; Collins, G. B.; Williams, E. G. Agrobacterium Induced Gall Formation in Bell Pepper (*Capsicum annuum* L.) and Formation of Shoot-like Structures Expressing Introduced Genes. *Plant Cell Rep.* **1990,** *9,* 360–364.

Loyola-Vargas, V. M.; Ochoa-Alejo, N. Somatic Embryogenesis. An Overview. In *Somatic Embryogenesis: Fundamental Aspects and Applications*; Springer International Publishing: USA, 2016; pp 1–8.

Madhuri, V.; Rajam, M. V. Apical Shoot Meristem Culture in Red Pepper (*Capsicum annuum* L.). *J. Plant Biochem. Biot.* **1993,** *2,* 67–68.

Maligeppagol, M.; Manjula, R.; Navale, P. M.; Babu, K. P.; Kumbar, B. M.; Laxman R. H. Genetic Transformation of Chilli (*Capsicum annuum* L.) with Dreb1A Transcription Factor Known to Impart Drought Tolerance. *Ind. J. Biotechnol.* **2016,** *15,* 17–24.

Mangang, R. J. *In Vitro* Callus Induction of Placental Tissues of *Capsicum chinense* Jacq. cv. 'Umorok' using Different Concentrations and Combinations of Growth Hormones. *Int. J. Interdiscip Multidiscip.* **2014,** *1,* 63–66.

Manoharan, M.; Vidya, C. S.; Sita, G. L. A Grobacterium-mediated Genetic Transformation in Hot Chilli (*Capsicum annuum* L. var. Pusa jwala). *Plant Sci.* **1998,** *131,* 77–83.

Manzur, J. P.; Penella, C.; Rodríguez-Burruezo, A. Effect of the Genotype, Developmental Stage and Medium Composition on the *In Vitro* Culture Efficiency of Immature Zygotic Embryos from Genus *Capsicum*. *Sci Hort.* **2013,** *161,* 181–187.

Matkowski, A. Plant *In Vitro* Culture for the Production of Antioxidants—A Review. *Biotechnol. Adv.* **2008,** *26,* 548–560.

Maxted, N.; Hawkes, J. G.; Guarino, L. Sawkins, M. Towards the Selection of Taxa for Plant Genetic Conservation. *Genet. Res. Crop. Ev.* **1997,** *44,* 337–348.

McCormack, P. L. Capsaicin Dermal Patch: in Non-diabetic Peripheral Neuropathic Pain. *Drugs* **2010,** *70,* 1831–1842.

Mihalka, V.; Fari, M.; Szasz, A.; Balazs, E.; Nagy, I. Optimized Protocols for Efficient Plant Regeneration and Gene Transfer in Pepper (*Capsicum annuum* L.). *J. Plant. Biotechnol.* **2000,** *2,* 143–149.

Mityko, J.; Andrasfalvy, A.; Csillery, G.; Fári, M. Anther-culture Response in Different Genotypes and F1 Hybrids of Pepper (*Capsicum annuum* L.). *Plant Breed.* **1995,** *114,* 78–80.

Montalvo-Peniche, M. D. C.; Iglesias-Andreu, L. G.; Mijangos-Cortés, J. O.; Nahuat-Dzib, S. L.; Barahona-Pérez, F.; Canto-Flick, A.; Santana-Buzzy, N. In Vitro Germplasm Conservation of Habanero Pepper (*Capsicum chinense* Jacq.). *HortScience* **2007**, *42*, 1247–1252.

Mulabagal, V.; Tsay, H. S. Plant Cell Cultures-An Alternative and Efficient Source for the Production of Biologically Important Secondary Metabolites. *Int. J. Appl. Sci. Eng.* **2004**, *2*, 29–48.

Munyon, I. P.; Hubstenberger, J. F.; Phillips, G. C. Origin of Plantlets and Callus Obtained from Chile Pepper Anther Cultures. *In Vitro Cell Dev. Biol.* **1989**, *25*, 293–296.

Mythili, J. B.; Rajeev, P. R.; Vinay, G.; Nayeem, A.; Synergistic Effect of Silver Nitrate and Coconut Water on Shoot Differentiation and Plant Regeneration from Cultured Cotyledons of *Capsicum annuum* L. *Indian J. Exp. Biol.* **2017**, *55*, 184–190.

Nair, R. A.; Jayakumar, K. S.; Pillai, P. P. Gene Banks and Bioprospecting. In *Bioresources and Bioprocess in Biotechnology*; 2017; pp. 347–373.

Negri, V.; Tosti, N.; Standardi, A. Slow Growth Storage of Single Node Shoots of Apple Genotypes. *Plant Cell Tiss. Org. Cult.* **2000**, *62*, 159–62.

Nowaczyk, P.; Kisiała, A. Effect of Selected Factors on the Effectiveness of *Capsicum annuum* L. Anther Culture. *J. Appl. Genet.* **2006**, *47*, 113–117.

Nowaczyk, L.; Nowaczyk, P.; Olszewska, D.; Niklas-Nowak, A. Effect of 2, 4-Dichlorophen-oxyacetic Acid Pretreatment of *Capsicum spp.* Donor Plants on the Anther Culture Efficiency of Lines Selected by Capsaicinoid Content. BioTechnologia. *J. Biotechnol. Comput. Biol. Bionanotech.* **2015**, *96*, 179–183.

Ochoa-Alejo, N.; Ireta-Moreno, L. Cultivar Differences in Shoot-forming Capacity of Hypocotyl Tissues of Chilli Pepper (*Capsicum annuum* L.) Cultured *In Vitro. Sci Hort.* **1990**, *42*, 21–28.

Orlinska, M.; Nowaczyk, P. *In Vitro* Plant Regeneration of 4 *Capsicum* spp. Genotypes Using Different Explant Types. *Turkish J. Biol.* **2015**, *39*, 60–68.

Otroshy, M.; Moradi, K.; Nekouei, M. K. Struik, P. C. Micropropagation of Pepper (*Capsicum annuum* L.) Through *In Vitro* Direct Organogenesis. *Asian J. Biotechnol.* **2011**, *3*, 38–45.

Palmer, J. D.; Soltis, D. E.; Chase, M. W. The Plant Tree of Life: An Overview and Some Points of View. *Am. J. Bot.* **2004**, *91*, 1437–1445.

Parveen, S.; Shahzad, A. Encapsulation of Nodal Segments of *Cassia angustifolia* Vahl. for Short-term Storage and Germplasm Exchange. *Acta Physiol. Plant* **2014**, *36*, 635–640.

Patel, N.; Rajput, T. B. S. Use of Simulation Modeling for Enhancing Potato Production Using Subsurface Drip. *Potato J.* **2010**, *37*, 21–27.

Pochard, E.; Dumas de Vaulx, R. Haploid Parthenogenesis in *Capsicum annuum* L. *The biology and taxonomy of the Solanaceae*; Hawkes, J. G., Lester, R. N., Skelding, A. D., Eds.; Academic Press for the Linnean Society: London, 1979; 455–472.

Prasad, B. C. N.; Kumar, V.; Gururaj, H. B.; Parimalan, R.; Giridhar, P.; Ravishankar, G. A. Characterization of Capsaicin Synthase and Identification of its Gene (csy1) for Pungency Factor Capsaicin in Pepper (*Capsicum* sp.). *Proc. Nat. Acad. Sci. USA* **2006**, *103*, 13315–13320.

Purohit, C. S. Aconitum Ferox Wall. ex Ser.-An Important Medicinal Plant of Sikkim. *Popular Kheti* **2013**, *1*, 71–75.

Raj, R. P.; Glint, V. D.; Babu, K. N. *In Vitro* Plant Regeneration in *Capsicum chinense* Jacq. (Naga Chili). *J. Appl. Biol. Biotechnol.* **2015**, *3*, 030–033.

Rajasekharan, P. E.; Ganeshan, S. Feasibility of Pollen Cryopreservation in *Capsicum* sp. *Capsicum* eggplant. *News Lett.* **2003**, *22*, 87–90.

Rakshit, A.; Rakshit, S.; Deokar, A.; Dasgupta, T. Effect of Different Explant and Hormones on *In Vitro* Callus Induction and Regeneration of Pepper (*Capsicum annuum* L.). *Asian J. Bio. Sci.* **2008,** *3*, 180–183.

Ramchiary, N.; Kehie, M.; Kumaria, S.; Tandon, P. Application of Genetics and Genomics Towards *Capsicum* Translational Research. *Plant Biotechnol. Rep.* **2014,** *8*, 101–123.

Ramirez-Malagón, R.; Ochoa-Alejo, N. An Improved and Reliable Chili Pepper (*Capsicum annuum* L.) Plant Regeneration Method. *Plant Cell Rep.* **1996,** 16, 226–231.

Rao, V. R. Groundnut Genetic Resources at ICRISAT, 1980.

Raveendar, S.; Jeon, Y. A.; Lee, J. R.; Lee, G. A.; Lee, K. J.; Cho, G. T.; ... Chung, J. W. The Complete Chloroplast Genome Sequence of Korean Landrace "subicho" Pepper (*Capsicum annuum* var. annuum). *Plant Breed. Biotechnol.* **2015,** *3*, 88–94.

Reddy, M. K.; Srivastava, A.; Lin, S. W.; Kumar, R.; Shieh, H. C.; Ebert, A. W.; ... Kumar, S. Exploitation of AVRDC's Chili Pepper (*Capsicum* spp.) Germplasm in India. *J. Taiwan Soc. Hortic. Sci.* **2015,** *61*, 1–9.

Renfiyeni, Y.; Trisno, J. Calli Induction of Some Chili Pepper (*Capsicum annuum* l.) Genotypes as Material for Genetic Transformation. *Int. J. Agr. Sci.* **2016,** *1*, 75–80.

Rizwan, M.; Sharma, R.; Soni, P.; Gupta, N. K.; Singh, G. Regeneration Protocol for Chilli (*Capsicum annuum* L.) Variety Mathania. *J. Cell. Tissue Res.* **2013,** *13*, 3513.

Rodeva, V.; Grozeva, S.; Todorova, V. *In Vitro* Answer of Bulgarian Pepper (*Capsicum annuum* L.). *Genetika* **2006,** *38*, 129–136.

Rodríguez-Arévalo, I.; Mattana, E.; García, L.; Liu, U.; Lira, R.; Dávila, P.;... Ulian, T. Conserving Seeds of Useful Wild Plants in Mexico: Main Issues and Recommendations. *Genet Resour. Crop Ev.* **2017,** *64*, 1141–1190.

Roshany, G.; Kalantarai, S.; Naderi, R.; Hassani, M. E. Callus Formation via Anther Culture in *Capsicum annuum* L. with Differences in Genotypes, Media and Incubation Temperature. *Tech. J. Engin. App. Sci.* **2013,** *3*, 3847–3853.

Roy, S. S.; Khan, M. S. I.; Pall, K. K. K. K. Nitrogen and Phosphorus Efficiency on the Fruit Size and Yield of *capsicum*. *J. Exp. Sci.* **2011,** *2*, 32–37.

Ruiz-González, C.; Niño-García, J. P.; Kembel, S. W.; del Giorgio, P. A. Identifying the Core Seed Bank of a Complex Boreal Bacterial Metacommunity. *ISME J.* **2011,** *11*, 2012–2021.

Samanta, A.; Sen, K.; Bakshi, P.; Sahoo, A. K. Screening of Some Chilli Germplasm Against Yellow Mite and Thrips in the Gangetic Plains of West Bengal. *J. Entomol. Zool. Stud.* **2017,** *5*, 881–884.

Santana-Buzzy, N.; López-Puc, G.; Canto-Flick, A.; Barredo-Pool, F.; Balam-Uc, E.; Avilés-Viñas, S.; ... Mijangos-Cortés, J. O. Ontogenesis of the Somatic Embryogenesis of Habanero Pepper (*Capsicum chinense* Jacq.). *HortScience* **2009,** *44*, 113–118.

Sanatombi, K.; Sharma, G. J. Micropropagation of *Capsicum annuum* L. *Notulae Botanicae Horti. Agrobotanici. Cluj-Napoca* **2007,** *35*, 57–64.

Sanatombi, K.; Sharma, G. J. Capsaicin Content and Pungency of Different *Capsicum* spp. Cultivars. *Notulae Botanicae Horti Agrobotanici Cluj-Napoca* **2008,** *36*, 89.

Santos, M. R. A. D.; Souza, C. A. D.; Paz, E. S. Growth Pattern of Friable Calluses from Leaves of *Capsicum annuum* var. annuum cv. Iberaba Jalapeño. *Rev. Cienc. Agron.* **2017,** *48*, 523–530.

Seguí-Simarro, J. M.; Corral-Martínez, P.; Parra-Vega, V.; González-García, B. Androgenesis in Recalcitrant Solanaceous Crops. *Plant Cell Rep.* **2011,** 30: 765–778.

Shahak, Y.; Yehezkel, H.; Matan, E.; Posalski, I.; Ratner, K.; Offir, Y.L; ... Ben-Yakir, D. Photoselective Netting Improves Productivity of Bell Peppers. *HortScience* **2007,** *42*, 851–851.

Sharaf, S. A.; Shibli, R. A.; Kasrawi, M. A.; Baghdadi, S. H. Slow-growth Preservation of Wild Shih (*Artemisia herba*-alba Asso.) Microshoots from Jordan. *J. Food Agric. Environ.* **2012**, *10*, 1359–1364.

Sharma, S.; Shahzad, A. Encapsulation Technology for Short-term Storage and Conservation of a Woody Climber, Decalepis hamiltonii Wight and Arn. *Plant Cell Tiss. Org. Cult.* **2012**, *111*, 191–198.

Shin, R.; Park, J. M.; An, J. M.; Paek, K. H. Ectopic Expression of Tsi1 in Transgenic Hot Pepper Plants Enhances Host Resistance to Viral, Bacterial, and Oomycete Pathogens. Mol. Plant Microbe Interact. **2002**, *15*, 983–989.

Shiva, V. *Monocultures of the Mind: Understanding the Threats to Biological and Cultural Diversity*; University of Guelph: Guelph, ON, CA, 1994.

Sibi, M.; Dumas de Vaulx, R.; Chambonnet, D. Obtention de plantes haploïdes par androgenèse *in vitro* chez le piment (*Capsicum annuum* L.). *Ann Amélior Plantes* **1979**, *29*, 583–606.

Siddique, I.; Anis, M. Thidiazuron Induced High Frequency Shoot Bud Formation and Plant Regeneration from Cotyledonary Node Explants of *Capsicum annuum* L. *Ind. J. Biotechnol.* **2006**, *5*, 303–308.

Silva Monteiro, C. E.; Pereira, T. N. S.; Campos, K. P. Reproductive Characterization of Interspecific Hybrids Among *Capsicum* Species. *Crop Breed Appl. Biotech.* **2011**, *11*, 241– 249.

Singh, N. K.; Pandey, A. Field Screening of Different Genotypes of Chilli Against Infestation of Thrips. *Progressive Hort.* **2015**, 47, 142–153.

Singh, R. V. Naik, L. B. Effect of Nitrogen, Phosphorus and Plant Spacing on Sweet Pepper (*Capsicum annuum* L.). *Haryana J. Hort. Sci.* **1990**, *19*: 168–172.

Singh, K. G.; Angrej, S.; Gulshan, M. Response of Sweet Pepper (*Capsicum annum*) to Irrigation and Fertigation Grown in Naturally Ventilated Polyhouse. *Indian J. Agr. Sci.* **2010**, *80*, 430–432.

Solís-Ramos, L. Y.; González-Estrada, T.; Nahuath-Dzib, S.; Zapata-Rodriguez, L. C.; Castano, E. Overexpression of WUSCHEL in *C. chinense* Causes Ectopic Morphogenesis. *Plant Cell Tiss. Org. Cult.* **2009**, *96*, 279–287.

Srivastava, M.; Purshottam, D. K.; Srivastava, A. K.; Misra, P. In Vitro Conservation of Glycyrrhiza Glabra by Slow Growth Culture. *Int. J. Adv. Biotechnol. Res.* **2013**, *3*, 49–58.

Stasolla, C.; Yeung, E. C. Recent Advances in Conifer Somatic Embryogenesis: Improving Somatic Embryo Quality. *Plant Cell Tiss. Org. Cult.* **2003**, *74*, 15–35.

Steinitz, B.; Küsek, M.; Tabib, Y.; Paran, I.; Zelcer, A. Pepper (*Capsicum annuum* L.) Regenerants Obtained by Direct Somatic Embryogenesis Fail to Develop a Shoot. *In Vitro Cell Dev. Pl.* **2003**, *39*, 296–303.

Steward, F. C.; Mapes, M. O.; Mears, K. Growth and Organized Development of Cultured Cells. II. Organization in Cultures Grown from Freely Suspended Cells. *Am. J. Bot.* **1958**, 705–708.

Subhash, K.; Christopher, T. Organogenesis and Transformation in *Capsicum baccatum*. *In Vitro.* **1997**, *33*, 54A.

Supena, E. D. J.; Suharsono, S.; Jacobsen, E.; Custers, J. B. M. Successful Development of a Shed-microspore Culture Protocol for Doubled Haploid Production in Indonesian Hot Pepper (*Capsicum annuum* L.). *Plant Cell Rep.* **2006**, *25*, 1–10.

Suthar, R. S.; Shah, D. Optimization of Callus and Cell Suspension Culture of *Capsicum annuum* L. *Int. J. Pharma. Bio. Sci.* **2015**, *6*, 664–671.

Swamy, S.; Krupakar, A.; Chandran, D. S.; Koshy, E. P. Direct Regeneration Protocols of Five *Capsicum annuum* L. Varieties. *Afr. J. Biotechnol.* **2014**, *13*, 307–312.

Szász, A.; Nervo, G.; Fári, M. Screening For *in vitro* Shoot-forming Capacity of Seedling Explants in Bell Pepper (*Capsicum annuum* L.) Genotypes and Efficient Plant Regeneration Using Thidiazuron. *Plant Cell Rep.* **1995**, *14*, 666–669.

Tandon, P.; Kumaria, S. Prospects of Plant Conservation Biotechnology in India with Special Reference to Northeastern Region. In *Biodiversity: Status and Prospects*; Tandon, P.; Kumaria, S., Eds.; Norasa Publishing House: New Delhi, 2005; pp 79–91.

Tang, H.; Sezen, U.; Paterson, A. H. Domestication and Plant Genomes. Curr. Opin. *Plant Biol.* **2010**, *13*, 160–166.

Taskin, H.; Büyükalaca, S.; Keles, D.; Ekbiç, E. Induction of Microspore-derived Embryos by Anther Culture in Selected Pepper Genotypes. *Afr. J. Biotechnol.* **2011**, *10*, 17116–17121.

Tautz, D.; Arctander, P.; Minelli, A.; Thomas, R. H.; Vogler, A. P. A Plea for DNA Taxonomy. *Trends Ecol. Evolut.* **2003**, 18, 70–74.

Thomas, D. T.; Jacob, A. Direct Somatic Embryogenesis of *Curculigo orchioides* Gaertn. An Endangered Medicinal Herb. *J. Plant. Biotechnol.* **2004**, *6*, 193–197.

Umamaheswai, A.; Lalitha, V. *In Vitro* Effect of Various Growth Hormones in *Capsicum annum* L. on the Callus Induction and Production of Capsaicin. *J. Plant Sci.* **2007**, *2*, 545–551.

Valadez-Bustos, M. G.; Aguado-Santacruz, G. A.; Carrillo-Castañeda, G.; Aguilar-Rincón, V. H.; Espitia-Rangel, E.; Montes-Hernández, S.; Robledo-Paz, A. In Vitro Propagation and Agronomic Performance of Regenerated Chili Pepper (*Capsicum* spp.) Plants from Commercially Important Genotypes. Developmental Biology/Morphogenesis. *In Vitro Cell Dev. Biol. Plant* **2009**, *45*, 650–658.

Venkataiah, P.; Christopher, T.; Subhash, K. Thidiazuron Induced High Frequency Adventitious Shoot Formation and Plant Regeneration in *Capsicum annuum* L. *J. Plant. Biotechnol.* **2003**, *5*, 245–250.

Venkataiah, P.; Bhanuprakash, P.; Kalyan, S. S.; Subhash, K. Somatic Embryogenesis and Plant Regeneration of *Capsicum baccatum* L. *J. Genet. Eng. Biotechnol.* **2016**, *14*, 55–60.

Verma, S.; Dhiman, K..; Srivastava, D. K. Efficient *In Vitro* Regeneration from Cotyledon Explants in Bell Pepper (*Capsicum annuum* L. cv. California wonder). Int. *J. Adv. Biotechnol. Res.* **2013**, *4*, 391–396.

Wang, Y. Y.; Ching-San, S. U. N.; Ching-Chu, W.; Nan-Fen, C. The Induction of the Pollen Plantlets of Triticale and *Capsicum annuum* from Anther Culture. *Sci. Sin* **1973**, *16*, 147–151.

Wang, W.; Yang, M.; Pan, N.; Chen, Z. H. Plant Regeneration and Transformation of Sweet Pepper (*Capsicum frutescens*). *Acta Bot. Sin.* **1991**, *33*, 780–786.

Wilson, S. A.; Roberts, S. C. Recent Advances Towards Development and Commercialization of Plant Cell Culture Processes for the Synthesis of Biomolecules. *Plant Biotechnol. J.* **2012**, *10*, 249–268.

Withers, L. A. Cryopreservation of Cultured Cells and Meristems. *Cell Cult. Somat. Cell Gen. Plants* **1985**, *2*, 253–316.

Xie, L. Y.; Kuang, H. Q.; Lai, Z. X.; Liu, S. C. Study on Callus Induction from *In Vitro Capsicum annuum* L. *Heilongjiang Agri. Sci.* **2013**, *11*, 007.

Yadav, R. K.; Kalia, P.; Choudhary, H.; BrihamaDev, Z. H. Low-cost Polyhouse Technologies for Higher Income and Nutritional Security. *IJAFST.* **2014**, *5*, 191–196.

Ye, Z.; Li, H.; Zhang, J.; Jing, Y. Genetic Transformation and Plant Regeneration in Pepper. *Acta. Bot. Sin.* **1993**, *35*, 88–93.

Zapata-Castillo, P. Y.; Flick, A. C.; López-Puc, G.; Solís-Ruiz, A.; Barahona-Pérez, F.; Santana-Buzzy, N.; Iglesias-Andreu, L. Somatic Embryogenesis in Habanero Pepper (*C. chinense* Jacq.) from Cell Suspensions. *HortScience* **2007**, *42*, 329–333.

Zhang, X. M.; Zhang, Z. H.; Gu, X. Z.; Mao, S. L.; Li, X. X.; Chadœuf, J.; ... Zhang, B. X. Genetic Diversity of Pepper (*Capsicum* spp.) Germplasm Resources in China Reflects Selection for Cultivar Types and Spatial Distribution. *J. Integ. Agric.* **2016**, *15*, 1991–2001.

Zhu, Y. X.; Ou-Yang, W. J.; Zhang, Y. F.; Chen, Z. L. Transgenic Sweet Pepper Plants from Agrobacterium Mediated Transformation. *Plant Cell. Rep.* **1996**, *16*, 71–75.

CHAPTER 18

Conservation Practices May Yield Sustainable Resource

S. M. JALIL*

Former Chief Conservator of Forest and President, Forestry & Environment Forum, Dhaka, Bangladesh

Corresponding author. E-mail: dr.jalilsm@gmail.com

ABSTRACT

We people on earth are after resource because our survival is absolutely dependent upon the resource and that resource must be a growing resource be it naturally renewable natural resource or nonrenewable natural or manmade resource. In any case, resource management policy and practice is vital for achieving our daily necessities. This policy decision through awareness build-up leads us to resort to conservation practice and that people-oriented conservation practice may yield sustainable resource—a saving/earning for today and tomorrow.

18.1 DEFINITION

18.1.1 DEFINITION OF CONSERVATION

A careful preservation and protection of something especially planned management of a natural resource to prevent exploitation, destruction, or neglect, water *conservation,* wildlife *conservation*, the preservation of a physical quantity and quality during transformations or reaction and interactions.

It may also be defined as the act of *conserving,* prevention of injury, decay, waste or loss, preservation, *conservation* of wildlife, co*nservation* of human rights, conservation of river systems, forests, soil and other natural resources in a wise manner, ensuring derivation of their highest sustainable economic return in order to preserve and protect them through prudent management.

18.1.2   DEFINITION OF CONSERVANCY

Conservancy is an organization dedicated to the conservation of resources including bio-resources. The government departments like local government engineering department, public health service, city or municipal corporation do have conservancy through wise management of resources. Similarly, department of forestry, environment, water and many other organizations have their responsibilities to conserve natural resources both living and nonliving. The Nature *Conservancy* is a charitable environmental organization, headquartered in Arlington, Virginia, United States. Its mission is to "conserve" the lands and all other resources including human resources. Brandywine *Conservancy* works with individuals, government agencies, and private organizations to permanently protect and conserve land, water, and many other necessary resources for protecting water, land, wildlife, and future.

Science-based solution to tackle the biggest threat to our ocean is the recent development of conservancy in blue economy. *Conservancy* to support, among other things, its performance of the valuable function of shining a bright light on the development history, may be the guarantee of our future. Practicing conservation is an instrument to save and built up a sustainable resource.

18.1.3   CONSERVATION PRACTICES

Conservation practices are materializing the concept of conservation of resources wisely such that resource base does not decrease rather it increases and build up stronger resource base. This way of uses of resources of any kind is likely to ensure sustainable development of resource base particularly the renewable one. They are living resources like forests, trees, plants, agricultural crop, and aquatic resources. The nonliving nonrenewable resources like oil, gas, minerals are also to be wisely used through conservation practices.

18.1.4   CONSERVATION PRACTICES FOR RENEWABLE RESOURCES

Renewable resources are trees, plants, herbs, shrubs, climbers, annual, biennial, perennial trees. Fungi, algae, and Seaweeds are also renewable resources. These are all terrestrial living resources. Solar, water and wind energy are also renewable. The aquatic renewable resources are all fishes, the sweet water one is more artificially cultivated, mammal, reptiles, amphibian like frog, tortoise, turtle, crab some birds, and so on.

18.1.5 CONSERVATION PRACTICES FOR NONRENEWABLE RESOURCES

Conservation practices of nonrenewable resources are more necessary as the same once is exhausted cannot be renewed. It has no scope of regenerating because they are nonliving. The only scope is of importing them from overseas at the expenses of foreign exchange, so conservation practices of nonrenewable resources like oil, gas, coal, stones, and many other minerals are more essential than even renewable one.

18.1.6 SUSTAINABLE GOAL

The resource base is the baseline that needs to be maintained strictly such that its regeneration capacity is sustained, when the population increases and consequently the demand/consumption increases, the production or the regeneration cannot keep pace with the consumption. Naturally, the resource base goes down. The goal is not to go down below the baseline, baseline needs to be uplifted for higher production/regeneration. The goal is then obtained if necessary by higher input. In fact, the higher is the input, the higher becomes the output. The higher is the output, it becomes easier to redress the increased demand or earn by saving. So, the practice of resource conservation is an important tool for resource build-up for future.

18.1.7 SUSTAINABLE USE

Sustainable use is the conservation practice where resource base instead of being declined, continues to increase and gradually build up strong resource base. Here the resource use is so wisely done, the resource gradually becomes healthy and production surpass the demand.

18.1.8 SUSTAINABLE YIELD

The yield that is accrued is sustained and it continues to yield and add to the base. This results in build up a fatty resource base and continues to yield more and make it a strong resource base.

18.1.9   SUSTAINABLE DEVELOPMENT

When the developed production rate continues to produce no less than achieved is sustainable development. Wise use of the resources may ensure sustainability and the future becomes all most risk free provided unwise use of resource does not take place.

18.2   RESOURCE CONSERVATION

Resource conservation being a wise use of any resource growing or static, we must for us, our future generation, make sure resource conservation at any cost otherwise we may find the future bleak. World communities are not only worried, they are aware of deteriorating resource base and thus they are trying to overcome any such crisis cropped up by a tentative time target of 2030 under the caption sustainable development goal (SDG). Ninth South Asia Economic Summit held in Dhaka on October 15–16, 2016 under the theme "Reimaging South Asia in 2030" organized by Centre for Policy Dialogue (CDP), Bangladesh in collaboration with IPS, RIS, SAWTEE, and SDPI. This summit stressed upon all the resource sectors including forestry where it focused upon protection, restoration, and promotion of sustainable use of terrestrial ecosystems, sustainable management of forests, combating desertification, and halting reversion of land degradation and biodiversity loss. Dhaka based Bangladesh Poribesh Andolon & Bangladesh Environment Network jointly organized Special Conference on Sustainable Development Goals & Environment. Many national and international organizations are also having program for resource conservation practices in the context of ever-growing demand.

18.2.1   BIO-RESOURCE CONSERVATION

Economists say—Bio-resources are important components for progress and economic activities of a nation but in fact, bio-resources are the determinant of the very existence of our planet—the only abode for mankind.

When we talk of bio-resource, it is vast, much of it is still unknown, undiscovered and again it is living, regenerating naturally, spontaneously, yet it is in dearth for human need. In fact, the growth rate of bio-resource cannot keep pace with the growth rate of human population and so is their consumption rate. In addition to that, the lifestyle or we may say, the living standard, may not be for all, has become and gradually becoming high and so the consumption of resources naturally goes up. One point here is necessary to impress upon is that the bioresources and non-bioresources are complementary to each other. If one is in dearth, the pressure goes upon the others. So, while talking one, the other should be talked about. When the question of management comes in, it becomes obligatory to manage both in order to maintain a balance in the system of ecosystem function for delivering goods and services to the society. This management must have the concept and applications of conservation principles. Therefore, conservation practices become the gateway to achieve protection, increased growth and growth rate, sustaining the growth and ensure fulfillment of future demand or consumption. This is how sustaining development goal may be achieved. United Nations development program aims at SDGs by 2030. In view of depleting trend of resources, most countries have their own resource conservation and sustainable development program. Of all the causes of resource depletion, human population growth and their changed lifestyle appear contributing more to the cause. Degeneration of forest resources appears jeopardized the ecology and economy, which the world communities could realize late. Earth Summit becomes the warning signals for the people on earth. Since then world communities began thinking and working on environment and development. Progress does not indicate any satisfactory achievement. As water resource is also severely decreasing, the expert's intuition is world war for water in near future. Cold war for water is already there between many countries. In fact, demand has increased so much and resource distribution is so disproportionate that the growth rate of growing resource cannot keep pace with the rate of consumption. Thus, this imbalance of all the resources leads to destroying harmony, peace, and tranquility.

To talk straightforward regarding bio-resource status all over the world, the present-day observation is that the bio-resource decreases with the increase in population and upgraded lifestyle. In fact, civilization has developed at the cost of bio-resources. Global warming, ozone layer depletion, or climate change, everything is changeable, changing. Nature itself is changing. It is dynamic. It is a natural phenomenon, a natural theory of evolution. The problem of bio-resource depletion is not the normal change, it is an enhanced rate of changes of bio-resources and so is the change of nature. This has happened and has been happening due to excess harvesting beyond the growth rate of the bio-resources and it is not the natural phenomenon. The problem lies in increased or accelerated rate of change and thus it has become a real problem creating gradually an alarming situation. These changes are directly and indirectly affecting the environment, the society, and the people's livelihood. The population of all life forms and their diversity is also affected. Knowingly well, this adverse situation is not definitely desirable but to someone in some cases, is welcome. It happens when the adverse situation creates an opportunity for someone for making some profitable business.

Forest being one of the most service-oriented bioresource, it is important to have a brief picture of global forest status for our action for overcoming the adverse situation. State of the World's Forests area in 2016 as estimated in 2005 was to be around 30% of the planet's land area just under 40 million km². This corresponds to an average 0.62 ha (6200 m²) per capita. Average forest area in Bangladesh is 0.053 ha per capita while in India, it is 0.58. Bioresource status in those countries is severely vulnerable. Based upon 228 countries, about half of the world forests are in America, one fourth in Europe and less than 20% in Asia. The largest forest areas are in Russian Federation, Brazil, Canada, USA, and China. Of all these five, Russia alone has 20%. Loss of forest from the planet was 130,000 km² per year during 1990–2005. Of course, efforts were made to regenerate the empty space by planting. Once the virgin forest is lost, it becomes difficult to recover them even by manual replanting. Therefore, the achievement is far behind the expectation. The net loss during that period was 89,000 km² per year. During the period of 2000 and 2005, the estimated loss was 73,000 km². per year equivalent to 200 km² per day. This loss of forests means loss of bioresources in addition to huge mined abiotic resources also. The trend of urbanization, industrialization, and civilization and the trend of bioresource depletion are intimately correlated. The disappearing and or depletion of the forests appear clearly the loss of bioresources. Further, the population growth and human activities are directly responsible for bioresources depletion. The more is the human activities, the more is the exploitation of natural resources. As result of more exploitation, the concept of sustainability of basic resources gets no importance and thus become unsustainable and the ecosystem of our environment becomes jeopardized.

Bioresource under such world trend of exploitation is naturally becomes an unavoidable necessity of the day but the quantity needs to be rationed. This act may help build up a reasonable justification of growth and consumption. In fact, this idea is not being conceived and thus the bioresources have reached a stage of vulnerability. This trend in the Asian region is likely to be in a horrible state where forest lie only 20% as against world average of 30%. Being an Asian country, Bangladesh is struggling hard to protect, to preserve her remnant forest resources but the trend of depletion of forest disheartening. When the world trend of forest resource depletion is likely to continue and the bioresource of countries like Bangladesh with huge population growth will naturally be at stake. This situation developed due to lack of conservation practices for forest resource or it may be for other resources.

18.2.1.1 NATURAL RESOURCES, FOREST, FISHERIES, AGRICULTURE, BIODIVERSITY

It is understood that people at one time were not really aware of the adverse impact of unregulated harvesting and using natural resources terrestrial and aquatic for meeting their ever increasing demand. Many of the countries today, cannot afford, though well aware of, but to use their natural resources under economic pressure. As a result, environmental deterioration like depletion of resources, pollution of air, water, soil and loss of productivity were going in the process over a long period of time. People aware of the science of natural resources have began to feel the pinch of what worse was going to happen with the natural resources. Salute to them for their initiative and endeavor for organizing a gathering of world leaders and scientists what it was termed Earth summit. Earth summit has taken step to awaken us from our carelessness about environmental degradation.

Universally accepted issue is our vulnerable nature and natural resources. Globally, people are worried for destruction of natural resources as and when they find shortage of necessary resources. Thus gradually they are becoming aware of the resource management for overcoming this world wide alarming situation. The Earth Summit in Rio held in 1992 was the awakening alarm for the mankind on earth. Since then, many countries are now to some extent aware and trying their best to protect, improve and make wise use of these natural resources. But this effort is yet to gain momentum in their activities. Many countries like Bangladesh at lower elevation is much more vulnerable to climate change impact. It is important that all trans-boundary issues are handled by the world communities for the sake of global interest. Many of the less developed countries are more vulnerable but unfortunately, cannot afford to accept challenge and combat adverse impact of climate change.

Environmental hazard, air, water, soil pollution are gradually becoming poisonous to human health but many countries are still continuing their uses of environment—unfriendly nonrenewable natural resources (NNRs). The adverse impact of all such uses are to be naturally shared by all the countries but to redress the adverse effect, the responsible incumbents are in many cases reluctant to share the cost of investment. Because of lack of knowledge about resource behaviors and necessary conservation technology, the conservation practice for resource protection, saving growth augment and built up were not introduced in the resource management plan.

18.2.1.2   MICROBIAL RESOURCES

It has a special emphasis on the utilization of biotechnology as a core technology to increase the value of commercial products, such as food and feed products, enzyme products, drug and bioactive compounds and bio control products. A wonderful world of micro-organisms is playing a vital role in delivering goods and services to mankind. There are many already discovered and yet there are many to discover. This resource management needs special knowledge for correct conservation practices.

18.2.1.3   AGRICULTURE

Forests and trees support sustainable agriculture. They stabilize soils, improve soil fertility level, regulate water flows, protect upland watershed, control soil erosion, and river bed sedimentation, regulate wind and sunlight, sequestrate atmospheric carbon dioxide and provide a habitat for pollinators and the natural predators of agricultural pests. They also contribute to the food security of hundreds of millions of people. The agriculture practices provide an absolute supply sources of food and farmers power and income. Besides, biologically diversified animals of herbivorous habit are solely dependent upon bioresources as food. Agriculture remains the major driver of deforestation globally. In the context of climate change, we need to see agriculture, forestry, horticulture, sericulture, apiculture, aquaculture by their weighted value and thereby a reasonable formulation of land use policy compatible to bioresource conservation policy and practice be achieved. Based on ecology and economy, the resource conservation policy and practice are likely to deliver environment-friendly goods and services.

18.2.1.4   DIVERSIFIED BIORESOURCES

Our planet supports roughly between 3 and 30 million species of plant systems, animals, fungi, single celled bacteria, and protozoans. They are interdependent, intricately linked in birth, death, and renewal. Human beings are just one small part of the vibrant component of the biological systems on the earth but human beings are the vital and key biological system and put tremendous amount of pressure on species and the environment and ecosystem functions. It interacts with and depends on the nonliving components of the planet such as atmosphere, oceans, freshwaters, rocks, and soils. Humanity depends totally on this community of life, the biosphere of which human populations are integral part. Of this, total biological systems, only about 1.4 million species have been identified and named so far. Little more than half the named species are insects which normally dominate terrestrial and fresh water communities worldwide. Biological balance and eco-system functions are largely governed by insect population. Pollination by insects is a great contribution to the success of agricultural sustainable yield. Predator insects are another group biologically control the harmful insects indirectly augment agriproduction. Many birds predate insect and protect crop while others feed upon crop. There are hundred and one of such example that ensures more or less biological balance. Because of wanton pressure over population some of the species get extinction. To my mind, it seems hardly few countries can manage well vastness of this diversified huge resources of biological species. Under some circumstances, some selective one may be tried in farming, captive breeding, rearing, and domesticated. This approach of resource conservation practice is the time need when we are all scared of rapid extinction of many species. (Prof. S. Kannaiyan, FNAAS, Email: skannaiyan@hotmail.com).

18.2.2 NONRENEWABLE RESOURCES—MINERALS, OIL, GAS, COAL, PEAT, AND SO ON

Many developed countries in the world are leading their modern way of living because they have achieved industrialization through utilization of natural resources—both biotic and abiotic. Their rich lifestyle is possibly by their unrestricted use of NNRs—fossil fuels, metals, and nonmetallic minerals—many of which are imported by some. These resources are subject to the geological limitations of a finite planet. Therefore, it would not be unwise to say that life style there in those developed countries is not granted sustainable. When this NNR base is depleted or exhausted, maintaining rich life style by many may become not only difficult, it may not be a surprise to face painful living. Some developed countries use 95% of their NNRs as raw material inputs to the economy each year. There is a record in 2006 that a country used over more than 6.00 billion tons of newly mined NNRs.

As life style is dependent upon both NNRs and renewable natural resources (RNRs), efficient management and utilization of both is necessary. They are complementary to each other i.e abundance of one release pressure upon other and on the contrary, scarcity of one creates pressure upon other one.

This is what has already been happening with many developed countries even. The less developed natural resource poor countries are more or less always remain naturally under pressure and need bound to over exploit bioresources. The access to the bioresources is also easy as they are open property. The developed countries at their dwindling trend of NNRs, are gradually becoming aware of this depleting situation of NNRs and therefore worried for their life style likely to be fallen down. The NNRs were used to be procured at cheaper rate and thus the cost of production was naturally more competitive and profitable. Obviously they were more inclined toward NNRs against the RNRs require costly intensive management. The cost of management of RNRs is much higher. Japan is bearing 66% land area under forests yet is highly dependent upon natural resource imports. They do import wood, wood products and huge import of coal for generating thermal power. This import policy of Japan appears wise enough not only to preserves her own natural resources, it ameliorates the environment and ecosystem functions in one hand and on the other hand, creates an unique opportunity in future of making profitable international timber trade and business.

Fossil fuels such as oil, gas, and coal and metals, and non-metallic minerals are the key sources of industrial revolution. Now the efforts around the world to reduce the use of coal have led some regions to switch to natural gas. Clean coal technology is still expensive but will be popular if it becomes cheaper.

Coal use in the world is still increasing though lot of arguments against the use is there. Some 659,645,000 to 7,238,208,000 ST of coal use has increased during the last 4 years and that is 15.6. The Environmentalists are very vocal against coal use. They understand well about harmful effect of coal burning. It tells upon health of most living being including human being. If coal use is banned, what would be the alternative to coal is a big question. Banning coal burning will cause depletion of bioresources which in turn reduce carbon sequestration and oxygen release into the atmosphere. The environmentalist should look into both sides of the coin and raise their voice according to the weighted value of use and no use of coal. The wise policy decision may come out through weighted value of the use and no use of coal in a particular area.

One thing here is very important to realize is that the very existence of the planet is dependent upon plant kingdom, that is, bioresource. Of course, symbiosis of biotic and abiotic resources ameliorates the total environment and in fact abiotic resource plays a great supplementary role in the delivery of goods and services through ecosystem functions. As we all know that NNRs are on the way of exhaustion, the world will depend absolutely upon bioresources. If it happens so, what would be the fate of the planet and the living being including human being?

Here, I may suggest that rich country may ban on use of coal upon them but not for the industry—poor countries. The industry poor country may be allowed to use coal for building up necessary industries and becomes weighted parallel with the rich countries. Then the application of ban for use of coal may be imposed for all worldwide. Resource conservation practices should be equally useful for all of us.

18.2.3 HERITAGE SITE CONSERVATION—FOREST RESOURCES LIKE SUNDARBANS WORLD HERITAGE SITE

A World Heritage Site is a place that is listed by the United Nations Educational, Scientific and Cultural Organization (UNESCO) as of special cultural or physical significance.

Conservation of world heritage site is as important as any other resources. The resource yield is as useful as any other useful resources. Two thirds of the world mangrove forests are replaced by urbanization, industrialization. The rest one third still exist under population pressure and they are on their way to exhaustion and extinction.

The Sundarbans mangrove forest, though not the highest area among the other mangrove rich countries, the Sundarbans of Bangladesh is one of the largest such forests in the world (140,000 ha), lies on the delta of the Ganges, Brahmaputra, and Meghna rivers on the Bay of Bengal. It is adjacent to the border of India's Sundarbans World Heritage site. Conservation practice must yield primarily the benefit to the people but the world-renowned mangrove forest/littoral forest at the coastal area has got special charm, special fascination for people of home and abroad. The sea breeze, plenty of pure oxygen, vastness of ever green forests, the royal Bengal tiger, the spotted deer and their friend monkey, the crawling red crab, birds are all visible special eye catching fascination. At time, culling of some deer, removal of some trees on silvicultural principle may be done for hygienic ground. This Conservation practice of heritage part is likely to yield more goods and services both tangible and intangible.

18.2.4 TALENT CONSERVATION

Talent conservation is nothing new. Intelligence boys and girls doing well in the school examination or otherwise are normally taken care by school teachers, guardian's neighbors, friends and known well-wishers. They desire that the intelligent boys and girls should obtain their highest academic degree and stay with them for rendering service to their people. Similarly, the country does also try to provide them within the country their befitting job. Sometimes it may so happen that the talented boys and girls are not provided their due facilities or opportunities, try to migrate other countries in search of better facilities. It may also so happen that the country cannot afford to extend necessary facilities, the talented one may migrate elsewhere leaving behind mother land. Sometimes the talented one being allured, left the country ignoring their responsibility toward the country. Sometimes some country may control the migration of the talent by imposing consti-tutional law. This undesirable migration is termed as brain drainage of a country and it is considered sad and loss of national interest.

Sometimes the talent is exported or it may be said lending for good mission. This one is beneficial to the nation. It is not a loss rather it is a gain to the nation as well. So, the country should accept this concept of talent conservation. A wise talent conservation practice may be adopted as a national talent conservation policy. In this policy guide lines, talent resource may be build up through a training program. This approach may be a commercial venture where plenty of unemployed adult are roaming. This is what is being practiced in many countries but the process needs to be upgraded to the international standard. Talent being a resource, its conserva-tion practice may yield sustainable resource for the nation.

18.3 RESOURCE CONSERVATION PRACTICES

"Wise saving is earning" is the best conservation practice of resource management.

There are many reasons in favor and against conservation practices for resource saving or build up. We have a common saying that is saving is earning. It is to be noted that if the saving is not wise or rational, that saving may harm otherwise or it may not work at all. This is the conservation prin-ciple applicable for all resources, be it bioresources or non-bioresources. Of course, the value of conservation practices may vary from one to another. For example, NNRs like oil, gas, coal, minerals are in deposit may exhaust any time and if they are exhausted, they would not be available any more from those sources unless a new deposit is discovered.

If we have lot of money earned, deposited in the bank and use them without following conservation practices, it is exhausted, it will not generate. If we follow the principle of conservation practices, spent money not more than the rate of interest in the Bank or elsewhere, the capital or basic investment is protected or conserved, while the expenditure is less than the increment, it is building up of resources, that is, we may have sustainable development through accretion by compound interest. In the case of natural resources like forest, horticulture, fish farming, forest farming, the growth rate is taken care of. Harvesting more than the increment, the growth will naturally lead to depletion of the resource base. In case of this natural living resource or we say bioresource, the growth rate, quality, quantity, rotation of cutting, and replanting, and so on are the determinant for prescribing the practicing principles. Here the silviculture and the silviculture of species of the crop is used to decide silvicultural system for conservation practice in order to obtain optimum yield from the crop being managed. The selection of silviculture system is again dependent upon objectives of the management. For example, production of paper pulpwood for running paper mills of the country with a view to reduce paper pulp import. Here, in our tropical climate, fast growing paper pulp producing ideal species, may be selected is *Eucalyptus camaldulensis* with rotation period of 12 years. The second choice may be *Acacia mangifera* with the same rotation.

18.3.1 AWARENESS OF CONSERVATION PRACTICES

Understanding conservation and conservation practice or being aware of conservation practice in the 21st century is so necessary that it becomes hard for mass people to survive without practicing conservation of resources or bioresources. This is because the ages are competition age in the context of rapid population growth, higher rate of consumption or utilization of resources and naturally depletion of re-sources. It is to be noted that you and I are not enough if we practice conservation of resources, it is in fact largely depend upon mass population. It will not be effective and bring about any positive change of the resources or economy until and unless mass people honestly and earnestly resort to conservation practices. Education, training of mass people is necessary so as to make them aware of importance of practicing conservation of resources, be it renewable or nonrenewable.

18.3.2   BOTTLENECKS IN CONSERVATION PRACTICES

It is not unusual to have bottleneck in any work. It is there in most of the cases particularly countries are not so well of in their resource base. Lacking education or unaware of conservation practices is one major bottleneck. Again, in this age of competition for upgrading living standard, saving though essential becomes very difficult particularly when one lives hand to mouth. In such a case, all out support needs to be extended to them along with the technology. One may earn plenty but there is no way of raising living standard or living better other than practicing conservation of the resource earned. It is a must for mass people. If one really mean business, must think and got down to the grass-root level with a basket of technical knowhow and teach them, motivate them, convince them about the useful-ness of practicing conservation of resources. National policy in this respect is very important and plays an effective role.

18.3.3   BALANCED CONSERVATION PRACTICES

Bioresource use is practically on the increase and it increases with the increase of human population. It is to be noted that rich or poor, all uses bioresources and the poor class is too much dependent upon bioresources. Bioresource use increases with the present trend of life style where demand is higher than the legal production and supply. The situation is such that in many countries, the growth rate cannot keep pace with the consumption. As a result, the basic bioresources are harvested legally or illegally to meet the bare minimum demand and therefore the scope for resource build up is shattered. This is just like eating the capital where interest or production decreases along with the decrease of capital value. As a result, the resource base is depleted and its eco system services degenerate.

Under such adverse situation of bioresource, how on earth it is possible to ensure balanced conservation practice? This is a question of survival of the people of today and tomorrow as well, when the trend of resource depletion is ongoing from time immemorial. The whole world is shaken by the wanton destruction of natural resources like forest resources and many others both in soil and sea. We know a stitch in time saves nine but here it is too late for many. When they live hand to mouth, how they do practice forest resource conservation. In countries like Bangladesh, moratorium or ban on felling of forest trees in the past did not work. This is forest dependent people live hand to mouth, cannot but to go for stealing forest trees. The forest conservation practice becomes almost impossible! In such a situation, Government is to come forward for help to the needy, ration of daily fuel wood or to provide free kerosene and also cash money so that they do not go to the forest. The greedy one should be prosecuted and deterrent punishment is desired so as to stop pilferage. This may be termed as gestation period and hopefully by that period the required level of forest resource is built up. Again another approach is to ban felling of forests and meet the national demand by import from other countries. This forest conservation practice depends upon the Government policy execution. Countries possessing adequate other resources may make this practice successful. But countries like Bangladesh, there are no guarantee of success by imposing moratorium on forest felling and or importing necessary forest produce. Balanced conservation practice for the resource poor countries is really difficult. As this living forest resource's contribution in ameliorating the trans-boundary environment, the world bodies like UNDP, UNEP, IUCN, WWF, and others may come forward for support.

18.4   SUSTAINABILITY

Sustainability has often been defined as how biological systems endure and remain diverse and productive. But, the 21st century definition of sustainability goes far beyond these narrow parameters. Today, it refers to the need to develop the sustainable models necessary for both the human race and planet Earth to survive. That is to ensure for present and future the abode, the food, the daily necessities for all living being. As we desire lasting peace, we depend upon lasting development of our resources. Sustainability in forest resources is more important in the sense that unless sustainability is ensured within the optimum time of reproducing capacities, the opportunity of ensuring sustainable development of forest resources becomes feeble. Forest resource, being a living regenerating entity, uses of the annual increment should never be more than the increment if the sustainability is expected. It is wise and appropriate to use the increment always less than the increment. This is something saving from the earning. The more is the saving from the earning the more is the stability of resources.

18.4.1   SUSTAINABLE DEVELOPMENT GOAL

SDG may be defined as desired achievement lasts more or less in perpetuity. It is natural that the goal or target when achieved remains everlasting or the development so achieved becomes sustainable. To make this development such, it is necessary to maintain an account book for income and expenditure from the basic or capital resources. In a forest, provision for similar forest management account book is maintained where the annual growth (increment or income) and the annual removal/tree felling (expenditure) is maintained. Now it becomes clear that if it is desired to have sustainable development of forest resources or any other business, expenditure must be less than the income. On the contrary, if the expenditure becomes more than the income, the business will show red light, the forest resource began dwindling. Unless this situation is not reversed within a reasonable time, the business, the forest resource will gradually get lost and there will be no point of return. Of course, by fresh investment, new business or new forest may be grown over a time with man, money, materials and time. So, conservation practice is wise, sensible, and economic as against wastage of man, money, materials and time. Here one is to understand through acquiring adequate knowledge for handling or managing the business efficiently. This achievement of SDG either in forest management or in any other business is a success of the business. Let everybody understand conservation practice and conservation practice will hopefully yield sustainable resource.

18.4.2   *SUSTAINABLE YIELD*

Sustainable yield is an optimum yield or production at a regular interval over a reasonable time period. Sustained Yield Use is a form of natural resource or forest management practice that aims at "not killing the goose that lays the golden egg." This means not to enjoy the present at the cost of future. To make sure solvency for future, sustained yield is necessary. This concept is mainly used for natural resources, particularly forestry and fishing, it can, however, also be applicable to all economic activities with a capital resource, production timeline, consumption, and surplus management. Sustained yield ensures the feasibility of continuous, long-term exploitation of available resources to obtain regular harvests.

18.5   CONCLUSIONS

Conservation practices may yield sustainable resource provided management prescription relating to the resources in question is well thought over documented and applied as prescribed in the management plan. Conservation practice is a careful use, preservation and protection of something especially planned management of any resource such as natural resources like vegetation, forests, agri-crops, air, water, minerals, oil, gas, and so on and to prevent exploitation, destruction, neglect, or overuse. The principle of conservation is normally followed by conservancy organizations such that any resources under management does not deplete rather it is expected to improve. Forests are valuable national assets and constitute multiple resources within a unit. There could be a variety of trees, wildlife, rivers, and leisure hot spots. Each of these constitutes a natural capital base, from which yields are extracted optimally, without jeopardizing the sustainability of each resource. The United States passed a Federal law in 1960 to manage and develop the renewable and maintainable resources of the national forests for multiple use and sustained yield. Sustainable yield in fisheries is the amount of fishing that can be done without reducing the population density of the species, that is, the surplus to maintain the ecosystem. The virgin population of the species decreases with fishing activity; hence it needs to be balanced with the time the species needs to breed and develop. The sustainable yield would be within the range of the population density and its capacity to reproduce. Concept of conservation practices in fishery may be maximum, optimal and annual sustainable yields depending upon nature of management objectives. The first is exactly half the carrying capacity of the species by the ecosystem. Population growth is highest at this stage. Optimal sustainable yield represents the highest difference between total revenue and cost. It is typically lower than maximum sustainable yield. The third is the harvest, which can be obtained without lowering original population numbers

According to FAO, 76% of the world's population rely on forests for their water supply. It is therefore important to make sure that the annual yield of water from a forest may be a sustained supply but lean period supply may not be same as wet season. It is therefore important to manage the forest of the watershed or the water producing forests such that lean period also produce and supply the same amount of water. Special treatment is necessary for water conservation practices. Water in the recent years has become more precious and in many places, water being a god gifted free commodity is unthinkable nowadays. In fact, water is life. Without water, there is no life. Forest is the mother of water.

As said, bioresource is intimately dependent upon water resources and not to speak of bioresources, the nonliving resources are also intimately related to water. The non-bioresources are also to maintain a percentage of moisture in them so that they are not destroyed or deteriorated. As forest is one of the most important bioresources and that it provides water in lean period, research on forest and water relationship is a matter of great urgency. As we all know that there is a global water crisis in spite of three-fourth of the earth is occupied by water, the land mass with all its belongings are subjected to suffer for want of water. The water crisis is due to replacement of one bioresource and that is forest. Forest/ Vegetation over the land is cleared for urbanization/ industrialization. This leads to a sort of distortion of chain action system of ecosystem functions for delivering goods and services. It is therefore becoming important issue deserves immediate study from all corners of the planet so that forest water relationship is well understood and ensures the very existence of both water and forest/vegetation. It is nothing uncommon history of world land use systems where over exploitation of land bearing soil, vegetation and water led to the destruction Maaya Civilization. Destruction of forest and ground water and faulty agriculture appeared to be the cause of such destruction. Time and again we need to remember that, we need to resort to a regular routine practice of resource conservation of any kind for building up a strong resource base—a security for future.

KEYWORDS

- **conservation**
- **natural resources**
- **nonnatural resources**
- **bioresources**
- **sustainability**

REFERENCES

Adhil, S. C. E. O. Bankbazzar.com-Wise Saving is Earning.
FAO. 76% World Population Rely on Forest for Water Supply.
History of the Maya Civilization. Faulty Irrigation Ruined Maya Civilization.
Kamaluddin, M. Clonalm Propagation of Eucalyptus & Acacia Hybrid Stem Cutting (BRAC).
    6. M. Hoskins (190/91)The Unasylva vol 160 "Forestry and Food security", 1996; pp 1.

Mellink. W. Y. S.; Rao, K. G.; MacDicken. *Agroforestry in the Asia Pacific*; RAPA Publication, 1991; p 5.

Ninth South Asia Economic Summit held in Dhaka, 15–16 October 2016, under the "Theme Reimaging south Asia 2030" organized by Centre for Policy Dialogue, Bangladesh.

Ogden. C. Building Nutritional Considerations into Forestry Development Efforts.

White, K. J. *Proceeding of the Regional Expert Consultation on Eucalyptus*; RAPA Publication, 1993/1995; Vol. 1 and 2, p 6.

CHAPTER 19

Phytochemistry of Medicinal Plants: Experimental Techniques

MARÍA JULIA VERDE-STAR[*] and CATALINA RIVAS-MORALES

Facultad de Ciencias Biológicas, Laboratorios de Fitoquímica y Química Analítica, Universidad Autónoma de Nuevo León, Av. Universidad s/n Cd. Universitaria, San Nicolás de los Garza, C.P. 66455, Nuevo León, Mexico

[*]*Corresponding author. E-mail: jverdestar@gmail.com*

ABSTRACT

This chapter compiles the research advances on phytochemical composition of medicinal plants used traditionally in Northeast Mexico for more than 30 years using standard phytochemical techniques.

Phytochemistry analysis is the scientific way to validate the popular knowledge about the therapeutic properties of the plants. The scientific study of toxic or medicinal plants used empirically as healing to diseases, seek of biological activity of the extracts, separate from an extract and identify the structure of secondary metabolites, find and test the active principles, constitute the target of our research team. More than 50% of the drugs used for the last three decades are directly or by chemical modifications obtained from the plants.

It is very important to mention that less than 15,000 of the nearly 250,000 known medicinal plants worldwide, have been studied in order to obtain their bioactive principles. This underlines the great potential of the plants in the search for new medicines. The present chapter highlights the importance of the chemotaxonomy and describes techniques of collection, identification and preparation of plant material, extraction techniques as well as the preliminary tests of the extracts trying to find their biological activity: antimicrobial, antioxidant, antifungal, antidiabetic, and the in vitro cytotoxic cell activity in tumor; and find the minimum concentration of active extract and also find the structure of the compounds, through chemical tube-tests and spectroscopy data.

19.1   INTRODUCTION

Through the human history, the man was trying to find cures for diseases in leaves, roots, bark, seeds, fruits, or flowers of wild plants, he also began to establish a relationship between the type of plant and the biological activity attributed to each one, based in external features and aromas, because still was not established what is known today as plant taxonomy.

From empirical knowledge of the benefits of the use of plants for therapeutic purposes, man knew for the first time, the synthetic drugs, such as aspirin, their structure and synthesis was inspired in the constituents of the bark of the white willow *Salix alba*, and the original structure was obtained by synthesis in pharmaceutical laboratories (Butler, 2004). The Herbalism and Ethnobotany have contributed to grow interest in the pharmacological study of plants and has allowed the development of the phytochemistry. An important difference between animal and vegetable Kingdom, is the capacity of the plants and fungi to produce substances that are not essential for the plants-survival; the determination of the presence of these substances and the analysis of their biological activity are the goal of the Phytochemistry (Sarker et al., 2005).

Chemotaxonomy is the relationship between the type of chemical compounds present in plants with their genus or families [*Journal of Medicinal Plants Studies 4* (2, 90–93)], these taxonomic relationships are also used in solving classification problems and allows increase the scientific interest about the medicinal plants and the relationship plant/activity, as taxonomic characteristics which allowed to distinguish algae, bacteria, fungi, Bryophytes, Pteridophytes, Gymnosperms, Angiosperms and classify families, genera, and species.

All the chemical compounds present in a plant are called metabolites and are classified as primary and secondary, nevertheless, cannot be distinguished based only and their chemical classification or biosynthetic map. A valid distinction between the two types of metabolites is not based on its structure or biochemistry, but on its function, thus is: primary metabolites are involved in nutrition and metabolic processes essential for the plant and secondary metabolites are those who allow ecological interactions of the plant with its environment (Dewick, 2002; Maplestone et al., 1992).

Primary metabolites examples in plants are mainly organic compounds as amino acids, carbohydrates, fatty acids, nucleic acids, amines, proteins, chlorophylls, which in turn produce secondary metabolites defined as substances that do not participate directly in the growth or development, that is, compounds that are not necessary for an organism, but they simply provide the plants an advantage to respond to stimuli of the environment, either as a defense mechanism against predators or as storage. David S-Y Wang says that secondary metabolite plays a role in reinforcement of tissue and tree body (e.g., cellulose, lignin), defense against insects, diseases, and plant regulation (plant hormones).

Higher animals rarely produce secondary metabolites and some exceptions only found in insects and some other mammals and invertebrates. some secondary metabolites are only present in certain species and have a specific function, for example, to attract insects to transfer pollen, or animals that eat the fruits and then disseminate their seeds; or also acting as natural pesticides of defense against herbivores or pathogens, or as allelopathic agents (substances that allow competition between plant species), can also synthesize secondary metabolites in response to damage in any plant tissue as well as against UV light and other aggressive physical agents, even act as signals for communication between plants with symbiotic microorganisms (Colegate and Molyneux, 2007) Chemotaxonomy is in other words the relationship that keeps a plant, in terms of their taxonomic classification and secondary metabolites containing.

For example, the relationship may be poppies: alkaloids, that is, allows to establish the hypothesis that plants belonging to the family Papaveraceae contains alkaloids. Most of secondary metabolites can be classified into three chemically groups: terpenes, phenols, and nitrogenated compounds (Vince, 2011). These three big groups include cyanogenic glycosides, terpenoids, sterols, phenolic flavonoids, coumarins, lignanes, cardiotonic glycosides, alkaloids, saponines, lactones (Valencia Ortiz, 1995).

Preservation of health is one of the important concerns of mankind mainly because the emergence of new diseases, this motivated man to seek a solution to these evils and plants and their secondary metabolites represent an opportunity. However, just 40 or 50 years ago began the scientific study of plants and their chemical constituents with medicinal properties or biological activities, which is the main objective of this chapter.

Methodology for the study of medicinal plants, comprises the following stages: (1) Bibliographic research: It is necessary to know the background to the plant to investigate; its origin, its uses, its toxic effects (if any), scientific papers about the plant or other plants of the genus or family. This stage must be continuous for all research. (2) Biological activity assays: checking scientific of therapeutic properties assays involving evaluation in vitro or in vivo. (3) Phytochemical study: through a bioassay, in order to determine qualitatively the main chemical groups in the plant extracts. (4) Toxicity and cytotoxicity evaluation on organisms or cells, the possible toxic effect of plant extract. (5) Developing a phytotherapeutic product: formulated with extracts or active compounds; a phytomedicine for clinical evaluation. After an ethnobotanical study of the plant and considering its chemotaxonomy, carry out the following procedure, for the study of the biological activity: (1) geographic location of the species, (2) collection of plant date and place, (3) taxonomic classification by experts obtaining its registration number for herbarium control (4) cleaning of the plant; eliminating visible impurities (earth, insects, etc.), (5) drying of the plant in the shade or stove, and (6) grinding on a mill and obtain extracts (Dominguez, 1988). The parts of the plant that will undergo an extraction are selected from popular and scientific reports and the method of extraction and solvent polarity type related to type of compounds to be isolated. One of the methods more simple and more attached to the background of traditional uses is through a decoction or infusion Other extractive methods most commonly used are: (1) maceration: cold or heat, (2) leaching, (3) Soxhlet, and (4) towed by steam.

Maceration is a solid–liquid extraction method where the plant material that is intended to extract contains the soluble compounds in the selected solvent. For this process the material is cut into small pieces or milled, fresh, or dry is placed in suitable containers, first add a nonpolar solvent like hexane (or petroleum ether), then with a more polar like chloroform and finally methanol or ethanol at rest or in an equipment with continuous agitation at room temperature (Bonatti, 1991). Lixiviation, in this method of extraction occurs a displacement of soluble substances by means of a liquid solvent, this process is used industrially to prepare elixirs; vegetable fresh material is placed in a container at room temperature for 3 days, with acetone or any other solvent or mixture of solvents.

After this time it is placed in a rotary evaporator (you can use other solvents or water) (Walton and Brown, 1999). Soxhlet extraction is a continue procedure in which a solid plant material, is placed inside a thimble of filter paper, then placed into the Soxhlet extractor, where will be the solvent continuously, this cycle can be repeated many times, for hours or days.

For the extraction of plant can be divided into: aerial parts (flowers, fruit, seeds, leaves, stem) and roots, phytochemical analysis can be to whole plant or one of its parts to a specific analysis. The dry and ground plant is placed in a Soxhlet with a nonpolar solvent as petroleum ether or hexane for 7 days at a temperature of 20–30°C. If there is a precipitate, filter it and eliminate the filtrate on a rotary evaporator and using the same solvent recover the precipitate by continue washing procedure, evaporate the filtrate again. Once the extract is ready in the flask, it is necessary evaporate the solvent and to do it quickly and recovering the solvent, it is very useful a rotary evaporator. This is a distillatory equipment with a hot water bath that reduces time to concentrate and obtain the dry extract of the vegetal material, the advantages are efficiency and selectivity (Huie, 2002).

19.2 ISOLATION AND IDENTIFICATION OF SECONDARY METABOLITES

19.2.1 THIN LAYER CHROMATOGRAPHY

Thin layer chromatography is an analytical method to separate and also isolate the compounds from a mix, it is a useful procedure to purify a compound isolated from a plant extract.

The test sample is deposited near one end of a glass plate which has been previously coated with a thin layer of adsorbent 0.1 mm thick (stationary phase). The sheet is then placed in a closed cuvette containing one or more mixed solvents (eluent or mobile phase). As the solvent mixture rises by capillarity through the adsorbent, there is a differential partition of the products present in the sample between the solvent and the adsorbent (SiO_2 or Al_2O_3).

The relationship between the distances traveled by the solute and the eluent from the origin of the plate is called front retainer (Rf), and has a constant value for each compound under particular conditions (adsorbent solvent, temperature, etc.), also for determining the degree of purity and track a chemical reaction.

The test sample is deposited near one end of a glass plate which has been previously coated with a thin layer of adsorbent 0.1 mm thick (stationary phase). The sheet is then placed in a closed cuvette containing one or more mixed solvents (eluent or mobile phase). As the solvent mixture rises by capillarity through the adsorbent, there is a differential partition of the products present in the sample between the solvent and the adsorbent (SiO_2 or Al_2O_3).

The relationship between the distances traveled by the solute and the eluent from the origin of the plate is called front retainer (Rf), and has a constant value for each compound under particular conditions (adsorbent solvent, temperature, etc.). To calculate the Rf of a compound, measure the distance from spot origin to the center of the spot and the following equation applies:

Rf = distance traveled by the compound (X)/
distance traveled by the eluent (Y)

Calculation front retention (Rf) eluents: to choose the eluents to be used in chromatography, it is necessary know the polarity of each solvent, in phytochemical analysis, are used, solvents from lower to higher polarity. Samples are deposited on the plate as spots, with a capillary tube: a point of extract of plant diluted, a point of a fraction obtained from a column. A small (3 × 7 cm) TLC plate takes just few minutes to run.

The analysis is qualitative, and it will show, how many compounds are present in the extract, how many in each fraction of the column, and how pure is a compound obtained from each fraction. For example: If it is eluted a thin layer chromatography of a sample of diluted extract or fraction of a chromatographic column or an insoluble precipitate or plant material, and so on.

First, dissolve a small quantity of sample in the adequate solvent and apply a sample with a capillary tube, approximately 1 cm from the lower end of the chromatographic plate, allow dry and place the plate in a glass vessel containing a mix of benzene: acetone 9:1. For example, if the chromatographic plate is 5 × 10 cm use a glass container of 250 mL with a lid and add 10 mL of eluent, in this case it would be: 9 mL benzene (B) and 1 mL of acetone (A), (0.5 cm before the upper end of the plate remove the plaque and dry) observe under ultraviolet light and spray with cobalt chloride solution (different developers subsequently described). If the sample in the TLC plate (Figs. 19.1 and 19.2), did not move up, then another solvent system is used: chloroform-methanol 9:1. In case the sample was not displaced from the application point in chromatographic plate, a third system of eluent is used; Butanol-acetic acid-water, in the ratio 7:2:1, if higher polarity is required, increase water volume, and decrease acetic acid, 7:1:2 and so on.

Chromatography is an effective isolation technique because the compounds on a mix travel different distance in the plate.

Each compound on a mix has a specific area on the plate because of its polarity and each one can be scraped away, to be analyzed and chemically identified. (Lewis, 1989) Revelators, most of the chromatographic plates have a fluorescent indicator that allows the active compounds be viewed under ultraviolet light (254 nm).

For compounds that do not absorb UV light, for chromatogram display, it is required to use a developer that reacts with adsorbates producing colored compounds:

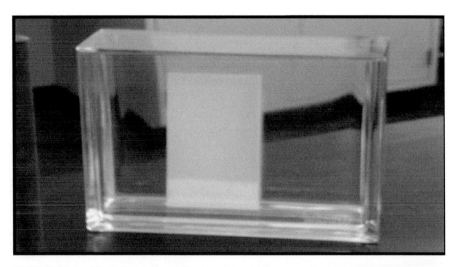

FIGURE 19.1   TLC plate and cuvette.

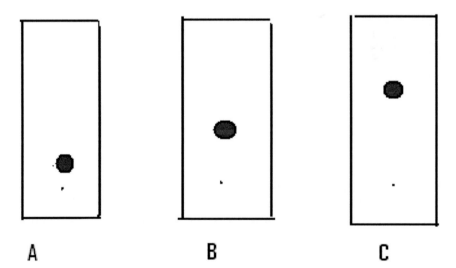

A   B   C

FIGURE 19.2   Thin layer chromatography with different elution systems

19.2.1.1   *COBALT CHLORIDE*

In 800 mL of distilled water add 20 g of $CoCl_2$ and 100 mL of concentrated sulfuric acid, gradually added sliding by the wall of the flask then add water until 1 L. This solution is sprayed to reveal a TLC.

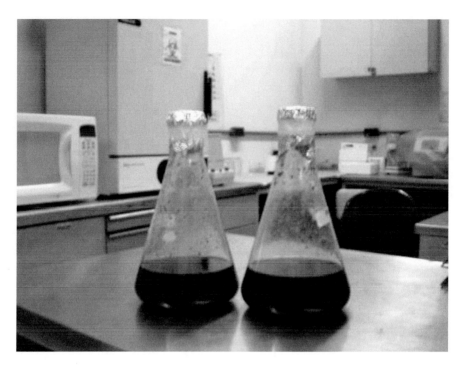

FIGURE 19.3   Plant extracts.

19.2.1.2   DRAGENDORFF REAGENT (MODIFIED) (SPECIFIC FOR ALKALOIDS)

Solution A is prepared dissolving 0.85 g of bismuth subnitrate in a mixture of 10 mL of glacial acetic acid and 40 mL of water. Solution B: 8.0 g of potassium iodide are dissolved in 20 mL of distilled water. Both solutions (A and B) are mixed just before the test: 5 mL of solution A and 5 mL Solution B is added 20 mL of glacial acetic acid, add distilled water to 100 mL (Domínguez, 1988)

19.2.1.3   EHRLICH (FURAN RINGS)

30 mg p-dimethylamino benzaldehyde are dissolved in 20 mL of ethanol, this reagent is used as revealing agent in chromatography by placing it in a camera with HCl for few minutes and compounds in TLC containing furan ring, will show purple, blue, or violet stains.

19.2.1.4 POLYOLS

Dissolve 200 mg vanillin in 50 mL of ethanol and at the time to be used is mixed with a solution of 3% perchloric acid ($HClO_4$) in water, this sand sprays the plate and 3 or 4 min allowed to dry. Pale blue stains will appear changing to pink and lilac color changes to gray.

19.2.1.5 MARQUIS (ALKALOIDS)

It is a mixture of sulfuric acid and formaldehyde in a ratio of 10:1.

19.2.1.6 QUINONES

100 mg of methylene blue are dissolved in 20 mL of ethanol, acetic acid (half milliliter), and 100 mg of zinc powder. Shake closed bottle and spray chromatography plate with that solution if color stains appear in few minutes indicating the presence of quinones.

19.2.1.7 SESQUITERPENLACTONES

Reagent is a mix of methanolic solution saturated with hydroxylamine, added with hydrochloric acid mixed with 2N sodium hydroxide (1:1), first spray with this solution the plate and then with a second reagent, which is prepared, mixing a solution of ferric chloride ($FeCl_3$)1% in methanol with 2N hydrochloric acid in a ratio (1:1).

19.2.1.8 SUGARS

Mixing 0.93 g of aniline with 1.66 g of o-phthalic anhydride and dissolved in 100 mL of butanol. The chromatographic plate is then sprayed and heated to 110°C, the recommended eluents for chromatography are: isopropanol–acetic acid–water in a ratio of 3:1:1 or butanol–water–acetic acid 7:2:1 (Dominguez, 1988).

19.2.1.9 ESSENTIAL OILS

30 mg of vanillin in 3 mL of ethanol then add 3 mL of water and 5 mL of concentrated sulfuric acid.

19.2.1.10   FLAVONOIDS

100 mg p-nitro aniline is dissolved in 15 mL of distilled water by adding 3 mL of hydrochloric acid and just to be used add 80 mg of sodium nitrite (for norhidroguaiaretic acid, NADG, orange or red spot appears reddish).

19.2.1.11   CARBONYL GROUP

3 g of 2,4-dinitrophenylhydrazine was solved in 30 mL of 85% phosphoric acid, heated to accelerate dissolution, dilute with 19.8 mL of absolute ethanol and filter the solution.

19.2.1.12   KELLER–KILLIANI TEST (CARDIAC GLYCOSIDES)

Solution A is prepared pouring 0.1 g of 3, 5 dinitrobenzoic acid in 10 mL of methanol, solution B: 0.5g of potassium hydroxide dissolved in 10 mL of methyl alcohol. In a test tube, we placed 20 mg of extract in methanol and added three drops of solution A and then three drops of solution B a reddish color appears (Garcia Gonzalez, 1992).

19.2.2   COLUMN CHROMATOGRAPHY

Column chromatography is a method used for separation, isolation and purification of various organic compounds in solid or liquid state.

The column for chromatography can be small or big depending on the quantity of vegetal material to be placed on it.

In column chromatography, it is very important to control the flow of solvent through the column to obtain the correct separation of fractions of the mix.

The stationary phase material must be moistened with mobile phase and packed correctly in the column to avoid empty spaces. The plant extract or sample to be separated is placed on the top of packed stationary phase. The mobile phase is added into the column over the sample. A collecting flask is placed at the bottom of column near the end to collect each fraction. The mobile phase go down through stationary phase (silica or alumina) leading the fractions elute out to be collected in a flask placed below. When the mobile phase descends, each compound of the extract travels at different speed through the stationary phase. This depends by the affinity of organic compounds with both stationary and mobile phases. The compounds of the extract more related to solvent polarity (mobile phase) descend fast and drop into the flask first. The fractions or compounds on the fraction more related to stationary phase will descend slow and reach bottom late. Column chromatography is a useful technique to isolate the compounds present in a mixture. Liquid chromatography using columns is a very useful procedure because almost every organic mixture can be separate using the specific polarity of the mobile phase, not only with single solvents but solvents mixed in calculated proportions.

The nonpolar or less polar compounds in a mixture will be the first compounds or fractions to drop into the collector flask, the more polar fractions or compounds are retained in the stationary phase, being necessary to use more polar solvents or mixes of two or more solvents of middle to high polarity. Retention time is the time a compound or fraction takes to travel through the column, and is specific for each compound, under the same conditions.

Eluents and agents use in chromatography column will be selected from those with better resolution on thin layer chromatography. The separation of each fraction of the extract or mixture can be monitored by the color developed in the descent of the extract through the adsorbent, this can be observed in form of colored rings at different heights of the column. The elution process can take more time depending the amount of mixture or extract, the column diameter, the mobile phase used and even if the mobile phase drops by gravity or accelerated using nitrogen gas or vacuum (flash chromatography). Crystallization is used for the purification of the obtained compounds and the criteria to follow considering that can be done with pure solvents or mixtures of them provided that they comply with the following requirements: to be very soluble at high temperature, impurities more soluble in cold temperature than solute, solvent volatile to be removed easily from crystals, and finally does not react with the solute.

19.3 OBTAINING, PURIFICATION, AND IDENTIFICATION OF SECONDARY METABOLITES

Once obtained the secondary metabolites of the fractionation done in the chromatography column, they must be purified by crystallization, making sure that each compound shows a single spot in TLC. The purity of an organic compound obtained by chromatography can be proved checking the physical constants of the compound as melting or boiling point, optic activity, Ultraviolet (UV), infrared (IR), and mass spectra (MS); and nuclear magnetic resonance (NMR), and by colored tests to identify functional groups.

19.3.1   DOUBLE BONDS C=C TEST OF TETRANITROMETHANE

1 mg of the sample is dissolved in chloroform and add 2 mL of dissolution of tetranitromethane in chloroform, the appearance of a yellow color indicates the presence of a nonterminal double bond; cyclopropanes and aromatic compounds give this positive test.

19.3.2   TEST OF BROMINE IN CARBON TETRACHLORIDE

1–2 mg of the sample is dissolved in 1 mL of CCl_4 and is added drop by drop this solution, the test is positive, if you notice a discoloration of the solution. Test of potassium permanganate: 1–2 mg of the sample is dissolved in 1 mL of water, acetone or methanol and added dropwise $KMnO_4$ solution 2% in water. The test is positive if appear discoloration or formation of a brown precipitate (manganese dioxide) in less than 1 min.

19.3.3   CARBOXYL GROUP TEST OF SODA BICARBONATE (NAHCO3)

Add few drops of the solution of 10% baking soda in water, to the sample (1–2 mg) dissolved in 1 mL of water or ethanol. The test is positive if bubbles of carbon dioxide appears. Carbonyl group: 1–10 mg of the sample is dissolved in ethanol, is added to a saturated solution of 2-4-dinitrophenylhidrazine in 6N HCl; if a yellow or orange precipitate appears then a carbonyl group is present.

19.3.4   FERRIC CHLORIDE TEST (PHENOLIC HYDROXYLS)

One or two mg of the sample is dissolved in 1 mL of ethanol and then add a few drops of ferric chloride 5% in ethanol. The appearance of a red precipitate, blue–violet or green is positive for phenolic hydroxyls.

19.3.5   STEROLS AND TRITERPENES LIEBERMANN-BURCHARD TEST

The reagent is prepared by adding 1 mL of acetic anhydride to 1 mL of chloroform and three drops of concentrated sulfuric acid. Then this reagent is added (one drop) to 1 mL of sample diluted in chloroform, sterols are present if a blue or purple color appears and triterpenes are present if appears reddish color. Test could take an hour.

19.3.6   SAPONINES

In a test tube is placed the sample (1–2 mg) dissolved in 1 mL of water, shaking and forms a lather generously, if this stays by 1 h, the test is considered positive.

19.3.7   CARBOHYDRATES TEST OF THE ANTHRONE

1–2 mg of sample dissolved in water are placed in a test tube, then leaves itself sliding down the walls of the tube a recent solution of Anthrone 0.2% in concentrated sulfuric acid; the test is positive if the interface shows a blue-green or purple ring.

19.3.8   COUMARINS

As the coumarins are lactones, they can dissolve in alkaline solutions aqueous or alcoholic with appearance of a yellow coloration, which disappears when acid. The presence of a furan group can be determined using the test of Ehrlich. Most of the coumarins, in thin layer, chromatography present blue fluorescence when observed under UV light and when sprayed with cobalt chloride, after heating the plate, is colored green or yellow. Dissolve 1–2 mg of the sample in a solution of sodium hydroxide 10% in water; if you see a yellow coloration, which disappears to acidify, the test is positive.

19.3.8.1   SESQUITERPENLACTONES BALJET TEST

Use two solutions that are mixed in equal volumes prior to use. A solution is prepared with 1 g of picric acid dissolved in 100 mL of ethyl alcohol.

Solution B is prepared with 10 g of sodium hydroxide in 100 mL of water. Performing the test, take 3–4 mg of the compound, add 3–4 drops of reagent, is positive if it forms dark orange or red coloration. A drop of solution in ethanol or Ethereal compound placed in 4 × 50 mm tube or in a micro-Crucible, add a drop of 2 N potassium hydroxides in methanolic solution. The mixture is heated with a lighter micro for 1–2 min. Immediately cools, add hydrochloric acid 0.5 N until acid pH, and add a drop of ferric chloride 1%; color purple is positive test, if the result is negative, you should dilute slightly and repeat the comment. Santonine gives a violet–pink color and alantolactone, dark violet. Coumarins, other lactones, and esters give positive this test. The simaroubolidanes and limonoids may also give positive the previous tests because they are lactones.

19.3.8.2 *FURANOCOUMARINES EHRLICH REAGENT*

A solution 1.5% of p-dimethylaminobenzaldehyde in ethanol is used. This solution is used as developer agent on the chromatographic plates with the sample. This plate is inserted into a chamber containing atmosphere of hydrogen chloride. A violet color is indicative for furan ring. Aromaticity The reagent is prepared just in the moment to be used, adding a drop of formalin (formaldehyde 37–40%) to 1 mL of concentrated sulfuric acid, placing it in a test tube and dissolved in a nonaromatic solvent, sample is added by the walls of the tube.

The formation of a colored ring at the interface, carmine red color to black, indicates the test is positive.

19.3.9 *NITRITES (NO$_2$)*

A bit of ferrous sulfate is dissolved in water then add the compound, passing through the walls of the tube a few drops of concentrated sulfuric acid, the test is positive when a ring of dark brown color is formed.

19.3.10 *CHLORIDES*

Dissolve 1 mg of silver nitrate in double distilled water and add a drop of this solution to the sample dissolved in double distilled water, the test for chloride is positive, when a milky white precipitate is observed.

19.3.11 HALOGENS—BEILSTEIN TEST

Wet a piece of copper wire in nitric acid or sulfuric acid, passes through the flame of a lighter, then the sample is taken and we direct it to the flame; chlorine gives a green coloration and bromine color blue.

19.3.12 CYANIDES

First solution is to soak the paper filter for the determination of cyanides. Solution: 200 mg of picric acid, plus 5 mL of ethanol add 5 mL of sodium hydroxide 1 N (5 g of NaOH in 125 mL of distilled water), this solution is to impregnate filter paper dry, which will yellow coloration. In a closed and clear container offers some vegetable material to be analyzed with a small amount of water and the filter paper inside the container but without gets wet, change from yellow to red, it is indicative for cyanides.

19.3.13 ALKALOIDS

19.3.13.1 MAYER REAGENT

Dissolve 1.36 g of $HgCl_2$ in 60 mL of water and 5 g potassium iodide in 10 mL of water. Join the two solutions and add water until total volume 100 mL. Single reagent should be added to previously acidified with diluted HCl or H_2SO_4 solutions. The solution must not contain acetic acid or ethanol, because they dissolve the precipitate. Only a few drops of reagent should be added because some alkaloids are soluble in excess of reagent.

19.3.13.2 SCHEIBLER REAGENT: (PHOSPHOTUNGSTIC ACID)

Dissolve in 50 mL of water 10 g of sodium tungstate and 7 g of disodium phosphate. The solution is acidified with nitric acid. The reagent is precipitated amorphous to mingle with alkaloids in dilute H_2SO_4 solutions. The precipitate is soluble in excess of reagent or in ethanol.

19.3.13.3 MARQUIS REAGENT

Add five drops of formalin to the sample being analyzed, add 5 mL of concentrated H_2SO_4, heroin and morphine immediately give a reddish-purple color and then it goes to violet color and finally to blue staining.

19.3.14   *FLAVONOIDS SHINODA TEST*

Dissolve 1–2 mg of sample in 1 mL of ethanol by adding a few drops of concentrated hydrochloric acid and one or two magnesium filings; If the solution turns a deep red color, the test is positive, other, orange, green, or blue color may be present, flavones, flavonones, flavonols, antioxidant xanthones When there are interference pigments not flavonoids, plant material can be tested directly; for example, if the white petals of a flower change to yellow in the presence of ammonia vapors, should contain flavones or flavonols. The chalcones and the aurones going from yellow to red.

The petals that contain anthocyanins change to red in the presence of ammonia. Antimony pentachloride in carbon tetrachloride, produces characteristic colors with flavonoids (Marini-Berttolo test). The chalcones form precipitates red dark or violet and flavones, precipitates yellow or orange. Flavones and Flavonols are dissolved in concentrated sulfuric acid and originate strongly yellow solutions. The flavanones give orange colors or cherry red to bluish red.

19.3.15   *QUINONES*

Quinones tend to give red or purple colors with concentrated alkali and sulfuric acid, which cane used to identify them. The presence of anthraquinones and naphthaquinones can be identified with the reaction of Borntrager, which consists in boiling for 10 min, some material with 2–5% potassium hydroxide. The solution cooled, is acidified and extracted with benzene. The benzene layer is separated and is tossed with a little of the potassium hydroxide solution. If the phase of benzene is discolored and the alkaline gets red, is positive for Quinones.

19.3.16   *CARDIOTONIC GLYCOSIDES*

Glucosides or glycosides are metabolites formed of two parts: one is a carbohydrate and the other no-sugar or aglycone. The link between the two is hydrolysable and must break which is activated compound; this rupture is catalyzed by enzymes containing the same plant. Glycosides are classified according to the structural characteristics of the aglycone:

19.3.16.1   RAYMOND REAGENT

Dissolve 1–2 mg of extract in 5–8 drops of ethanol at 50% then add 1–2 drops of 1% of m-dinitrobenzene in ethanol and then add 2–3 drops of an aqueous solution NaOH 20%. A violet color is formed. Legal test: Treat the extract with pyridine and add alkaline sodium nitroprusside solution, blood red color appears. Tollens test: In a small, clean test tube 5–10 mg of extract dissolve in 5–8 drops of pyridine and add 4–6 drops of very recent Tollens reagent. (Mix 0.5 ml of 10% AgNO3 and 0.5 mL of NaOH 10%; after ammonium hydroxide is added dropwise to complete dissolve of the precipitate.) This reagent must decompose before one hour, since explosive nitrides are formed. Positive if is formed a mirror on the tube.

19.4   CONCLUSIONS

The general techniques have been described in this chapter applied to phytochemical analysis of a plant whose therapeutic or toxic properties have been described by the ethnobotanic and through an analytical procedure and applying the scientific method is it aims to validate the hypothesis of herbalists. The main objective is the pursuit of secondary metabolites that possess biological activity and the description of the main extraction methods and techniques of separation and structure elucidation of these compounds.

The phytochemical screening is a tool that guides us for the separation and purification of compounds and through a bioassay determine the biological activity and identify by spectroscopic methods the bioactive compounds, validating scientifically its use in traditional medicine; This information would provide knowledge for the pathways of biosynthesis of the active principles isolated, and their further use as a drug of natural origin.

KEYWORDS

- **medicinal plants**
- **phytochemistry**
- **extraction techniques**
- **biological activity**
- **antioxidant**
- **chemotaxonomy**
- **identification techniques**

REFERENCES

Bonatti, A. Formulation of Plant Extracts into Dosage Form. In *The Medicinal Plant Industry*; Wijesekera, R. O. B., Ed.; CRC Press: London, 1991; pp 106–107.

Butler, M. S. The Role of Natural Product Chemistry in Drug Discovery. *J. Nat. Prod.* **2004,** *67*, 2141–2153. http://doi.org/10.1021/np040106y.

Colegate, S. M.; Molyneux, R. J. *Bioactive Natural Products: Detection, Isolation, and Structural Determination*, 2nd Ed.; CRC Press, 2007.

Der Marderosian, A.; Beutler, J. A. The Review of Natural Products: The Most Complete Source of Natural Product Information. Facts & Comparisons, Saint Louis, USA, 2005, 1343.

Dewick, P. M. *Medicinal Natural Products: A Biosynthetic Approach*; John Wiley & Sons: New Jersey, USA 2002.

Dominguez, X. A. *Metodos de investigacion fitoquimica*; Limusa, 1988.

Garcia Gonzalez, S. *Estudio Quimico de Cnidoscolus urens*; Instituto Tecnologico y de Estudios Superiores de Monterrey, 1992.

Harborne, A. J. Phytochemical Methods A Guide to Modern Techniques of Plant Analysis; Springer Science & Business Media, 1998.

Lambert, J.; Srivastava, J.; Vietmeyer, N. *Medicinal Plants: Rescuing a Global Heritage*; World Bank, 1997.

Lewis, H. W.; Christopher, J. Moody. *Experimental Organic Chemistry: Principles and Practice (Illustrated ed.)*; WileyBlackwell, 1989; pp 159–173. ISBN 978-0-632-02017-1.

Luque de Castro, M. D.; Priego-Capote, F. Soxhlet extraction: Past and Present Panacea. *J. Chromatogr. A* **2010,** *1217* (16), 2383–2389. http://doi.org/10.1016/j.chroma.2009.11.027.

Maplestone, R. A.; Stone, M. J.; Williams, D. H. The Evolutionary Role of Secondary Metabolites—A Review. *Gene* **1992,** *115* (1–2), 151–157.

Mishra, B. B.; Tiwari, V. K. Natural Products: An Evolving Role in Future Drug Discovery. *Eur. J. Med. Chem.* **2011,** *46* (10), 4769–4807. http://doi.org/10.1016/j.ejmech.2011.07.057.

Paech, K.; Tracey, M. V. *Modern Methods of Plant Analysis/Moderne Methoden der Pflanzenanalyse*; Springer: Berlin Heidelberg, 2012.

Sarker, S. D.; Latif, Z.; Gray, A. I. *Natural Products Isolation*; Humana Press, 2005.

Verde-Star, Maria Julia; Rivas-Morales, Catalina; Garcia, Gonzalez Sergio. *Metodologia cientifica para el estudio de plantas medicinales*. In *Investigacion en plantas de importancia medica*, 1a Ed.; OmniaScience, 2016; p37. ISBN: 978-84-944673-7-0.

Vogel, A. I.; Tatchell, A. R.; Furnis, B. S.; Hannaford, A. J.; Smith, P. W. G. *Vogel's Textbook of Practical Organic Chemistry*, 5th ed. ISBN 0-582-46236-3.

Walton, N. J.; Brown, D. E. *Chemicals from Plants: Perspectives on Plant Secondary Products*; Imperial College Press, 1999.

CHAPTER 20

Phytoplankton and Toxic Threats

AHMED IBRAHIM JESSIM*

Ministry of Higher Education, Scientific Research, Science and Technology, Treatment and Disposal of Chemical, Biological and Military Hazardous Wastes, Center of Research and Development, Baghdad, Iraq

Corresponding author. E-mail: ahm_jas71@yahoo.com

ABSTRACT

The microscopic planktonic algae are a critical food or different filter-feeding planktonic bivalves, such as shellfish (oyster, mussels, scallops, and clams), also for larvae of commercially important crustaceans and finfish. Moreover, among the 5000 existing marine algal species, approximately sometimes a significant number of these creatures can occur in such a high number (blooming) that they obviously discolor the surface of the lagoons, coastal areas, and the contaminated shore of seas. The term "Bloom" usually is used to indicate massive growth of any of these organisms, which they are may vary in color from the commonly cited red so they called "Red tides" for different shades of blue, brown, green, and yellow depending on the type of algae, their depth, and concentration. The conditions of the algal bloom are not fully elucidated yet but the phenomenon probably is influenced by hydrographic circumstances and climate change. Sometimes, the massive growths appear during changes of weather conditions but an important contributing cause may be variations in upwelling's temperature, transparency, turbulence or salinity of the water, concentrations dissolved nutrients, illumination of the surface, and the wind. But the importance of this case is there are many species of planktonic algae can produce toxins, such as Paralytic shellfish toxins, namely Diarrheic shellfish toxins, Amnesic shellfish toxins, Neurotoxin shellfish toxins, and Azaspiracid shellfish toxins. These toxins are called marine biotoxins and there were other different types of toxins in the freshwater ecosystem; however, marine biotoxins can impact the health of human and his food resources in seas. Actually, this phenomenon needs efforts to face the real challenge of Marine (biotoxins). Different phytoplankton species can produce different types of toxins or else different species can produce one type of toxin, for example, toxic plankton as a species *Dinophysis sacculus* and as a genus *Gyrodinium, protoperidinium* and *Prorocentrum.* All these toxins are producible from phytoplankton mostly in warm time especially in spring, therefore, many countries depend on early mentoring to keep people safe especially at summer when they spend time on the beaches, but unfortunately knowledge about phytoplankton is day by day increasing and it is found that the range of its spreading in the world via trade ships as one of probable factor which can clarify toxic phytoplankton as exotic species may be in noneffected shores or aquatic basin and lagoons in coastal areas. Several projects on aquaculture and bivalves' cultures have a threat of toxicity by marine toxins when they import mothers of bivalves and larvae of wild fish to develop them and produce seafood, actually by valves are accused to transfer toxic phytoplankton from effected basin or bivalves farm to noneffected one. The answer is why these creatures are toxic? Or is it not nontoxic before activities, here we can say we need rearrangement or reducing the quantity of pollutants inputs which were and are increasing day after day to at least to control managing real solutions of this global phenomenon, because it is one of the bioresources at this planet.

20.1   INTRODUCTION

20.1.1   COASTAL ENVIRONMENT

Many countries have a long distance of coasts, such as India (Verlecar and Desai, 2004). This environment is usually a significant part, also or significant element, and this environment varies from one place to another, depending upon the extent to which it affects or is directly affected by coastal processes and the management issue. It includes three distinct areas, but they are interrelated: The coastal marine area, the active coastal zone, and the land backdrop (Jessim, 2009). Therefore, for diagnosis of the environment or assessment for the impacts of urban activities now is a general concern and also it gives a good evaluation to represent a real hard challenge. Through the last decades, the identification of indicators that represent stress upon phytoplankton population has been searched through intensive efforts. Generally, there are several signs that should be taken in consideration for health assessment of an aquatic ecosystem, for example, species diversity, biotic of community structure, length of the food chain, and stability of population (Gianesella et al., 1999). The term Phytoplankton is referring to the number of species, such as Diatoms, Dinoflagellates, Blue–green algae, Silicoflagellates, Cocolithophors, etc., representing about 59% from the primary products in the oceans and considered as first ring of the food chain. Then, secondary production Zooplankton depends on phytoplankton, then third production, such as fish, shellfish, mammals and other, depends on productions of marine (Verlecar and Desai, 2004).

The development of phytoplankton population depends upon certain micronutrients that are required in high enough concentration to support population growth of phytoplankton. In marine environment, nitrogen (n) generally is considered to be a limiting nutrient, although, phosphorus (p) and silicon (Si) also require in varying quantities from certain phytoplanktonic groups (Hydes et al., 2004), In addition, due to human activities, coastal areas were and are a real subject of eutrophication that comes from increasing the inputs of inorganic elements, like phosphorus (P), which is with another 16 elements are essential for growth of plant, also the organic compounds, such as Urea, which is available from dissolved organic nitrogen in the marine environment (Fouko et al., 2006). Increase of phosphorus at the surface of water comes from high-soil phosphorous, anthropogenic inputs (agricultural and industrial) in addition the conditions that can transport phosphorus to the surface of the water (Mullins, 2001). Then, Silicon (Si) is a control and effective element and most common that limits primary production at both coastal and freshwater ecosystem (Tallberg, 1999). Si found as a nutrient governing the total primary production, globally, of the world's oceans and it has been emphasized that possibly Si drawdowns carbon dioxide (Tallberg, 2000). Lately, the studies now have gone intensively in the relationship and interactions between Si and the other elements, particularly P, at particle surfaces the effects have given a little attention (Tallberg, 2000). Later Morre et al. (2006) referred to iron (Fe) as a supplied by dust deposition has shown to be an important factor control dynamics of phytoplankton development at spring blooms. In addition to nutrients, physical factors can affect strongly phytoplankton development, like wind and temperature in coastal lagoons (Pilkaitytė and Razinkovas, 2006). Blooms can occur and develop over a wide range of salinity but, actually, there is an optimal salinity for high cellular densities, significant and problematic growth of phytoplankton species that are able to synthesize a toxic bioactive compound to humans (Fauchot et al., 2005; Delia et al., 2015). In other studies, researchers found the growth of pulses of toxic species affected and are associated with high solar radiation, low speeds of wind, and shallow mixed layer (Bleiker and Schanz, 1988; Häder et al., 2015).

At coastal lagoons and coastal areas, eutrophication environments receiving high- nutrient inputs from anthropogenic sources and from autochthonous origin that keeps primary production high, for both as benthic and planktonic. The environmental features of lagoons shallow waters, a strong seasonal gradient of temperature, salinity, and wind or tidal effects, were studied well and found very high variable compared with short spatial and temporal scales (Nuccio et al., 2003; Bonilla-Gómez et al., 2013). In addition to above, there are also relation of the chemical and physical factors that can cause eutrophication of coastal waters, one of most important ecological consequences of aquatic pollution, which is a main reason of occurrence for massive growth of toxic algal blooms [harmful algal blooms (HABs)], often called red tides. This massive growth of phytoplankton mostly represents dinoflagellates and may produce highly toxic products that can cause illness and even death for aquatic organisms as well as humans (Andersone et al., 2002; Santi Delia et al., 2015).

20.1.2   HARMFUL ALGAL BLOOMS

HABs is a term that refers to a heterogeneous development of events that share two characteristics caused by microalgae and they have a negative impact on human health and activities. Algal blooms occur when phytoplankton grows at a rate that is harmful and detrimental to the other living forms.

Ecophysiological requirements for the most harmful species need more studies to be known well and need further laboratory studies to learn more about this field. Unfortunately, results from laboratory studies are not sufficient to predict the succession of phytoplankton species and blooms of specific harmful organisms in the sea. Indeed, the net growth performance of the species is affected by complex interactions with other organisms, which are scarcely reproducible in laboratory experiments. These include a negative interaction, such as grazing competition, viral infections, and positive feedback from predator excretions, bacterial nutrients regeneration, and viral lysis. In fact, the evidence of phytoplankton life strategies and their interactions with surrounding environment has increased and may reach a degree of unexpected complexity for unicellular organisms. The capability of the species to adapt with an environmental condition apparently not matching their optimal range is notably expanded and its occurrence is more difficult to predict (Zingone and Enevoldsen, 2000).

The term "Bloom" has been defined as "the rapid growth of one or more species in the same area of water that leads to a nuisance increase in the biomass of the species" (Smayda, 1997; Richardson, 1997; Arroyo and Bonsdorff, 2016).

HABs are an increasing phenomenon because of the massive growth of phytoplankton throughout coastal waters worldwide (Gastrich, 2000; Piuz et al., 2008). Globally, concern over an apparent increase of HABs, especially toward blooms occurring near the shores and affecting important fisheries and marine culture operations, has prompted research to control HABs and mitigation in an effort to reduce the ecological and economic impacts that they cause (Archambalut et al., 2002; France and mozetič, 2006). There are many questions about toxic phytoplankton when they bloom and become HABs. What is a harmful bloom? How abundant do a harmful species have to be harmful? Are its harmful effects density-dependent? Blooms have been regarded as a significant massive increase in the number of individuals of the phytoplankton population without concern over magnitude or impacts. Recognition that harmful species can represent a broad spectrum of antagonistic properties relative to the blooms of other species that has been stimulated efforts and distinguished formally between such different bloom types while this has broadened insights into the nature of phytoplankton blooms, also it has revealed widespread confusion concerning (What is a bloom) also how it is to be defined, this becomes even more problematic when efforts to defined a bloom in the terms of abundance are linked to a descriptor, such as an exceptional bloom (Smayda, 1997; Maso and Garce, 2006). HABs pose a serious threat and impact negatively the commercial fisheries and aquaculture, human health, and coastal aesthetics because of the water discoloration and accumulation of foam and mucilage on the coast producing unpleasant odors (Anderson, 1997; Anderson et al., 2001; Boesch et al., 1997; Beaulieu et al., 2005). HABs include a microscopic species, which is usually single cell, eukaryotes that live in estuarine and marine waters. Among 5000 marine phytoplankton recorded species, approximately 300 can occur in such high numbers (blooming) which obviously discolor the surface of the sea, the so-called "red tides" (Hallegraeff et al., 1995; Lindahl, 1998). Visible red tides may contain phytoplankton individuals from 20,000 to >50,000 cell mL^{-1} of seawater; however, concentrations as low as 200 cell mL^{-1} may produce toxic shellfish (Connell, 2007; Smith, 1992). When the conditions of temperature, light, nutrients, and salinity of water are appropriate, the cysts of dinoflagellates, which is one of red tide members, for example, germinate and causes swimming cells, then reproduces by simple division within few days. If the conditions remain optimal, cells will continue growing exponentially, so from one cell up to 6000–8000 cells can be produced in a week. When the appropriate environmental conditions are no longer available, growth rates are gradually reduced and the gametes are formed, two gametes join to form a cell that develops into a zygote and then into a new cyst that falls to the ocean bottom, ready to germinate when conditions permit (Daranas et al., 2001), HABs' increase worldwide has been related to increase in aquatic nutrient concentrations from human activities (Tango et al., 2003; Sengco and Anderson, 2004). The data indicate that these phenomena are on the rise worldwide, hence estuarine and near coastal researchers have begun to invest an increasing amount of time and other resources in efforts to characterize this phenomenon and understand what causes them (Scatasta et al., 2001). All world sites including Middle and South Tyrrhenian Sea waters, Australasian Region, Danish waters, the North Sea, South Africa, northeast American coasts, northwest American coasts, and Vietnam with detailed lists of harmful algal species have been published. Despite notable differences in size among the areas considered, the total numbers of harmful species are comparatively high. Harmful microflora is varying among these sites obviously, more than nontoxic species are concerned. Furthermore, in these types of studies, the diversity of harmful microflora parallels the pattern generally observed for the whole phytoplankton diversity at single site and also with the micro floral diversity where a significant number of cosmopolitan species found in addition to species which are more restricted. As already postulated by earlier authors, they proved that there are many species of phytoplankton are cosmopolitan but not all of them are identified or diagnosed at many places yet, which resulted in nonactive local microflora (Zingone et al., 2006; Congestri et al., 2006). In the Arabian area, the countries located near waters bodies and Arabian sea, have experienced massive marine mortality that caused as natural phenomenon or by manmade due to anthropogenic inputs like domestic and industrial wastes. HABs have been associated with some of the frequent episodes of seafood contamination, sometimes with very serious consequences for human health and associated with economic losses, such as in Kuwait and Iran at the period of 1999–2001, Oman in 1999–2002, Saudi Arabia in 2003, and Qatar during 2008. Particularly, in Qatari waters, benthic HABs events have been recorded due to the development of *Coolia monotis, C. tropicalis, Gambierdiscus toxicus, Lingulodinium polyedrum, Ostreopsis lenticularis, Prorocentrum balticum, P. convacum,* and *P. emarginatum.* At same waters, *Dinophysis miles* and *D. caudata*, were described as dominant species together with *Ceratium furca, Prorocentrum sigmoides,* and *P. micans*, but the *Trichodesmium erythraeum* was found usually to persist for a long period and *Perodinium bahamenes*, also *V. compresum,* was found in a large number of samples (Al-Muftah, 2008). During September–October, blooms of *Karenia* sp. were implicated in the mortality of 30 tons from wild mullets and 150 tons from caged sea bream fish at a cost of $7 million (Subba Rao et al., 2003), during the year 2000 A.D. Two red-water episodes have occurred that were ephemeral and massive, about two billion cells L^{-1} with patches were extending from 50 m^2 to 15×104 m^2. Here, the dominant species differed each time, for example, *Prorocentrum* spp., *Pseudo-nitzschia seriata, Nitzschia longissimi, Leptocylindrus sp.,* and *Trichodesmium erythraeum*. Experimental growth studies, an eoliak dust rich in essential micronutrients for the growth of phytoplankton had a positive effect on summer growth of phytoplankton, which is similar to the red tied proportions (Subba Rao et al., 2003). Researchers described and isolated into culture new species of potentially harmful algae from HABs in United Arab Emirates area, as *Ostreopsis labens, Prorocentrum norrisianum, P. faustiae, P. arabianium, P. reniformis, Pfiesteria shumwayiae, Protoperidinium ponticum,* and *Ostreopsis tholus* (Morton et al., 2002). Omani waters had shown a wide range of two HABs groups of phytoplankton, diatoms, and dinoflagellates. The diatom group included *Coscinodiscus marginatus, C. oculus irids, Biddulphia aurita, Asteromphalus cleveanus, A. flsbellatus, Melosira radiate, M. coronate, Planktoniella sol, Thalasssiosira decipiena, Nitzschia* ap., *Pleurosigma directum, Chaetoceros* ap., *Rhizosolenia* sp., *R. imbricate, R. alata, Guinardia flaccida, Fragilaria oceanica,* and *Bcteriastrum hyalinum*, and *dinoflagellate* group including *Noctiluca scintollans, Ceratium furca, C. fusus, C. massiliense* var. *protuberans, C. massiliense* var. *massiliense, C. falcatiforme, C. tripos, C. belone, C. trichoceros, Amphisolenia bidentate, Gymnodinium* sp., *Prorocentrum micans, Pyrophacus horologicum, Dinophysis caudata, D. cuneus,* and *Gonyaulax diegensis* (Thangaraja et al., 2007).

20.2 TOXIC PHYTOPLANKTON SPECIES

Approximately there are from 4000 (Lin et al., 2016) to 5000 species of identified microalgae (Daranas et al., 2001; Santi Delia et al., 2015; Hallegraeff et al., 1995; Lindahl, 1998). Naturally, some bloom-forming species, basically harmless, cause water discolorations, on the other hand, another species can bloom densely, under exceptional conditions in sheltered water bodies, especially those used for fish farming; they indiscriminately kill fishes and invertebrates because of oxygen depletion. Other species of phytoplankton can be harmful to the fish and invertebrates especially in the intensive aquaculture systems due to damaging or clogging their gills. Moreover, there are microalgal species which have the ability to produce potent toxins, named phycotoxins which can find their way through levels of food chain, for example, Mollusks, Crustaceans, and finfish that are ultimately consumed by humans causing a variety of gastrointestinal and neurological illnesses (Al-Ghelani et al., 2005; Zaccaroni and Scaravelli, 2008; Berdalet et al., 2016).

20.2.1 GROUPS OF TOXIC SPECIES

There are three major groups depending on the problem they cause. The first group is formed by nontoxic species that discolor the water, includes *Trichodesmium thiebautii, Skeletonema costatum, Chaetoceros sociale, Thalasiossiara mala, Eucampia zodiacus, Prorocentrum sigmoides, P. micans, Dinophysis caudata, Noctiluca scintillans, Ceratium tripos, C. furca, C. fusus, Gymnodinium sanguineum, G. mikimotoi, Cochlodinium polykrikoides, Lingulodinium polyedrum, Protoceratium reticulatum, Gonyaulax polygramma, Alexandrium affine, Peridinium quinquecorne, Heterocapsa triquetra, Heterosigma akashiwo, Scrippsiella trochoidem, Heterocapsa circulasqiama, Fibrocapsa japonica,* and *Chattonella antiqua* (Fukuyo, 2000).

However, under some conditions, growth is very high that it generates anoxic conditions which result in indiscriminate killing of both fish and invertebrates. Depletion of oxygen (O) can be due to high respiration by algae community at the night or in dim light during the day, with another cofactor which considered more commonly is resulting from the respiration of bacteria during the decay of the bloom.

Examples of microalgae that can cause these problems are some species of the dinoflagellates *Gonyaulax, Noctoluca,* and *Scrppsiella* (Daranas et al., 2001).

Recently, there is a second group recognized and has become apparent only as a result of our increasing interest in intensive aquaculture systems, some species of algae can damage gills of fish mechanically and seriously or due to production of hemolytic substances while wild fish stocks have the freedom and ability to avoid such areas of problem, and the caged fish are appearing to be vulnerable to HABs. Recently, studies refer to potent ichthyotoxins named Prmymnsin-1 and prymnesin-2 have been isolated from *Prymnesium parvum* cultures (Manning and La Claire, 2010), the Prmymnsin-1 has been known for the last three decades (Sasaki et al., 2006; La Claire et al., 2015). Due to extreme difficulty in purification, the chemical nature of the toxin was not known for a long time. Also, in this group, it can be considered hemolysin isolated from *Amphidinium carterae* cultures which structures are glyceroglycolipids. Other species within this group of HABs are diatoms, like *Chaetoceros convolutes,* dinoflagellates like *Gymnodinium mikimotoi,* prymnesiophytes—*Chrysochromulina polylepis, Prymnesium patelliferum,* and raphidophytes-*Heterosigma carterae* or *Chatonella antiqua* that they were impacted and killed caged yellowtail fish at the Seto Island Sea in 1972, causing losses estimated about 500 million US dollars (Daranas et al., 2001).

The third group, collect those species that produce potent toxins, which they can easily find their way to humans via the food chain, also these toxins impact humans and cause a variety of gastrointestinal and neurological illnesses after ingestion.

In fact, among all the existing marine algal species, there are 75 diagnosed as phycotoxins producers and responsible for blooms (Ade et al., 2003; IOC-UNESCO, 2009). Besides the numbers of dinoflagellates, the diatoms are also responsible of toxicity, and toxic threats of diatoms should not be neglected, because diatoms form the major individuals of the phytoplankton community, and they tend to dominate under neutral high nutrient concentration. The diatoms are the main biochemical cycles of macronutrients N, P, Si, and Fe, also tend to dominate export production (Sarthou et al., 2005). There are several toxic species of diatoms have been recorded and classified as a toxic species, like *Amphora coffeaeformis. Nitzschia navis-varingica, Pseudo-nitzschia australis, P. calliantha, P. cuspidata, P. delicatissima, P. fraudu-lenta, P. galaxiae, P. multiseries, P. multistriata, P. pungens, P. seriata,* and *P. turgidula* (IOC-UNESCO, 2009). The toxic species of *Pseudo-nitzschia* bloom may occur and become a recurring phenomenon, it is very important to determine if there is any seasonal or spatial predictability that is what has been reported by Congestri et al. (2006, 2008) and Villac et al. (1993). There are important factors, like climate change and warming of oceans, helped a lot in spreading affected coastal zones with neurotoxins of domoic acid (DA), which is produced by *Pseudo-nitzschia* (McKibben et al., 2017). High cell numbers up to 4×10^4 cell L^{-1} of toxic species *P. delicatissima, P. delicatissima,* and *P. pseudodelicatissima* that have been recorded in the gulf Naples and along with Latium coasts (Congestri et al., 2006; Montresor et al., 2000). Due to many studies, some algal species are recorded as toxin producers at a low abundance of several or some hundreds of cells L^{-1}, while other species must occur in some millions of cells L^{-1} to cause any harm. The taxonomic diversity of HABs species was suggesting that each species is adapted to some of the environmental conditions or in ecological terms, for a defining niche. Once ecological requirements for each species separately are known, it may or easy to predict its occurrence (Zingone and Enevoldsen, 2000; Wells et al., 2015). Actually, most of the harmful algal species have restricted distribution pattern but some harmful species have a worldwide distribution (Hallegraeff, 2010; Fu et al., 2012). However, the impacts of HABs depends upon the concentration to appear harmful effects, but in fact, the most harmful species are widespread also become hazardous only when their concentration exceeds a certain threshold for sufficiently high toxic dose (Berdalet et al., 2016; Zingone and Enevoldsen, 2000). Toxins that produced by phytoplankton can harm Invertebrates too and developed higher trophic level organisms such as fish, marine birds, and mammals because of the accumulation of toxins and/or due to varying degrees of physiological damage. Different accumulated types of potent toxins are produced during the bloom's development of several HABs species in suspension-feeding shellfish and also affect human consumers and is resulting in outbreaks of paralytic, neurotoxic, amnesic, azaspiracid, and diarrheic shellfish poisoning (DSP) as reported in (Table 20.1). Direct effects on suspension-feeding bivalves include the valve (Archambalut et al., 2002).

There are many toxic algal species, such as dinoflagellates, were recorded internationally via IOC-UNESCO in 2009, and cited by Jessim (2009) (Table 20.2).

Some of these species were mentioned to them by Kaladharan et al. (2011) along the Karnataka coast, for example, Gymnodiniales, Peridinales, and Prorocentrales.

20.2.2   TOXIC SPECIES OF DINOFLAGELLATES

There are several toxic species dinoflagellates diagnosed as toxic, which is mentioned in this chapter depending on (FAO, 2004) as in follow.

20.2.2.1   PARALYTIC SHELLFISH TOXIN PRODUCERS

The first recorded group of species of phytoplankton as producer of paralytic shellfish toxin, which cause paralytic shellfish poisoning syndrome (PSP), are Alexandrium, which was named formerly *Gonyaulax or Protogonyaulax,* and identified as contaminators in shellfish. These species are *Alexandrium tamarensis, A. minutum* (syn. *A. excavata), A. catenella, A. fraterculus, A. fundyense, A. cohorticula, Gymnodinium catenatum, and Pyrodinium bahamense.*

20.2.2.2   DIARRHEIC SHELLFISH TOXIN PRODUCERS

The second group was recorded as diarrheic Shellfish toxin can cause DSP syndrome, production of DSP toxins has been identified and confirmed in seven identified species of Dinophysis species *D. fortii, D. acuminata, D. acuta, D. norvegica, D. mitra, D. rotundata D. tripos,* and *Phalacroma*

TABLE 20.1 Some Vectors of Algal Toxins and Related Human Syndromes.

Toxin	Vector	Short-term health consequences	Long-term consequences of toxin
Ciguatoxins	Reef fish	Ciguatera fish poisoning: Abdominal pain, nausea, vomiting, diarrhea; paresthesias, temperature dysesthesia, pain, weakness, bradycardia, hypotension	Long duration (months to years) of symptoms, Chronic
Okadaic acid and its derivatives	Shellfish	Diarrhetic shellfish poisoning: Nausea, vomiting, diarrhea, vomiting, diarrhea, abdominal pain accompanied by chills, headache, fever	Gastrointestinal tumor promoter in laboratory animals
Yessotoxins, Pectenotoxins	Shellfish	Not documented as toxic in humans, but co-occur with DSP and are highly toxic to mice	Unknown
Azaspiracids	Shellfish	Azaspiracid shellfish poisoning: nausea, vomiting, severe diarrhea, stomach cramps	Unknown
Brevetoxin	Shellfish	Neurotoxic shellfish poisoning: Numbness of lips, tongue, and throat, muscular aches and pains, fever, chills, abdominal cramping, nausea, diarrhea, vomiting, headache, reduced heart rate, pupil dilation	Unknown
	Inhalation	Acute eye irritation, respiratory distress, asthma exacerbation	Unknown
Saxitoxins	Shellfish	Paralytic shellfish poisoning: Tingling, burning, numbness, drowsiness, incoherent speech, respiratory paralysis leading to death	Unknown
	Puffer Fish	Saxitoxin puffer fish poisoning tingling, burning, numbness, drowsiness, incoherent speech, respiratory paralysis leading to death	Unknown

Source: Reprinted from Archambault, et al., 2002.

TABLE 20.2 List of toxic dinoflagellates and their harmful effects according to IOC-UNESCO 2009.

Dinophysiales	*Dinophysis acuminata*	OA
	D. acuta	OA, Dinophysis toxin-1
	D. caudata	OA, Pectenotoxin-2
	D. fortii	OA, DTX-1, PTX-2
	D. miles	OA, DTX-1
	D. mitra	DTX-1
	D. norvegica	OA, DTX-1
	D. rapa	OA
	D. rotundata	DTX-1
	D. sacculus	OA
	D. tripos	DTX-1
Peridiniales	*Alexandrium catenella*	Paralytic Shellfish Poisoning toxins
	A. Andersonii	PSP toxin
	A. balechii	Fish mass mortality
	A. catenella	PSP toxin and fish mass mortality
	A. fundyense	PSP toxins
	A. hiranoi	Producer of antifungal substance
	A. minutum	PSP t and fish mass mortality
	A. monilatum	Fish mortality-causing, haemolytic compounds
	A. ostenfeldii	PSP toxin, macrocyclic imine. a neurotoxin
	A. tamarense	PSP toxin
	A. tamiyavanichii	PSP toxin
	Coolia monotis	Cooliatoxin
	Gambierdiscus australes	Ciguatoxin, maitotoxin-like toxins
	G. pacificus	Ciguatoxin, maitotoxin-like toxins
	G. toxicus	

TABLE 20.2 *(Continued)*

G. yasumotoi	Ciguatoxins 4A, 4B and 3C and maitotoxins-1, -2 and -3
Ostreopsis lenticularis	Maitoxin-like compound, lethal to mice
O. mascarenensis	Neurotoxins, ostreotoxin-1 and -3
O. ovata	Palytoxin analogues, mascarenotoxin-A and –B
O. siamensis	Toxic butanol-soluble compound
Protoceratium reticulatum	Ostreocin D Yessotoxin
Pyrodinium bahamense	PSP toxin
Prorocentrales	*Prorocentrum arenarium*	OA
	P. belizeanum	OA
	P. cassubicum	Diarrhetic Shellfish Poisoning (DSP)
	P. emarginatum	OA, DTX-1
	p. faustiae	OA
	p. hoffmannianum	OA, Fast Acting Toxins (FAT)
	p. minimum	OA, Prorocentrolide B, FAT
	p. lima	OA, DTX-1 DTX-2, FAT
	p. arabianum	Cytotoxic compounds
	p. brobonicum	Probably neurotoxic lethal to mice
	p. rhathymum	Toxic to mice, ingested cells can cause detrimental effects in molluscs. Some strains excrete substances toxic to *Artemia nauplii*. Water soluble acetone precipitate is toxic to mice
Gymnodiniales	*Amphidinium carterae*	Haemolysins
	A. operculatum	Compounds with haemolytic and antifungal properties (amphidinols), may be toxic to fish
	Cochlodinium polykrikoides	Serious fish killer, PSP toxin
	Gymnodinium catenatum	Fish killer

TABLE 20.2 (*Continued*)

Species	Description
Gyrodinium corsicum	Produces brevetoxin in culture. Marine animal mortalities, Neurologic Shellfish Poisoning (NSP), respiratory irritation.
Karenia bicuneiformis	Animal and plant mortalities, human respiratory distress, eye and skin irritations
K. brevis	Believed to cause NSP and respiration distress in humans
K. brevisulcata	Found to produce brevetoxin in culture
K. concordia	Killing of fish, and cultured seaweed (*Porphyra tenera*) also affected
K. cristata	
K. digitata	A cytotoxic polyether, Gymnocin-A from a Japanese culture
K. papilionace	Spiroimine gymnodimine producer in culture
K. selliformis	Fish kills in Tasmania, killing rainbow trout and salmon Fish mortality
K. umbrella	Fish kills, killing rainbow trout and salmon.
Karlodinium armiger	Fish mortality
K. veneficum	Toxic to a range of marine invertebrates and fish, karlotoxins producer that exhibits a broad-spectrum of lytic effect on membranes from very diverse cell types
Takayama cladochroma	Mortality of fish and invertebrate

Source: Reprinted from IOC-UNESCO, 2009.

rotundatum. Diarrheic shellfish toxin can be found in benthic dinoflagellates which are *Prorocentrum lima, P. concavum,* or (*P. maculosum*), and *P. redfieldi* that were also recorded as producers of DSP toxins, also the isolated benthic species *P. arenarium* from the reef ecosystem of Europa Island (Mozambic channel, France) and isolated *P. belizeanum* from Belizean coral reef ecosystem also were found produce OA. Other studies reported suspected three other dinophysis species that are *D. caudata, D. hastate,* and *D. sacculus* and also suspected as producers of OA. (Hallegraeff et al., 1995). According to (Jessim, 2009) *D. sacculus* one of OA. producers. (Giacobbe et al., 2000) reported that *D. saccilus* contained OA. and DTX1 with maximum (DSP) toxins (OA. + DTX1 = 455 fg/cell) were found at early spring blooms. On the other hand, the detection of DSP toxins presence in the heterotrophic dinoflagellates *Protoperidinium oceanicum* and *P. pellucidum* may reflect their feeding on Dinophysis (Hallegraeff et al., 1995).

20.2.2.3 DOMOIC ACID PRODUCERS

Third group is collect diatoms, these diatoms are the main resource of DA that are responsible about amnesic shellfish poisoning syndrome, this group contain several species of Diatoms, and they are *Amphora coffeaeformis, Pseudo-nitzschia pungens f. multiseries, P. pseudodelicatissima, P. delicatissima* (syn. *Nitzschia actydrophila*), *P. seriata, P. fraudulenta, P. turgidula,* and *Nitzschia navis-varingia.*

20.2.2.4 NEUROLOGIC SHELLFISH TOXINS PRODUCERS

The fourth group is containing the species who produce Neurologic Shellfish Toxins that cause neurologic shellfish poisoning (NSP) syndrome; this group collects *G. breve* also named *Ptychodiscus breve,* since 2000 called *Karenia brevis,* which executed as a producer of several neurotoxins, they are *Chattonella antiqua, Fibrocapsa japonica,* and *Heterosigma akashiwo.*

20.2.2.5 AZASPIRACID SHELLFISH TOXIN PRODUCERS

The fifth group suggests that *Protoceratum crassipes* is the Azaspiracid Shellfish toxin producer producing Dinoflagellates. There is other reported that an organism belonging to the genus *Protoperidinium* suggests as the source organism.

20.2.2.6   *MARINE TOXINS THE WATER-SOLUBLE MAITOTOXINS AND THE FATE-SOLUBLE CIGUATOXINS*

The sixth group contains *Gambierdiscus toxicus* that is reported as a responsible organism for about 2 types of marine toxins, water-soluble maitotoxins, and fat-soluble ciguatoxins, researches have reported a benthic dinoflagellates *Ostreopsis lenticularis* was shown to be a vector of Ciguatera fish poisoning, mentioned that other dinoflagellates, which may play a role in the production of toxins associated with ciguatera poisoning, like *P. rorocentrum concavum, P. meicanum, P. rhathytum, Gymnodinium sanguineum,* and *Gonyaulax polyedra.*

20.3   QUALITATIVE AND QUANTITATIVE IDENTIFICATION OF PHYTOPLANKTON

In order to give early monitoring, the responsible person or team most cover the area each time to discover early effects, normally HABs can contain toxins via producing by phytoplankton and these toxins can harm invertebrates and trophic level of organisms, like fish and marine birds, and mammals via accumulation of toxins and/or variable degrees of physiological and ecological damage. We can recognize important thing, potent toxin produced via some HAB species that accumulate in suspension-feeding shellfish and affect consumers at the end of food chain which is human, these types of toxins are resulting in outbreaks of paralytic, neurotoxic, amnesic, azaspiracid, and diarrhetic shellfish poisoning (Archambalut et al., 2002). Before resulting HABs of toxic phytoplankton, cities have coastal areas or coastal cities, must have developed early alarm system for early monitoring depend on early signs of died birds and fish mortality, also the number of cells at the body water (Anderson et al., 2001). There are many methods, some of them need a period of time and depending on light microscope as qualitative and quantitative identification (Karlson et al., 2010).

20.3.1   *MOLECULAR AND MICROSCOPIC IDENTIFICATION*

Actually, the words may not cover the title, but the schismatic Figure 20.1 will explain everything belong to identification of Phytoplankton, which depends on both molecular and microscopic identification. However, now results are more accurate depending on molecular studies and give degree of relatives among the identified species (Karlson et al., 2010).

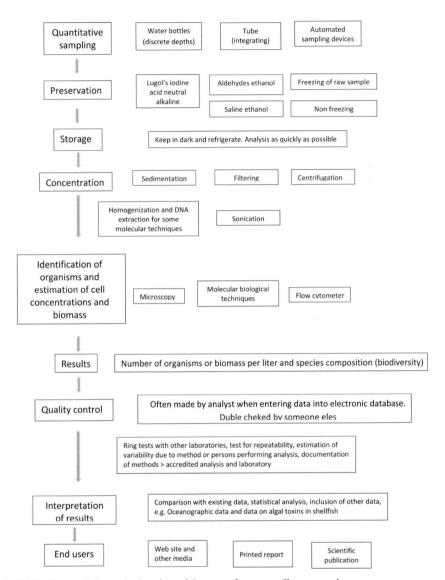

FIGURE 20.1 Schematic drawing of the steps from sampling to results.
Source: Reprinted from Karlson, et al., 2010.

20.3.2 UTERMÖHL METHOD

The second method was named Utermöhl method (Utermöhl, 1931, 1958), this method has an advantage over other methods of phytoplankton analysis and in this method, the algal cells can be both identified and enumerated.

Through this method, it is also possible to determine individual cell size, form, biovolume, and resting stage. This method is based on the assumption that cells are toxic and distributed in the counting chamber and on the sedimentation of an aliquot water sample in counting chamber. Because of gravity, phytoplankton cells go down to settle on the bottom of the chamber, then settled cells on the bottom of the chamber can be identified and enumerated using an inverted microscope. To quantify results as cells per liter a conversion factor must be determined, this method depends on if the sample must identify immediately or after a few days. Plastic vials may be used and the examiner should notice that the preservatives may be absorbed by the plastic. For a long time to store samples, glass of bottles of samples should be used for minimizing any chemical reactions with preservative. Clear glass bottles allow the state of Lugol's iodine preservation to be easily monitored. Samples must store in a dark place to prevent the degradation of Lugol's iodine in light. It is very important to tight bottle cap to avoid spillage of samples and evaporation of preservative.

Utermöhl noted that the bottle is filled to 75–80% from total volume and homogenizes of samples before disposing into the sedimentation chamber. The agents of preservation must be chosen depending on the objective of the study. The most commonly used is potassium iodine; Lugol's iodine solution: Acidic, neutral, or alkaline. If the samples are stored for a long period, they may be preserved with formaldehyde (Edler and Elbrächter, 2010). For counting, researcher use an inverted light microscope for counting and as shown in Figure 20.2. Where counting is for whole chamber bottom with parallel eyepiece threads indicating the counted area, as in Figure 20.3. Counting of diameter transect according to Edler and Elbrächter (2010).

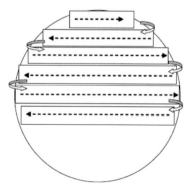

FIGURE 20.2   Counting of the whole chamber bottom with parallel eyepiece threads indicating counted area.

Source: Reprinted from Edler et al., 2010.

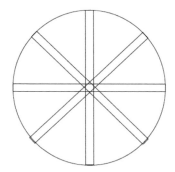

FIGURE 20.3   Counting of diameter transect.

Source: Reprinted from Edler et al., 2010.

Many studies it has been decided that counting of 50 units of the dominant species, giving a 95% confidence limits of 28% is sufficient. For the increasing of the precision, for example, to 10–20% would need a dramatic increase in the counted units, 100 and 400 respectively (Venrick, 1978; Edler, 1979). The precision is given by the following equation:

$$\text{Precision } \% = 2 \times 100 / \sqrt{\text{number of counted cells}}.$$

It is not possible for counting 50 units of all species in the samples clearly because some species may not sufficiently abundant which will decrease the over precision for an acceptable precision the entire sample a total of at least 500 units should be counted (Edler and Elbrächter, 2010). For microscopic counting transformation or to the density of phytoplankton of desired water volume which is usually one liter or one milliliter can achieve using the following equations:

Cells $L^{-1} = N \times (A_t/A_c) \times 1000/V,$
Cells $mL^{-1} = N \times (A_t/A_c) \times 1/V,$

where V: Volume of the counting chamber (mL),
      At: Total area of the counting chamber (mm^2),
      Ac: Counted area of the counting chamber (mm^2),
      N: Number of units (cells) of counted specific species,
      C: Concentration (density) of the specific species.

Utermöhl method for testing and identification of phytoplankton communities is probably most used widely for the quantitative analysis of phytoplankton, both of microscopic and sedimentation chambers along the years, have developed considerably, it is the taxonomic skill of the analyst that sets the standard of the results (Edler and Elbrächter, 2010). There were other methods that can be used along with those two methods mentioned above, which are settlement bottle method for quantitative phytoplankton analysis—hemocytometer, this method is a modified Utermöhl method (McDermott and Raine, 2010), and counting chamber methods for quantitative phytoplankton analysis—haemocytometer, Palmer–Maloney cell and Sedgewick Rafter cell, this method is established for counting methods, these three are common types of counting chambers to enumerate phytoplankton are Sedgewick-Rafter counting slide, the Palmer–Maloney counting slide and the hemocytometer counting slide, these methods are easy to learn and use and just require preserved sample, good quality microscope, and counting slide. The capability of the Sedgewick–Rafter and the Palmer–Maloney for viewing the whole community of phytoplankton including the presence of harmful species (LeGresley and McDermott, 2010).

20.4   RESULTS AND DISCUSSION

The Bloom events the toxic algal species may result in extensive and unprecedented closures of aquaculture of fish farming and near beaches also harvesting areas of shellfish that prevent poisoning syndromes in human via consuming sea products. The Residents in coastal areas which may be affected with *Karenia* and *Ostreopsis* blooms by inducing respiratory irritation in beachgoers. Decomposition for dead animals and algal cells may cause an anoxia of bottom water, which may spiral into multiple species unusual mortality events in thousand square of mails in the sea bottom. Environmentally sound techniques to reduce HAB impacts that should be based on effective methodologies for rapid field detection of several types belong to phytoplankton, to develop early warning systems, response plans, and methods for reducing public health, ecological, social, and impacts of HABs. Therefore, there is acritical need for cost-effective and user-friendly monitoring tools that which can be used by, local environmental groups, and the sates agencies for monitoring toxins concentrations (Albertano et al., 2008, Gualtieri and Parshykova, 2008). For development of early warning protocols, electrochemical SPE-immunosensors, may presently contribute for routine application. On different animal matrices, further studies might reveal the fat of phycotoxins and their amplification along the whole food chain and thus contribute to assessing an extent of the impact of toxic bloom events on human health and environment. One of the used strategies include use of resins that can absorb lipophilic toxins in situ SPATT at different places of countries, such as Canada, Galicia, and Scotland, to act as early warning systems when the number of *Dinophysis* cells are high. Here appears crucial questions and will be to determine if the toxins are librated actively by healthy cells of *Dinophysis*, and in which state (free or attached to adsorbing the particles), phenomenon of water-borne toxins can be detected by SPATT occur. The observation is that a large proportion of toxins can be liberated by cells during common (nets, pumps) concentration procedures (Reguera, 2006). Actually, successful management of the coastal environment and marine ambient requires a sound knowledge of biological, chemical, and physical processes governing growth, retention, dispersion, and transport of water constituents, including phytoplankton. The growing problem posed by existence of phytoplankton species currently demands thorough comprehension of life histories and population's dynamics of theses toxic organisms. Without knowledge of above, managers can neither assess the impact of anthropogenic activity on the environment and biota nor do they understand the relationship among species of harmful phytoplankton and HABs events that are caused by them and the climate. Without this comprehension and understanding, the desirable goals of harmful events are unattainable (Patrick et al., 2005).

20.5 CONCLUSIONS

Decreasing of nutrients in aquatic ambient and terrestrial, which come via urban activities, including agricultural fertilizing, and those which come from another bath, must be the first aim of many aims because these nutrients are the main source of eutrophication and increase of HABs, among these HABs, some of them can increase threats of toxicity in water bodies. Rarely, we need the knowledge to control and manage biological recourses, it is very important to reduce all threats, one of these threats are toxic phytoplankton. Globally, all organizations and associations must work as one hand team to reduce pollutants, otherwise, this problem will enlarge and grow up more and more, second thing, technology of communications and satellites should be also used to the fullest extent possible.

For science and technology in this field a major role to monitor variables of environment, especially which related with satellite and modern transmit signals wirelessly due to hard impact of toxins economically, human health and seafood, this should start from first signs of toxic phytoplankton development to the end of HABs phenomenon, these efforts should be considered for finding out how to reduce toxic threats at least if we cannot treat it permanently.

KEYWORDS

- **coastal environment**
- **phytoplankton population**
- **harmful algal blooms**
- **algal toxins**
- **organisms**

REFERENCES

Ade, P.; Funari E.; Poletti, R. Risk to Human Health Associated with Marine Toxic Algae. *Annali Istituto Superiore Sanità.* **2003,** *39,* 53–68.

Albertano, P.; Congestri, R.; Micheli, L.; Moscone, D.; Palleschi, G. Development of Sensors to Trace Toxins from Dinoflagellates and Other Algae in Seafood. In *Algal Toxins, Nature, Occurrence, Effect, and Detection*; Evangelista, V., Barsanti., Frassanito, A. M., Passarelli, V., Gualtieri, P., Eds; Springer: Dordrecht (NL), 2008; pp 301–310.

Al Ghela, H. M.; Alkindi, A. Y. A.; Amer, S.; Al Akhzami, Y. K. Harmful Algal Blooms: Physiology, Behavior, Population Dynamics and Global Impacts—A Review. *SQU J. Sci.* **2005,** *10,* 1–30.

Al Muffttah, A. Harmful Algae Species off Qatari Water. Qatar Biodiversity Newsletter, 2, 1–4.

Anderson, D. M. Diversity of Harmful Algal Blooms in Coastal Waters. *Limnol. Oceanograph.* **2008,** *42,* 1009–1022.

Anderson, D. M.; Glibert, P.; Burkholder, J. Harmful Algal Blooms and Eutrophication: Nutrient Sources, Composition, and Consequences. *Estuaries.* **2002,** *25,* 704–726.

Anderson, D. M.; Anderson, V. M.; Bricelj, J. J.; Cullen, J. J.; Rensel, J. E. Monitoring and Management for Harmful Algal Blooms in Coastal Waters, APEC #201-MR-01.1, Asia Pacific Economic Program, Springer and Intergovernmental Oceanographic Commission Technical Series, Paris, 2001, 59.

Archambault, M. C.; Bricelj, V. M.; Grant, J.; Anderson, D. M. Effects of Clay, Used to Control Harmful Algal Blooms, on Juvenile Mercenaria mercenaria. *J. Shellfish Res.* **2002,** *21,* 395–396.

Arroyo, N. L.; Bonsdorff, E. The Role of Drifting Algae for Marine Biodiversity. In *Marine Macrophytes as Foundation Species*; Olafsson, E., Ed.; CRC Press, Tylor and Francis Group, 2016, 100–123.

Beaulieu, S. E.; Sengco M. R.; Anderson D. M. Using Clay to Control Harmful Algal Blooms: Deposition and Resuspension of Clay/Algal Flocks. *Harm. Algae.* **2005,** *4,* 133–138.

Berdalet, E.; Fleming, L.; Gowen, R.; Davidson, K.; Hess, P.; Backer, L.; Enevoldsen, H. Marine Harmful Algal Blooms, Human Health and Wellbeing: Challenges and Opportunities in the 21st Century. *J. Mar. Biol. Assoc. U.K.* **2016,** *96,* 61–91.

Bleiker, W.; Schanz, F. Influence of Environmental Factors on the Phytoplankton Spring Bloom in Lake Zürich. *Aqua. Sci.* **2015,** *51*, 158.

Boesch, D. F.; Anderson, D. M.; Horner, R. A.; Shumway, S. E.; Tester, P. A.; Whit ledge, T. E. Harmful Algal Blooms in Coastal Waters Options for Prevention Control and Mitigation, NOAA Coastal Ocean Program, Decisin Analysis, NOAA Coastal Ocean Office, USA, 1997, 10.

Bonilla, G. J. L.; Badillo, M.; López, K.; Gallardo, A.; Galindo, C.; Arceo, A.; Chiappa, C. Environmental Influences on the Abundance of Dominant Fishes in a Very Shallow Tropical Coastal Lagoon in Northwestern Yucatan Peninsula, Mexico. *Mar. Sci. Rese. Dev.* **2013,** *3*, 1–11.

Congestri, R.; Polizzano, S.; Albertano, P. Toxic *Pseudonitzschia* from the Middle Tyrrhenian Sea (Mediterranean Sea, Italy). In *Algal Toxins: Nature, Occurrence, Effect and Detection*; Evangelista, V., Barsanti, L., Frassanito, A. M., Passarelli, V., Gualtieri, P., Eds.; Springer: Netherlands, 2008; pp 197–210.

Congestri, R.; Sangiorgi, V.; Bianco, I.; Cappuci, E.; Albertano, P. Ilfitoplancton delle coste laziali dal 1997 ad oggi: struttura della comunià, taxa dominate e specie tossiche, Biologia Marina Mediterranea. **2006,** *13*, 54–60.

Connell, E. O.; Lyons, W. B.; Sheridan, C.; Lewis, E. Development of a Fibre Optic Sensor for Detection of Harmful Algae Bloom and in Particular Domoic acid. Technology Conference-IMTC. Instrumentation and Measurement, Warsaw, Poland, 2007.

Daranas, A. H.; Norte, M.; Fernàndez, J. J. Toxic Marine Microalgae. *Toxicon.* **2001,** *39*, 1101–1132.

Delia, A. S.; Caruso, G.; Melcarne, L.; Caruso, G.; Parisi, S.; Lagnà, P. Biological Toxins from Marine and Freshwater Microalgae. In *Microbial Toxins and Related Contamination in the Food industry. Hand Book*; Caruso, G., Lagnà, P., Santi Delia, A., Parisi, S., Barone, C., Melcarne, L., Mazzù, F., Eds.; 2015; Vol. 2, p 18.

Edler, L.; Elbrächter, M. The Utermöhl Method for Quantitative Phytoplankton Analysis. In *Microscopic and Molecular Methods for Quantitative Phytoplankton Analysis*; Karlson, B., Godhe, A., Cusack, C., Bresnan, E., Eds., Chapter 2, Intergovernmental Oceanographic Commission Manuals and guides, 2010; Vol. 55, pp 13–20.

Edler, L. Recommendations for Marine Biological Studies in the Baltic Sea. Phytoplankton and Chlorophyll. *Bdrzc Mar. Biol.* **1979,** *5*, 1–38.

FAO. Food and Agriculture Organization. Food and Nutrition Paper, Rome, Italy, 2004, Pages 18, 66, 105, 145, 176 and 192.

Fauchot, J.; Levasseur, M.; Roy, S.; Gagnon, R.; Weiese, A. M. Environmental Factors Controlling Alexandrium tamarenes. (Dinophyceae) Growth Rate During a Red Tide Event in the St. Lawrence estuary (Canada). *J. Phycol.* **2005,** *41*, 263–272.

Fauoko, T.; Nishijima, T. T.; Fukami, K.; Adachi, M. Contribution of Urea to Occurrence of Phytoplankton in the Eutrophic Costal Environment Uranouchi Inlet. *Bull. Phytoplankton Soc. Jpn.* **2006,** *53*, 77–86.

France, J.; Mozetič, P. Ecological Characterization of Toxic Phytoplankton Species (Dinophysis spp., Dinophyceae) in Slovenian Mariculture Areas (Gulf of Trieste, Adriatic sea). And the Implications for Monitoring. *Mar. Pollut. Bull.* **2006,** *52*, 1504–1516.

Fu, F. X.; Tatters, A. O.; Hutchins, D. A.; Global Change and the Future of Harmful Algal Blooms in the Ocean. *Mar. Ecol. Prog.* **2012,** *470*, 207–233.

Fukuyo, Y. Red Tide Microalgae. WESTPAC/IOC/UNESCO, HAB., Harmful Algal Bloom Program, Tokyo, Japan, 2000.

Gastrich, M. D.; Harmful Algal Blooms in Coastal Waters of New Jersey. New Jersey Department of Environmental Protection, Division of Science Report, 2000.

Giacobbe, M. G.; Penna, A.; Ceredi, A.; Milandri, A.; Poletti, R.; Yang, X. Toxicity and Ribosomal DNA of the Dinoflagellate *Dinophysis sacculus* (Dinophyta). *Phycologia* **2000,** *39,* 177–182.

Gianesella, S. M. F.; Kutner, M. B. B.; Saldanha, C. F. M. P.; Pompeu M. Assessment of Plankton Community and Environmental Conditions in São Sebastião Channel Prior to the Concentration of a Produced Water Outfall. *Rev. Bras. Oceanogr.* **1999,** *47,* 29–46.

Gualtieri, P.; Parshykova, T. Comparative Estimation of Sensor Organisms Sensitivity for Determination of Water Toxicity. In (eds). *Algal Toxins, Nature, Occurrence, Effect and Detection*; Evangelista, V.; Barasanti, L.; Frassanito, A. M.; Passarelli, V.; Gualtieri, P. Springer: Dordrecht (NL), 2008; pp 221–233.

Häder, D. P.; Williamson, C. E.; Wängberg, S. A.; Rautio, M.; Rose, K. C.; Gao, K.; Walter, H. E.; Sinhah, R. P.; Worresti, R. Effects of UV Radiation on Aquatic Ecosystems and Interactions with Other Environmental Factors. *Photochem. Photobiol. Sci.* **2015,** *14,* 108–126.

Hallegraeff, G. M.; Anderson, D. M.; Cembella, A. D. Manual on Harmful Marine Microalgae. IOC Manuals and Guides, UNESCO: France, 1995; Vol. 33, pp 283–317.

Hallegraeff, G. M. Ocean Climate Change, Phytoplankton Community Responses, and Harmful Algal Blooms: A Formidable Predictive Challenge. *J. Phycol.* **2010,** *46,* 220–235.

Hydes, D. J.; Gowen, R. J.; Holliday, N. P.; Shammon, T.; Mills, D. External and Internal Control of Winter Concentrations of Nutrients (N, P and Si) in North-west European Shelf Seas, Estuarine. *Coast. Shelf Sci.* **2004,** *59,* 151–161.

IOC-UNESCO Taxonomic Reference List of Harmful Microalgae, 2009. http://www.marinespecies.org/hab/aphia.php?p=taxlist&pid=148899&tRank=220&rComp=%3D&context_in=30&vOnly=1

Jessim, A. I. Investigation of Dinoflagellates Populations and Okadaic Acid Detection in a Costal Lake (Middle Tyrrhenian Sea), Ph. D. Thesis, University of Rome Tor Vergata, 2009, 1.

Kaladharan, P.; Zacharia, P. U.; Vijayakumaran, Coastal and Marine Floral Biodiversity Along the Karnataka Coast. *J. Mar. Biol. Ass. India.* **2011,** *53,* 121–129.

Karlson, B.; Godhe, A.; Cusack, C.; Bresnan, E. Introduction to Methods for Quantitative Phytoplankton Analysis. In *Microscopic and Molecular Methods for Quantitative Phytoplankton Analysis*; Karlson, B., Godhe, A., Cusack, C., Bresnan, E., Eds.; Chapter 1, Intergovernmental Oceanographic Commission Manuals and Guides, **2010,** *55,* 5–12.

Karlson, B.; Godhe, A.; Cusack, C.; Bresnan, E. Microscopic and Molecular Methods for Quantitative Phytoplankton Analysis. Intergovernmental Oceanographic Commission Manuals and Guides, 2010, Vol. 55, pp 8–107.

La Claire, J. W.; Manning, S. R.; Talarski, A. E. Semi-quantitative Assay for Polyketide Prymnesins Isolated from Prymnesium parvum (Haptophyta) Cultures. *Toxicon* **2015,** *102,* 74–80.

Le Gresley, M.; Mc Dermott, G. Counting Chamber Methods for Quantitative Phytoplankton Analysis-heamocytometer, Palmer-Maloney Cell and Sedgewick-Rafter Cell. In *Microscopic and Molecular Methods for Quantitative Phytoplankton Analysis*; Karlson, B.; Godhe, A.; Cusak, C.; Brenan, E., Eds.; Chapter 4, Intergovernmental Oceanographic Commission Manuals and guides, 2010, Vol. 55, pp 24–30.

Lin, C. J.; Wade, T. J.; Sams, E. A.; Dufour, A. P.; Chapman, A. D.; Hilborn, E. D. A Prospective Study of Marine Phytoplankton and Reported Illness among Recreational Beachgoers in Puerto Rico, 2009. *Environ. Health Perspect.* **2016,** *124,* 477–483.

Lindhal, O. Occurrence and Monitoring of Harmful Algae in the Marine Environment. In *Mycotoxins and Phycotoxins–Developments in Chemistry, Toxicology and Food Safety*, Miraglia, M., Van Egmond, H., Brera, C., Gilbert, J., Eds.; Proceedings of the IX International IUPAC Symposium on Mycotoxins and Phycotoxins, Fort Collins: Colorado, Alaken Press, 1998, pp 409– 423.

Manning, S. R.; La Claire, J. W. Prymnesins: Toxic Metabolites of the Golden Alga, *Prymnesium parvum* Carter (Haptophyta). *Mar. Drugs.* **2010**, *8*, 687–704.

Moore, C. M.; Mills, M. M.; Milnes, A.; Langlois, R.; Achterberg, E.; Lochte, K.; Geider, R. J.; La Roche, J. Iron Limits Primary Productivity During Spring Bloom Development in the Central North Atlantic. *Glob. Change Biol.* **2006**, *12*, 626–634.

Masó, M.; Gracés, E. Harmful Microalgae Blooms (HAB); Problematic and Conditions that Induce Them. *Mar. Pollut. Bull.* **2006**, *53*, 620–630.

McDermott, G.; Raine, R. Settlement Bottle Method for Quantitative Phytoplankton Analysis Method. In *Microscopic and Molecular Methods for Quantitative Phytoplankton Analysis*; Karlson, B.; Godhe, A.; Cusack, C.; Bresnan, E. Chapter 3. Intergovernmental Oceanographic Commission Manuals and Guides. **2010**, *55*, 21–24.

McKibben, S. M.; Peterson, W.; Wood, A. M.; Trainer, V. L.; Hunter, M.; White, A. E. Climatic Regulation of the Neurotoxin Domoic Acid. *Proc. Nat. Acad. Sci. U.S.A.* **2017**, *114*, 239–244.

Mullins, G. Phosphorus, Agriculture and the Environment. Virginia Tech, Virginia Polytechnic Institute and state University. USA, 2001, pp 1–12.

Montresor, M.; Sarno, D.; Zingone, A. Can we Peacefully Live Together with Harmful Phytoplankton? The Case of the Gulf of Naples. Proceedings of the 9th Conference on Harmful, 2000.

Algal, B.; In Morcillo, Y.; Porte C. Tasmania Abstract. Evidence of Endocrine Disruption in Calms – Ruditapes Decussate Transplanted to a Tributyltin-polluted Environment. *Environ. Pollut.* **2000**, *107*, 47–52.

Nuccio, C.; Melillo, C.; Massi, L.; Innamorati, M. Phytoplankton Abundance, Community Structure and Diversity in the Eutrophicated Orbetello lagoon (Tuscany) from 1995 to 2001. *Oceanologica Acta 26*, 15–25.

Patrick, G.; Percy, D.; Hidekatsu, Y.; Robin, R.; Beatriz, R.; Thomas, O. Harmful Algal Blooms in Stratified Environments. *Oceanography.* **2003**, *18*, 171–183.

Pilkaitytė, R.; Razinkovas, A. Factors Controlling Phytoplankton Blooms in a Temperate Estuary: Nutrient Limitation and Physical Forcing. *Hydrobiologia.* **2006**, *555*, 41–48.

Piuz, A.; Kluser S.; Peduzzi, P. Human Induced Har mful Algal Blooms. *Environ. Alert Bull.* UNEP. **2008**, *12,* 1–4.

Reguera, B. Dinophysis News. *Harmful Algal News* 2006, 32, 1–4.

Richardson, K. Harmful or Exceptional Phytoplankton Blooms in the Marine Ecosystem. *Adv. Mar. Biol.* **1997**, *31*, 301–385.

Santi, D. A.; Caruso, G.; Melcarne, L.; Parisi, S.; Laganà, P. Biological Toxins from Marine and Freshwater Microalgae. In *Microbial Toxins and Related Contamination in the Food Industry.* Springer Nature: Switzerland, 2015, 13–55.

Caruso, G.; Caruso, G.; Laganà, P.; Santi, D. A.; Parisi, S.; Barone, C.; Melcame, L.; Mazzù, F. Microbial Toxins and Related Contamination in the Food Industry. *Chemistry of Foods;* Springer Nature: Switzerland, 2015; Vol. 2, pp 15–17.

Sarthou, G.; Timmermans, K. R.; Blain, S.; Tréguer, P. Growth Physiology and Fate of Diatoms in Ocean: A Review. *J. Sea Res.* **2005**, *53*, 25–42.

Sasaki, M.; Takeda, N.; Fuwa, H.; Watanabe, R.; Satake, M.; Oshima, Y. Synthesis of the JK/LM-ring Model of Prymnesins, Potent Hemolytic and Ichthyotoxic Polycyclic Ethers Isolated from the Red Tide Alga Prymnesium parvum: Confirmation of the Relative Configuration of the K/L-ring Juncture. *Tetrahedron Lett.* **2006**, *47*, 5687–5691.

Scatasta, S.; Stolte, W.; Granèli, E.; Weikard, H. P.; Vanierland, E. Harmful Algal Blooms in European Marine Waters: Some Case Studies for Socio-economic Analysis. Second Deliverable for the Project. Ecoharm: The Socio-economic Impact of Harmful Algal Blooms in European Waters Contract n. EVK3-CT-2001-8003, 2001.

Sengco, R. M.; Anderson, D. M. Controlling Harmful Algal Blooms Through Clay Flocculation. *J. Eukar. Microbiol.* **2004**, *51*, 169–172.

Smayda, T. J. Bloom Dynamics: Physiology, Behavior, Trophic Effects. What is a Bloom? A Commentary. *Limnol. Oceanogr.* **1997**, *42*, 1132–1136.

Smith, R. L. The Physical Processes of Coastal Ocean Upwelling Systems. In *Upwelling in the Ocean: Modern Processes and Ancient Records*; Summerhayes, C. P., Emeis, K.-C., Angel, M. V., Smith, R. L., Zeitzschel, B., Eds.; John Wiley and Sons Ltd.: Chichester, UK, 1992; pp 39–64.

Subba Rao, D. V.; Al Hassan, J. M.; Al Yamani, F.; Al Rafaie, K.; Ismal, W.; Nageswara, R. C. V.; Al Hassan, M. Elusive Red Tides in Kuwait Coastal Waters. *Harm. Algae News* **2003**, *24*, 9–10.

Tallberg, P. The Magnitude of Si Dissolution from Diatoms at the Sediment Surface and its Potential Impact on P mobilization. *Arch. Hydrobiol.* **1999**, *144*, 429–438.

Tallberg, P. Silicon and its Impacts on Phosphorus in Eutrophic Freshwater Lakes. Ph. D. Thesis, Department of Limnology and Environmental Protection, University of Helsinki: Yliopistopaino, Helsinki, 2000, pp 1–57.

Tango, P.; Butler, W.; Wazniak, C. Assessment of Harmful Algal Bloom Species in the Maryland Coastal Bays. In *Maryland's Coastal Bays: Ecosystem Health Assessment.* Maryland Department of Natural Resources, Annapolis, USA, **2003**, *7*, 11–27.

Utermöhl, H. Zur Vervollkommnung der quantitativen Phytoplankton Methodik. Mitteilung Internationale Vereinigung fuer Theoretische und Amgewandte Limnologie. **1958**, *9*, 1–38.

Utermöhl, H. Neue Wege in der quantitativen Erfassung des Planktons (mit besonderer Berücksichtigung des Ultraplanktons). *Verh. Int. Ver. Theor. Angew. Limnol.* **1931**, *5*, 567–596.

Thangaraja, M.; Al Aisry, A.; Alkharusi, L. Harmful Algal Blooms and Their Impacts in the Middle and Outer ROPME Sea Area. *Int. J. Oceans Oceanogr.* **2007**, *1*, 85–98.

Villac, M. C.; Roelke, D. L.; Villareal, T. A.; Fryxell, G. A. Comparison of Two Domoic Acid-producing Diatoms; A Review. *Hydrobiologia.* **1993**, *269/270*, 213–224.

Verlecar, X. N.;, Desai, S. Phytoplankton Identification Manual. National Institute of Oceanography. Dona Paula, Goa, 2004, pp 30–40.

Venerick, E. L. How Many Cells to Count? In *Phytoplankton Manual*; Sournia, A., Ed.; UNESCO: Paris, 1978; pp 167–180.

Villac, M. C.; Roelke, D. L.; Villareal, T. A.; Fryxell, G. A. Comparison of Two Domoic Acid-producing Diatoms: A Review. *Hydrobiologia* **1993**, *269*, 213–224.

Wells, M. L.; Trainer, V. L.; Smayda, T. J.;, Karlson B. S.; Trick, C. G.; Kudela, R. M.; Ishikawa, A.; Bernard, S.; Wulff A.; Anderson, D. M.; Cochlan, W. P. Harmful Algal Blooms and Climate Change: Learning from the Past and Present to Forecast the Future. *Harmful Algae.* **2015**, *1*, 68–93.

Zaccaroni, A.; Scaravelli, D. Toxicity of Algal Toxins to Humans and Animals. In Algal Toxins, Nature, Occurrence, Effect, and Detection; Evangelista, V., Barsanti, L., Frassanito, A. M., Passarelli, V., Gualtieri, P., Eds.; Springer: Dordrecht (NL), 2008; pp 91–158.

Zingone, A.; Enevoldsen, H. O. The Diversity of Harmful Algal Blooms: A Challenge for Science and Management. *Ocean Coast. Manag.* **2000,** *43*, 725–748.

Zingone, A.; Raffaele, S.; D'Alelio, D.; Sarno, D. Potentially Toxic and Harmful Microalgae from Coastal Waters of the Campania Region (Tyrrhenian Sea, Mediterranean Sea). *Harmful Algae* **2006,** *5*, 321–337.

PART IV
Animal Resources Management

CHAPTER 21

Protected Area Effectiveness for Fish Spawning Habitat in Relation to Earthquake-Induced Landscape Change

SHANE ORCHARD[1*] and MICHAEL J. H. HICKFORD[2]

[1]*Waterways Centre for Freshwater Management, University of Canterbury and Lincoln University, Christchurch, New Zealand*

[2]*Marine Ecology Research Group, University of Canterbury, Christchurch, New Zealand*

Corresponding author. E-mail: s.orchard@waterlink.nz

ABSTRACT

We studied the effectiveness of spatial planning methods for the conservation of *Galaxias maculatus,* a riparian spawning fish, following earthquake-induced habitat shift in the Canterbury region of New Zealand. Mapping and GIS overlay techniques were used to evaluate three protection mechanisms in operative or proposed plans in two study catchments over 2 years. Method 1 utilized a network of small protected areas around known spawning sites. It was the least resilient to change with only 3.9% of postquake habitat remaining protected in the worst-performing scenario. Method 2, based on mapped reaches of potential habitat, remained effective in one catchment (98%) but not in the other (52.5%). Method 3, based on a habitat model, achieved near 100% protection in both catchments but used planning areas far larger than the area of habitat actually used. This example illustrates resilience considerations for protected area design. Redundancy can help maintain effectiveness in face of dynamics and maybe a pragmatic choice if planning area boundaries lack in-built adaptive capacity or require lengthy processes for amendment. However, an adaptive planning area coupled with monitoring offers high effectiveness from a smaller protected area network.

Incorporating elements of both strategies provide a promising conceptual basis for adaptation to major perturbations or responding to slow change.

21.1   INTRODUCTION

For many species, critical life-history phases create obligate habitat require-ments. These may be vulnerable points in the life cycle, especially where relatively specific biophysical conditions are required (Lucas et al., 2009). The vulnerability may be associated with both periodic events and longer-term change involving natural and anthropogenic processes (Turner et al., 2003). A particular concern is where human activities reduce the quality or availability of existing habitat unless counterbalanced by compensatory actions, such as the creation of suitable habitat elsewhere (Faith and Walker, 2002). The concept of resilience provides a focus on thresholds in system properties that are important to their persistence (Holling, 1973). In linked socioecological systems it is related to adaptive capacity (Gallopín, 2006) and actual responses to changed hazard exposure and/or sensitivity (Turner et al., 2007). Since resilience assessment is concerned with identifying the conditions required to maintain a desirable state (Gunderson et al., 2010), it may be readily applied to habitat management.

Protected areas (PAs) describe the desired state defined by clear objec-tives. They are a cornerstone of global efforts to halt biodiversity loss (UN, 2011). The IUCN recognizes six categories of PAs defined by differences in management approaches (Stolton et al., 2013). Category IV PAs aim to protect particular species or habitats (Table 21.1). They are often relatively small and are designed to protect or restore: (1) Flora species of international, national, or local importance; (2) fauna species of international, national, or local importance including resident or migratory fauna; and/or (3) habitats (Dudley, 2008).

Effective conservation involves managing risks yet biodiversity declines are continuing (Butchart et al., 2010). Management effectiveness evaluation is an essential activity to assess the strengths and weaknesses of the protec-tion mechanisms in place and to consider alternatives (Stolton et al., 2007). A key area of focus is the extent to which PAs actually deliver on objectives such as the protection of important values (Hockings, 2003). Under condi-tions of environmental change, evaluation is especially important to address whether the areas involved are functioning as an effective conservation strategy (Leverington et al., 2010). Various methodologies have been used, many of which were originally developed to support adaptive management of PA sites and systems (Coad et al., 2015). Range shifts are a topic of particular importance since they may undermine the effectiveness of existing PA networks. In this setting, human agency is inextricably linked to the trajectory of the values identified for protection. This may require amendment of the protection mechanism itself to ensure continued performance over time.

TABLE 21.1   Aspects of IUCN Category IV Protected Areas (Dudley, 2008).

Role in the landscape/seascape

Category IV protected areas frequently play a role in "plugging the gaps" in conservation strategies by protecting key species or habitats in ecosystems.

They could, for instance, be used to:

- Protect critically endangered populations of species that need particular management interventions to ensure their continued survival;
- Protect rare or threatened habitats including fragments of habitats;
- Secure stepping-stones (places for migratory species to feed and rest) or breeding sites;
- Provide flexible management strategies and options in buffer zones around, or connectivity conservation corridors between, more strictly protected areas that are more acceptable to local communities and other stakeholders.

Issues for consideration

- Many category IV protected areas exist in crowded landscapes and seascapes, where human pressure is comparatively greater, both in terms of potential illegal use and visitor pressure.
- The category IV protected areas that rely on regular management intervention need appropriate resources from the management authority and can be relatively expensive to maintain unless management is undertaken voluntarily by local communities or other actors.
- Because they usually protect part of an ecosystem, successful long-term management of category IV protected areas necessitates careful monitoring and an even greater-than-usual emphasis on overall ecosystem approaches and compatible management in other parts of the landscape or seascape.

Diadromous fishes have specific habitat requirements across several stages of their life histories, involving both freshwater and marine environments (Gross et al., 1988). In some species, these may be separated by vast distances and associated with significant migrations (Metcalfe et al., 2002). There may be different conservation issues affecting each critical habitat requiring a wide range of management responses (McDowall, 1999). *Galaxias maculatus* (Jenyns, 1842) or 'īnanga' is a diadromous species currently listed as 'at risk-declining' under the New Zealand

Threat Classification System (Goodman et al., 2014). Adult fish are found in lowland coastal waterways with the upstream distribution limited by relatively poor climbing ability (Baker and Boubee, 2006; Doehring et al., 2012). Spawning occurs in estuarine waterways with the exception of some populations that have become landlocked in lakes (Chapman et al., 2006). The locations used are highly specific as the result of specialized reproductive behavior associated with the migration of adult fish toward river mouths at certain times of the year (Benzie, 1968a). Spawning events are strongly synchronized with the spring high tide cycle with an apparent association between spawning site distribution and the salinity regime (Burnet, 1965). The majority of spawning sites have been found within 500 m of the inland limit of saltwater (Richardson and Taylor, 2002; Taylor, 2002). In addition, spawning sites occupy only a narrow elevation range located on waterway margins just below the spring tide high-water mark (Taylor, 2002). As tidal heights drop toward the neap tides these sites are no longer inundated at high-water and for most of their development period the eggs are in a terrestrial environment (Benzie, 1968a, 1968b). Egg survival rates are highly dependent on the condition of the riparian vegetation in these locations until hatching in response to high water levels, usually provided by the following spring tide (Hickford et al., 2010; Hickford and Schiel, 2011).

The degradation of spawning habitat has been identified as a leading factor in the species' decline (McDowall, 1992; McDowall and Charteris, 2006). This has been linked to land-use intensification on coastal waterway margins (Hickford et al., 2010), as is a common trend worldwide (Kennish, 2002). Protection mechanisms must often address contested-space contexts characterized by incompatible activities. Multiple-stressor situations are common with grazing, vegetation clearance, mowing, grazing, flood protection, and channelization being examples that have contributed to degradation (Hickford and Schiel, 2011; Mitchell and Eldon, 1991). Habitat protection is a requirement of national legislation under the Conservation Act (1987) and the Resource Management Act (1991). The implementation relies on the identification of areas for protection enforced by appropriate rules and documented in plans or management strategies prepared under the relevant Acts (Orchard, 2016). In many cases, spatially explicit planning methods (e.g., maps) are used to delineate the protected areas. Although these provide a practical approach to address the conservation objective, they require reliable habitat information. In dynamic environments challenges include recognizing spatiotemporal variance and accommodating it in design of the protection mechanisms used (Bengtsson et al., 2003).

In 2010 and 2011, a sequence of major earthquakes affected the Canterbury region of New Zealand. It included several large destructive events and numerous aftershocks centered beneath the city of Christchurch (Beavan et al., 2012). The magnitude of physical effects necessitated a long-term socioecological response associated with new ecological trajectories and a variety of land-use planning needs. Topographic and bathymetric measurements identified enduring changes in ground levels, especially in the vicinity of waterways (Quigley et al., 2016). Ecohydrological effects have been a particular focus in light of changed water levels on the landscape (Hughes et al., 2015), and alterations to estuarine dynamics (Measures et al., 2011; Orchard and Measures, 2016, 2017). *G. maculatus* spawning was recorded at locations never previously utilized in comparison to prequake records (Orchard and Hickford, 2016). Vulnerability assessments identified anthropogenic threats at many of these locations and recommended a review of protection methods in the operative statutory plans (Orchard et al., 2018). This context presented a unique opportunity to evaluate conservation planning options in light of landscape-scale change whilst informing the practical needs of postquake adaptation processes. The objectives of this paper are to (1) evaluate the efficiency and effectiveness of contemporary protection mechanisms, and (2) identify recommendations for conservation planning to address earthquake-induced landscape change.

21.2 MATERIALS AND METHODS

21.2.1 STUDY AREA

The study area is the Avon Heathcote Estuary (Ihutai) located at 43.5°S, 172.7°E in the city of Christchurch (Fig. 21.1). The estuary is located between the Waimakariri River and the southern end of a large sandy bay (Pegasus Bay) where it is a prominent local feature (Kirk, 1979). It is a barrier enclosed tidal lagoon type estuary (Hume et al., 2007) with high ecological and social values including cultural significance for Māori (Jolly and Ngā Papatipu Rūnanga Working Group, 2013; Lang et al., 2012).

The Avon and Heathcote are the two major rivers of the estuarine system, both of which provide *G. maculatus* spawning habitat. These are spring-fed lowland rivers waterways with average base flows of approx. 2 and 1 cumecs, respectively (White et al., 2007). They are also among the most well-studied spawning locations in New Zealand with surveys having been conducted periodically since 1988 (Taylor et al., 1992).

21.2.2 GEOSPATIAL ANALYSES

We analyzed spawning site data from postearthquake studies comprising of seven independent surveys conducted over two years during the peak spawning months using a census-survey methodology designed to detect all spawning in the catchment (Orchard and Hickford, 2018). The areas surveyed were approximately 4 km reaching in each river extending from the saltmarsh vegetation zone (downstream) to 500 m upstream of the inland limit of saltwater (Fig. 21.1). The dataset of 188 records provided details of 121 spawning occurrences in the Avon and 67 in the Heathcote. Each record included upstream and downstream coordinates of the spawning site, mean width of the egg band, and area of occupancy (AOO) of eggs with each site being defined as a continuous or semicontinuous patch of eggs.

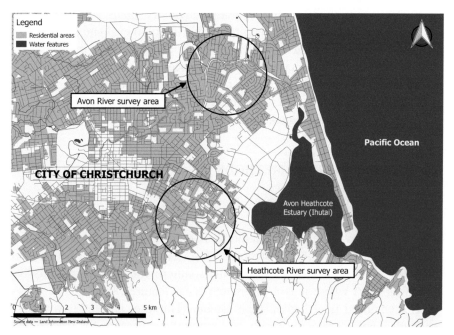

FIGURE 21.1   Location of postearthquake survey areas for *G. maculatus* spawning habitat in the Avon and Heathcote River catchments, city of Christchurch, New Zealand.

Three spatially explicit protection mechanisms were identified in an analysis of proposed and operative resource management plans (Table 21.2). In this paper, we use the term 'protected areas' to denote spatially explicit areas identified in planning methods to address conservation objectives in statutory

TABLE 21.2 Protected Area Mechanisms for *G. maculatus* Spawning Habitat Evaluated in this Study.

Method	Protected area mechanism	Delineation method in plans	Information source	Planning documents
1	Network of small protected areas based on known spawning sites.	20-m diameter areas centered on point data coordinates of known spawning sites, identified in schedule to the plan.	Point data and descriptions from NISD[†] and historical reports (Maw and McCallum-Clark, 2015).	Environment Canterbury (2015) Environment Canterbury (2016)
2	Mapped reaches of potential spawning habitat on a catchment basis.	Reaches identified in planning maps and referenced in the plan.	NISD point data and historical reports coupled with field surveys of riparian vegetation to identify potential habitat (Margetts, 2016).	Environment Canterbury (2014)
3	Mapped polygons of predicted spawning habitat coupled with a text description of where in the polygon the protection requirements apply.	Polygons identified in planning maps and GIS layer referenced in the plan.	GIS-based model of predicted spawning habitat (Greer et al., 2015).	Environment Canterbury (2017)

[†]National Īnanga Spawning Database.

policies and plans. The areas evaluated in this study are consistent with the IUCN definition of Category IV protected areas being 'areas to protect particular species or habitats, where management reflects this priority' (Dudley, 2008). The size of these areas is often relatively small with varying management arrangements depending on protection needs (Stolton et al., 2013).

Protected area and spawning site data were visualized in QGIS v2.8.18 (QGIS Development Team, 2016) and reach lengths (RL) calculated in relation to the centerlines of waterway channels digitized from 0.075 m resolution postquake aerial photographs (Land Information New Zealand, 2016). Three comparable RL metrics were calculated to reflect (1) the RL protected under each planning method, (2) extent of occurrence (EOO) of spawning sites, and (3) the total AOO of spawning sites (Table 21.3).

The effectiveness of each protection mechanism was evaluated as the percentage of postearthquake RL^{AOO} located within the PA. Efficiency was considered using two ratios: RL^{EOO} to $RL^{protected}$ and RL^{AOO} to $RL^{protected}$. These reflect the size of the area set aside for protection (in terms of reach length) versus the extent of the spawning reach, and the size of the areas actually utilized for spawning, respectively. Each calculation was made on a catchment basis at a yearly temporal scale (i.e., 2015 and 2016) and also using the combined data from both years of postearthquake surveys.

TABLE 21.3 Metrics Calculated to Evaluate the Effectiveness and Efficiency of Protected Area Mechanisms for *G. maculatus* Spawning Habitat.

Metric	Definition	Calculation method
$RL^{protected}$	Reach length protected areas within a catchment.	Combined length of waterway channels falling within protected areas, as calculated from channel centrelines on a catchment basis.
RL^{EOO}	Reach a length of the extent of occurrence (EOO) of spawning within each catchment during the timeframe under consideration.	Total length of waterway channels between the upstream and downstream limits of spawning, as measured along channel centrelines on a catchment basis.
RL^{AOO}	Reach a length of the area of occupation (AOO) of all spawning sites within each catchment during the timeframe under consideration.	Total length of all individual spawning sites, as measured along channel centrelines on a catchment basis.

21.3 RESULTS

The three protected area mechanisms provided considerably different $RL^{protected}$ values reflecting their spatial basis (Table 21.4). However, for each mechanism, the RL^{protected} was comparable between catchments. An overlay of each protection mechanism on combined postquake spawning site data is provided for each of the study catchments in Figure 21.2.

TABLE 21.4 Reach Length (RL) Protected by each of the Three Protected Area Mechanisms Evaluated in the Two Study Catchments.

Method	Description of protected area mechanism	Reach length protected (m)	
		Avon river	**Heathcote river**
1	The network of small protected areas based on known spawning sites.	120	80
2	Mapped reaches of potential spawning habitat on a catchment basis.	3230	3098
3	Mapped polygons of predicted spawning habitat coupled with a text description of where in the polygon the protection requirements apply.	19.100	16,600

Method 3 was highly effective at protecting spawning habitat, achieving 92.7% protection in the Avon and 100% in the Heathcote using the combined postquake data (Table 21.5). The anomaly in the Avon relates to a few spawning sites that occurred outside of the mapped polygon in the vicinity of a small tributary and this occurred in both years. In the Avon, the effectiveness of method 2 was similar with close to 100% achieved (Table 21.4). However, in the Heathcote, only 69.9% of spawning habitat fell within the protected area and 45.6% in 2016. This reflected the occurrence, in both years, of spawning downstream of the protected area (Fig. 21.2d). In comparison, the effectiveness of method 1 was low. The percentage of habitat protected ranged from 3.9–14.2% (Table 21.4). This reflected the extent to which spawning occurred at previously known sites which formed the basis for delineation of the PAs (Fig. 21.2a,b).

In the efficiency evaluation, all of the protection mechanisms were relatively inefficient in terms of land use allocation when the evaluation metric was RL^{AOO}. For all methods, more than half of the RL^{protected} was allocated to areas that were not utilized for spawning habitat over the study period, even when the areas allocated were very small and targetted at previously known spawning sites. The highest percentage overlap with RL^{AOO} was 47.5% achieved by method 1 in the Avon in 2016. However, when the evaluation metric was RL^{EOO} the percentage overlap results changed considerably. Method 1 achieved a 100% overlap in the Avon in both years but in the Heathcote only 12.5%. Method 2 achieved 67.6% overlap in the Avon

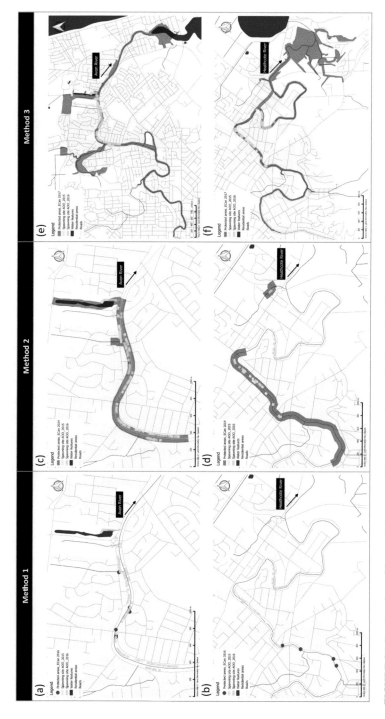

FIGURE 21.2 Overlay of the spatial extent of three protection mechanisms found in conservation plans on the footprint of post-earthquake *G. maculatus* spawning sites recorded in 2015 (*n* = 85) and 2016 (*n* = 103). (a) Method 1, Avon river, (b) Method 1, Heathcote river, (c) Method 2, Avon river, (d) Method 2, Heathcote river, (e) Method 3, Avon river, (f) Method 3, Heathcote river.

(2016) and 48.7% in the Heathcote (2016), whilst method 3 achieved 11.5% in the Avon (2016) and 17.6% in the Heathcote (2016).

TABLE 21.5 Effectiveness of Three Protected Area Mechanisms for *G. maculatus* Spawning Habitat Following Earthquake-induced Landscape Change.

Protection mechanism	Time period	Percentage of habitat protected (% RL^{AOO})	
		Avon river	Heathcote river
Method 1	2015	5.4	7.5
	2016	14.2	6.3
	2015+2016	9.3	3.9
Method 2	2015	96.9	69.9
	2016	99.0	45.6
	2015+2016	98.0	52.5
Method 3	2015	96.9	100
	2016	96.5	100
	2015+2016	97.2	100

Comparing these results, method 3 was the least efficient in terms of land use allocation for the purposes of protection in all comparisons in the Avon. However, in the Heathcote method 1 was even less efficient in terms of RL^{EOO}. This reflected that the protected areas identified were not well located in relation to the areas utilized for spawning (Fig. 21.2). In the Avon, the PAs under method 1 was much better located with all PAs overlapping the RL^{EOO}. In terms of RL^{AOO} method 1 also performed better in the Avon versus the Heathcote as a result of the PAs coinciding several of the areas actually utilized. However, even here the efficiency of the PA mechanism was rather variable with 47.5% of the RL^{protected} overlapping with spawning sites in 2016 but only 17.5% in 2015. This variability is associated with the repeated use of some, but not all, previously used spawning sites between years (Fig. 21.2).

Overall, method 2 produced relatively consistent results in the efficiency comparisons between years. This reflects that the RL^{EOO} was similar in both catchments between years and also located in a similar position in the catchment versus the reaches mapped for protection. Within the RL^{EOO} the total RL^{AOO} was also very similar between years (Avon 386 m^2 and 410 m^2, Heathcote 133 m^2 and 158 m^2 for 2015 and 2016, respectively) despite considerable variation in the location of the sites used each year (Fig. 21.2).

21.4   DISCUSSION

21.4.1   ADDRESSING SPATIOTEMPORAL VARIATION

Several aspects of *G. maculatus* spawning site ecology are potential sources of spatiotemporal variation. The reported relationship with salinity results in horizontal structuring along the axis of waterway channels in relation to saltwater intrusion (Richardson and Taylor, 2002; Taylor, 2002). This may drive variability in the position of spawning reaches on a catchment scale when coupled with dynamism of river discharges and tidal forcing. Despite that previous studies have highlighted the use of the same spawning sites for multiple years (Taylor, 2002), this case was characterized by habitat shift in both catchments in comparison to all known records. Although the potential effects of salinity changes have seldom been highlighted in the literature, this study indicates that they may important in relation to perturbations from extreme events or to incremental changes, such as sea level rise. However, a lack of historical salinity data for the reaches of interest makes the degree of variation difficult to confirm directly in our study area, and this is generally case elsewhere.

In addition, the timing of spawning on or soon after the peak of the tide, combined with a preference for shallow water depths, leads to vertical structuring of the habitat in relation to water level heights (Benzie, 1968a; Mitchell and Eldon, 1991). Interaction between the waterline and floodplain topography also influences the distance between spawning sites and the alignment of (i.e., perpendicular to) waterway channels. This variation may be considered where the topography is relatively flat and is a further consideration for effective PA design.

21.4.2   EVALUATING PA EFFECTIVENESS FOR DYNAMIC HABITATS

There are at least three aspects of this study that are likely to be applicable to the design and evaluation of Category IV PAs elsewhere. They include the question of PA boundary setting in relation to the habitat to be protected, the need for data to inform this and monitoring strategies to support future evaluations, and practical considerations for identifying boundaries on the ground as required by stakeholders.

Clearly, accuracy is important when setting boundaries for Category IV PAs, yet spatiotemporal variation may hamper acquisition of the necessary data in practice. For *G. maculatus* strong temporal trends are a particular consideration. Variation has been reported in relation to the peak days of activity within a tidal sequence, the tidal sequences preferred in different parts of the country and months of most spawning activity in the year (Taylor, 2002). International studies have also reported large-scale variation in traits associated with spawning (Barbee et al., 2011). In combination, these aspects suggest that spatiotemporal variability could arise at multiple scales creating practical difficulties for both empirical data collection and model-based approaches for determining habitat distribution. In this case, the study catchments are New Zealand's best-studied spawning areas yet surveys have only been periodic and seldom comprised more than one month in any given year (Taylor, 2002). Consequently, the times of peak spawning activity may not have been captured in the survey record. Identification of the spawning distribution has, therefore, relied on the compilation of multi-year data despite the potential for confounding factors associated with both short- and long-term change.

Albeit that the postearthquake context represents a major perturbation, the impacts of spatiotemporal variance on PA effectiveness are clearly seen in planning methods 1 and 2. These methods were developed using the planning authority's up to date information on spawning habitat in both catchments. Particularly in the Heathcote, earthquake-induced habitat shift rendered these methods relatively ineffective. Despite this, regular monitoring and amendment of the same protection mechanism could provide a strategy for maintaining effectiveness and addressing change. However, for method 1 the data collection requirements would be onerous to achieve this in practice. This partly reflects reliance on a network of small PAs but also that the detection of spawning sites is difficult (Orchard and Hickford, 2018). The number of PAs identified appears woefully inadequate in light of the postquake data, yet fairly represents results of the monitoring effort that was in place prequake. Increasing this to the level of a census-survey for peak spawning months represents a considerably scaling-up of the monitoring program.

In comparison, method 3 was based on considerably larger PAs and was much more resilient to earthquake change. In that case, a degree of redundancy was seen as a desirable aspect of resilience (Greer et al., 2015). However, from the perspective of PA evaluation, the three PA mechanisms share similar monitoring requirements. This arises since the demonstration of PA management effectiveness requires information on the values to be protected (Stoll-Kleemann, 2010). Given that monitoring resources are inevitably limited, dynamic environments demand particular attention. In turn, this illustrates the need for research on monitoring strategies to inform priorities for data collection and frequency (Teder et al., 2007). Moreover, it exemplifies the need for more management-driven science to close the gap between conservation policy and practice (Knight et al., 2008).

Potential strategies include using abiotic proxies for conservation objectives for which data acquisition is easier thus reducing the burden of repeat measurement (Lawler et al., 2015). Method 3 provides an example of this approach, using a predictive model based on elevation above sea level (Greer et al., 2015). However, the results indicate that its efficiency as a planning method is relatively low since much of the area set aside did not help achieve the stated objectives and it could not be used as a proxy for outcomes monitoring against the relevant policy objectives. From an ecosystem-based perspective, inefficient planning methods may also hinder other potential uses of the areas involved, leading to unnecessary trade-offs (Southworth et al., 2006). The practical aspects of this relate to the rules that apply within the PA and are designed to confer protection. Where a degree of sustainable use is envisaged within PAs, the specific arrangements for management need to be well matched to intended objectives.

Efficiency may be a particularly important consideration for Category IV PA evaluation where the management context is characterized by high land-use intensity in adjacent areas (Dudley, 2008). In this case method 2 offered an alternative approach that identified the known EOO and additional areas considered be 'potential' habitat and included these in the areas delineated for protection (Margetts, 2016). Essentially this created a buffer around the mapped EOO that served to address limitations in the information available for quantifying known habitat, as well as a providing a degree of redundancy, to improve resilience. Although in the Heathcote the post-quake habitat was found to have shifted outside of these areas, they were effective in accommodating the smaller magnitude of change observed in the Avon (Fig. 21.2). Management effectiveness evaluation of methods 2 and 3 primarily requires information on EOO as could be obtained by regular census-surveys of spawning habitat (Orchard and Hickford, 2018). The combination of an evaluation-informed adaptive approach and degree of redundancy could offer an effective and efficient PA strategy for the dynamic habitat with regards to land use allocation.

Lastly, this case highlights some practical issues for the visualization of PA boundaries. In our evaluation, spatial co-occurrence was based on coordinates describing the upstream and downstream extent of spawning sites and polygons describing PAs. In many instances, the spawning site locations were very close to the PA boundaries as mapped. Unless they were clearly outside of the boundaries, such sites were assessed as being protected with the result being an optimistic view of the spatial coverage of the PA mechanism. In reality these boundaries may not be so clear. However, it is important that they are clear for the benefit of all stakeholders (Langhammer et al., 2007), and this depends considerably on design and communication of the planning methods. In this case the areas delineated by method 1 were interpreted by stakeholders using a location description and schedule of coordinates (Table 21.2). This is considered to offer a relatively clear mechanism for implementation of the PA requirements in practice.

Under method 2, the areas for protection were first visualized as lines in Council planning documents (Margetts, 2016) and then subsequently incorporated into 'Sites of Ecological Significance' (SESs) in a recent statutory plan (Christchurch City Council 2015), which is now operative. The visualization method for plan users is a set of polygons annotated on planning maps appended to the plan (Fig. 21.S1a). These SESs have, therefore, become the PAs of interest and method 2 (as assessed in this study) can be interpreted in relation to *G. maculatus* objectives within these larger areas. However, at the scale of the mapping provided it is difficult to see exactly where the PA boundaries lie in the riparian zone, requiring considerable guesswork by plan users (Fig. 21.S1b).

Under method 3 the situation is improved by the provision of PA polygons as a public dataset with an online GIS viewer available, in addition to planning maps appended to the relevant plan (Environment Canterbury, 2017). Nonetheless, similar boundary issues arise with regards to the exact location of the PA in relation to the spatial extent of spawning habitat. The GIS analysis revealed a few spawning sites that were clearly outside of the PA boundary in the Avon, as reflected in effectiveness results of <100% in both years (Table 21.5) and, in general, many of the actual spawning locations were again very close to the PA boundary. Furthermore, the habitat may shift a considerable distance from the low flow channel on high water spawning events, and these circumstances are difficult to detect by operators (e.g., management contractors) in the field. Indeed spawning sites were found to have been destroyed by the City Council's own reserve management contractors subsequent to notification of the relevant statutory plan (Orchard et al., 2018). This suggests that better guidance materials, such as interactive maps, may be required to improve PA effectiveness in practice, as was recommended in a recent management trial that aimed to avoid such damage to spawning sites (Orchard, 2017). These results also indicate that a buffer should be considered as an aspect of PA design.

21.4.3   ASSUMPTIONS AND LIMITATIONS

Several assumptions have been made in this evaluation consistent with a focus of the protection of dynamic habitats and the objective of identifying

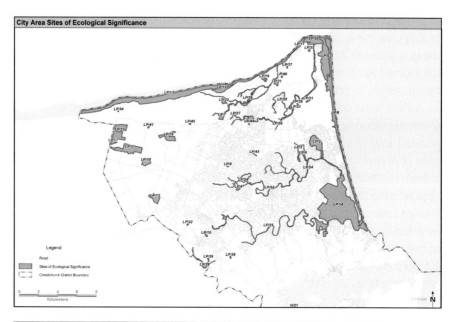

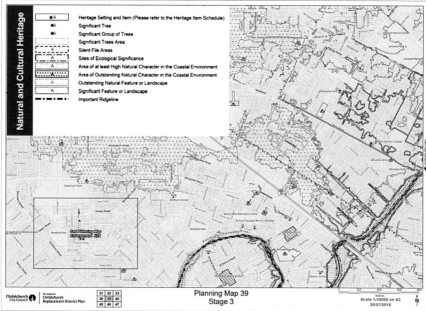

FIGURE 21.S1 Planning maps showing Sites of Ecological Significance (SESs) in the Christchurch City area (Christchurch City Council 2015). (a) Schedule Reference Map. (b) Example of detailed planning map. No enlargements are provided for SESs in riparian zones. For brevity, only an excerpt of the full legend is shown.

learning from the unique postearthquake situation. Most importantly, the focus has been restricted to the spatial basis of protection mechanisms for critical habitat as found in planning documents. In all cases, they were assumed to confer protection where spatial overlap occurred. In reality, this also depends considerably on the design of the rules that apply within the PA and aspects such as the provision of compliance monitoring. Also, a conservative approach has been taken in the mapping of PA boundaries and protection assumed to be effective. In the case of method 2, the width of the riparian zone protected could not be accurately identified and all spawning sites with the protected reach were assumed to be covered. Other limitations of the study include the spatial coverage of postquake surveys in relation to method 3 since the full extent of those PAs was not directly surveyed. Despite this the spatial coverage of the surveys was extensive in both catchments and the methodology was designed to capture the upstream and downstream extents of the full habitat distribution (Orchard and Hickford, 2018). Different evaluation results can also be expected in light of new information. In particular, the number of spawning events captured in the postquake survey record is limited. Further spatiotemporal variation may arise from effects, such as differing water heights outside of the sampled range, future vegetation change, river engineering impacts, the potential for further ground-level changes, and the ongoing influence of sea-level rise.

21.5 CONCLUSIONS

This evaluation was conceived to challenge PA thinking. Firstly, our evaluation extends the discussion of PA management effectiveness toward that of resilience. Although management actions within existing PAs may help increase the resilience of natural resources, the realities of global change create a fundamental challenge that demands a range of approaches (Baron et al., 2009). In this case, the PAs involved are small and are best thought of as PA networks under the management of local and regional government entities. Yet in all respects, they meet the definition of Category IV PAs and are found nationwide in recognition of their statutory role and origins. Although a focus on critical habitats is just one dimension of protected areas management, it is an important function in terms of their role as a management tool and wider contribution to spatial planning. Importantly, attention to relatively fine scales may offer practical opportunities for integrating PA systems into the wider land and seascape (Guarnieri et al., 2016). For example, small and dynamic PAs have the potential to help fill representation gaps in

PA networks as is a critical need in lowland river and floodplain systems (Tockner et al., 2008). In addition, an understanding of the role of PAs in climate change adaptation has been steadily developing but there is much work to be done. For example, new questions to assess the effects of climate change on PAs have only recently been employed in management effectiveness tracking tool evaluations despite its long history and widespread use (Stolton and Dudley, 2016). Through investigation of change following an extreme event this study provides insights into similar considerations. Our findings suggest that adaptive networks of well-targeted and relatively small PAs could produce an effective mechanism for responding to change, thereby, contributing to system resilience. Whether new or traditional PAs networks can be adapted along these lines deserves further research. We predict this will become a key topic for environmental planning and conservation management in the years ahead.

ACKNOWLEDGMENTS

We thank Environment Canterbury and Christchurch City Council staff for information on planning methods and riparian management activities. Funding was provided by the Ngāi Tahu Research Centre and a New Zealand Ministry of Business, Innovation and Employment grant (C01X1002) in conjunction with the National Institute of Water and Atmospheric Research.

KEYWORDS

- **dynamic environments**
- **landscape change**
- **spatial planning**
- **protected areas**
- **conservation management**
- **resilience**
- *Galaxias maculatus*

REFERENCES

Baker, C. F.; Boubee, J. A. T. Upstream Passage of Inanga Galaxias Maculatus and Redfin Bullies *Gobiomorphus huttoni* Over Artificial Ramps. *J. Fish Biol.* **2006**, *69*, 668–681.

Barbee, N. C.; Hale, R.; Morrongiello, J.; Hicks, A.; Semmens, D.; Downes, B. J.; Swearer, S. E. Large-scale Variation in life history traits of the widespread diadromous fish, Galaxias maculatus, reflects geographic differences in local environmental conditions. *Mar. Fresh. Res.* **2011**, *62*, 790–800.

Baron, J. S.; Gunderson, L.; Allen, C. D.; Fleishman, E.; Mc Kenzie, D.; Meyerson, L. A.; Stephenson, N. Options for National Parks and Reserves for Adapting to Climate Change. *Environ. Manag.* **2009**, *44*, 1033–1042.

Beavan, J.; Motagh, M.; Fielding, E. J.; Donnelly, N.; Collett, D. Fault Slip Models of the 2010-2011 Canterbury, New Zealand, Earthquakes from Geodetic Data and Observations of Postseismic Ground Deformation. *New Zealand J. Geol. Geophys.* **2012**, *55*, 207–221.

Bengtsson, J.; Angelstam, P.; Elmqvist, T.; Emanuelsson, U.; Folke, C.; Ihse, M.; Sveriges, l. Reserves, Resilience and Dynamic Landscapes. *Ambio* **2003**, *32*, 389–396.

Benzie, V. Some Ecological Aspects of the Spawning Behaviour and Early Development of the Common Whitebait Galaxias *Maculatus attenuatus* (Jenyns). *Proc. New Zeal. Ecol. Soc.* **1968**, *15*, 31–39.

Benzie, V. Stages in the Normal Development of Galaxias maculatus attenuatus (Jenyns). *New Zeal. J. Mar. Fresh. Res.* **1968**, *2*, 606–627.

Burnet, A. M. R. Observations on the Spawning Migrations of Galaxias attenuatus. *New Zeal. J. Sci.* **1965**, *8*, 79–87.

Butchart, S. H. M.; Walpole, M.; Collen, B.; van Strien, A.; Scharlemann, J. P. W.; Almond, R. E. A.; Watson R. Global Biodiversity: Indicators of Recent Declines. Sci. **2010**, *328*, 1164–1168.

Chapman, A.; Morgan, D. L.; Beatty, S. J.; Gill, H. S. Variation in Life History of Land-Locked Lacustrine and riverine Populations of *Galaxias maculatus* (Jenyns 1842) in Western Australia. *Environ. Biol. Fishes* **2006**, *77*, 21–37.

Christchurch City Council. The Proposed Christchurch Replacement District Plan. Chapter 9 Natural and Cultural Heritage. Notified 25 July 2015. Christchurch: Christchurch City Council, 2015, 145.

Coad, L.; Leverington, F.; Knights, K.; Geldmann, J.; Eassom, A.; Kapos, V.; Hockings, M. Measuring Impact of Protected Area Management Interventions: Current and Future Use of the Global Database of Protected Area Management Effectiveness. *Philos. Trans. Royal Soc. B: Biol. Sci.* **2015**, *370*.

Doehring, K.; Young, R. G.; McIntosh, A. R. Facilitation of Upstream Passage for Juveniles of a Weakly Swimming Migratory Galaxiid. *New Zeal. J. Mar. Fresh. Res.* **2012**, *46*, 303–313.

Dudley, N. *Guidelines for Applying Protected Area Management Categories*; IUCN: Gland, Switzerland, 2008; p 86.

Environment Canterbury. Resource Consent CRC146620. Christchurch: Environment Canterbury, 2014, 8.

Environment Canterbury Land and Water Regional Plan. Christchurch: Canterbury Regional Council, 2015, Vol. 1, p 383.

Environment Canterbury. Plan Change 4 to the Canterbury Land and Water Regional Plan. 31. Christchurch: Canterbury Regional Council, 2016, p 77.

Environment Canterbury. Canterbury Land and Water Regional Plan. Updated 24. Christchurch: Canterbury Regional Council, 2017, Vol. 1, p 470.

Faith, D. P.; Walker, P. A. The Role of trade-offs in Biodiversity Conservation Planning: Linking Local Management, Regional Planning and Global Conservation Efforts. *J. Biosci.* **2002,** *27*, 393–407.

Gallopín, G. C. Linkages Between Vulnerability, Resilience, and Adaptive Capacity. *Glob. Environ. Change* **2006,** *16*, 293–303.

Goodman, J. M.; Dunn, N. R.; Ravenscroft, P. J.; Allibone, R. M.; Boubée, J. A. T.; David, B. O.; Rolfe J. R. *Conservation Status of New Zealand Freshwater Fish*, 2013. New Zealand Threat Classification Series, Wellington: Department of Conservation, 2014, 12.

Greer, M.; Gray, D.; Duff, K.; Sykes, J. Predicting Inanga/whitebait Spawning Habitat in Canterbury. Report No. R15/100, Christchurch: Environment Canterbury, 2015, 12.

Gross, M. R.; Coleman, R. M.; Mc Dowall, R. M. Aquatic Productivity and the Evolution of Diadromous Fish Migration. Sci. **1988,** *239*, 1291–1293.

Guarnieri, G.; Bevilacqua, S.; Leo, F. D.; Farella, G.; Maffia, A.; Terlizzi, A.; Fraschetti, S. The Challenge of Planning Conservation Strategies in Threatened Seascapes: Understanding the Role of Fine Scale Assessments of community Response to Cumulative Human Pressures. *PLoS One.* **2016,** *11*.

Gunderson, L. H.; Allen, C. R.; Holling, C. S. *Foundations of Ecological Resilience*; Island Press: Washington, DC, 2010.

Hickford, M. J. H.; Cagnon M.; Schiel, D. R. Predation, Vegetation and Habitat-specific Survival of Terrestrial Eggs of a Diadromous Fish, Galaxias maculatus (Jenyns, 1842). *J. Exp. Mar. Biol. Ecol.* **2010,** *385*, 66–72.

Hickford, M. J. H.; Schiel, D. R. Population Sinks Resulting from Degraded Habitats of an Obligate Life-history Pathway. *Oecologia* **2011,** *166*, 131–140.

Hockings, M. Systems for Assessing the Effectiveness of Management in Protected Areas. *Bioscience* **2003,** *53*, 823–832.

Holling C. S. Resilience and Stability of Ecological Systems. *Ann. Rev. Ecol. Evol. S.* **1973,** 4, 1–23.

Hughes, M. W.; Quigley, M. C.; van Ballegooy, S.; Deam, B. L.; Bradley, B. A.; Hart, D. E.; Measures, R. The Sinking City: Earthquakes Increase Flood Hazard in Christchurch, New Zealand. *GSA Today* **2015,** *25*, 4–10.

Hume, T. M.; Snelder, T.; Weatherhead, M., Liefting, R. A Controlling Factor Approach to Estuary Classification. *Ocean Coast. Manag.* **2007,** *50*, 905–929.

Jolly, D.; Ngā Papatipu Rūnanga Working Group. Mahaanui Iwi Management Plan, 2013. Mahaanui Kurataiao Ltd. Ōtautahi Christchurch, 2013.

Kennish, M. J. Environmental Threats and Environmental Future of Estuaries. *Environ. Conserv.* **2002,** *29*, 78–107.

Kirk, R. M. Dynamics and Management of Sand Beaches in Southern Pegasus Bay. Morris and Wilson Consulting Engineers Limited, Christchurch, 1979.

Knight, A. T.; Cowling, R. M.; Rouget, M.; Balmford, A., Lombard, A. T.; Campbell, B. M. Knowing but Not Doing: Selecting Priority Conservation Areas and the Research-Implementation Gap. *Conserv. Biol.* **2008,** *22*, 610–617.

Land Information New Zealand. Christchurch 0.075m Urban Aerial Photos (2015–2016). 2016 from 6993 GeoTIFF sources in NZGD2000/New Zealand Transverse Mercator 2000, 2016.

Lang, M.; Orchard, S.; Falwasser, T.; Rupene, M.; Williams, C.; Tirikatene, N. N.; Couch, R. State of the Takiwā 2012 -Te Āhuatanga o Te Ihutai. Cultural Health Assessment of the Avon-Heathcote Estuary and its Catchment. Christchurch: Mahaanui Kurataiao Ltd. 2012, 41.

Langhammer, P. F.; Bakarr, M. I.; Bennun, L. A.; Brooks, T. M.; Clay, R. P.; Darwall, W.; Tordoff, A. W. *Identification and Gap Analysis of Key Biodiversity Areas: Targets for Comprehensive Protected Area Systems*; IUCN: Gland, Switzerland, 2007; p 116.

Lawler, J. J.; Ackerly, D. D.; Albano C. M.; Anderson, M. G.; Dobrowski, S. Z.; Gill, J. L.; Weiss, S. B. The Theory Behind, and the Challenges of, Conserving Nature's Stage in a Time of Rapid Change. *Conserv. Biol.* **2015**, *29*, 618–629.

Leverington, F.; Costa, K. L.; Pavese, H.; Lisle, A.; Hockings, M. A Global Analysis of Protected Area Management Effectiveness. *Environ. Manag.* **2010**, 46, 685–698.

Lucas, M. C.; Bubb, D. H.; Jang, M. H., Ha, K.; Masters, J. E. G. Availability of and Access to Critical Habitats in Regulated Rivers: Effects of Low-head Barriers on Threatened Lampreys. Fresh. Biol. **2009**, *54*, 621–634.

Margetts, B. I. Statement of Evidence of Dr Belinda Isobel Margetts for the Christchurch City Council. 29. Christchurch City Council, 2016, 21.

Maw, P.; Mc Callum, C. M. Plan Change 4 (Omnibus) to the Partially Operative Canterbury Land and Water Regional Plan Section 42A Report. Report Number R15/148. Prepared for Environment Canterbury, 2015, 196.

Mc Dowall, R. M. Particular Problems for the Conservation of Diadromous Fish. *Aquat. Conserv. Mar. Fresh. Ecosyst.* **1992**, *2*, 351–355.

Mc Dowall, R. M. Different Kinds of Diadromy: Different Kinds of Conservation Problems. *ICES J. Mar. Sci.* **1999**, *56* (4), 410–413.

Mc Dowall, R. M., Charteris S. C. The Possible Adaptive Advantages of Terrestrial Egg Deposition in Some Fluvial Diadromous Galaxiid Fishes (Teleostei : Galaxiidae). *Fish Fisheries* **2006**, *7*, 153–164.

Measures, R.; Hicks, M. D.; Shankar, U.; Bind, J.; Arnold, J.; Zeldis, J. Mapping Earthquake Induced Topographical Change and Liquefaction in the Avon-Heathcote Estuary. Environment Canterbury Report No. U11/13. Christchurch: Environment Canterbury, 2011, 28.

Metcalfe, J. D.; Arnold, G. P.; Mc Dowall, R. M. Migration. In *Handbook of Fish Biology and Fisheries*; Hart, P. J. B., Reynolds, J. D., Eds.; Fish Biology. Blackwell Publishing: Oxford, **2002**, *1*, 175–199.

Mitchell, C. P.; Eldon, G. A. *How to Locate and Protect Whitebait Spawning Grounds*; Freshwater Fisheries Centre: Rotorua, 1991, 49.

Orchard, S. Identifying Īnanga Spawning Sites in Plans: Options for Addressing Post-quake Spawning in Ōtautahi Christchurch. Report prepared for Christchurch City Council and Environment Canterbury. Christchurch: University of Canterbury, 2016, 14.

Orchard, S. Response of Īnanga Spawning Habitat to Riparian Vegetation Management in the Avon & Heathcote Catchments. Report prepared for Christchurch City Council, 2017, 35.

Orchard, S.; Hickford M. Spatial effects of the Canterbury earthquakes on īnanga spawning habitat and implications for waterways management. Report prepared for IPENZ Rivers Group and Ngāi Tahu Research Centre. Waterways Centre for Freshwater Management and Marine Ecology Research Group. Christchurch: University of Canterbury, 2016, 37.

Orchard, S.; Hickford, M. J. H. Census Survey Approach to Quantifying Īnanga Spawning Habitat for Conservation and Management. New Zeal. J. Mar. Fresh. Res. **2018**, *52*, 284–294.

Orchard, S., Hickford, M. J. H., & Schiel, D. R. Earthquake-induced habitat migration in a riparian spawning fish has implications for conservation management. *Aquatic Conservation: Marine and Freshwater Ecosystems,* **2018**, *28*(3), 702–712. doi:10.1002/aqc.2898.

Orchard, S.; Measures, R. Development of a Fine-scale Salinity Model for the Avon Heathcote Estuary Ihutai. Report prepared for Brian Mason Scientific & Technical Trust. Christchurch: University of Canterbury & NIWA, 2016, 22.

Orchard, S.; Measures, R. Sea Level Rise Impacts in the Avon Heathcote Estuary Ihutai. Salinity Intrusion and Īnanga Spawning Scenarios. Report prepared for Christchurch City Council, 2017, 56.

QGIS Development Team. QGIS Geographic Information System. Open Source Geospatial Foundation Project, 2016.

Quigley, M. C.; Hughes, M. W.; Bradley, B. A.; van Ballegooy, S.; Reid, C.; Morgenroth, J.; Pettinga, J. R. The 2010–2011 Canterbury Earthquake Sequence: Environmental Effects, Seismic Triggering Thresholds and Geologic Legacy. *Tectonophysics.* **2016,** *672–673,* 228–274.

Richardson, J.; Taylor, M. J. A Guide to Restoring Inanga Habitat. NIWA *Sci. Technol. Ser.,* **2002,** *50,* 1–29.

Southworth, J.; Nagendra, H.; Munroe, D. K. Introduction to the Special Issue: Are Parks Working? Exploring Human–environment Tradeoffs in Protected Area Conservation. *Appl. Geo.* **2006,** *26,* 87–95.

Stoll, K. S. Evaluation of Management Effectiveness in Protected Areas: Methodologies and Results. *Basic Appl. Ecol.* **2010,** *11,* 377–382.

Stolton, S.; Dudley, N. *METT Handbook: A Guide to Using the Management Effectiveness Tracking Tool (METT)*; WWF: UK, 2016; p 74.

Stolton, S.; Hockings, M.; Dudley, N.; Mackinnon, K.; Whitten, T.; Leverington, F. *Management Effectiveness Tracking Tool. Reporting Progress at Protected Area Sites*; World Wide Fund for Nature: Gland, Switzerland, 2007; Vol. 2, p 22.

Stolton, S.; Shadie, P.; Dudley, N. *IUCN WCPA Best Practice Guidance on Recognising Protected Areas and Assigning Management Categories and Governance Types*; Best Practice Protected Area Guidelines Series No. 21; IUCN: Gland, Switzerland, 2013; p 31.

Taylor, M. J. The National Inanga Spawning Database: Trends and Implications for Spawning Site Management. Science for Conservation 188, Wellington: Department of Conservation. 2002, 37.

Taylor M. J., Buckland A. R., Kelly G. R. South Island inanga spawning surveys, 1988-1990. New Zealand Freshwater Fisheries Report No. 133. Ministry of Agriculture and Fisheries. Christchurch. 1992.

Teder, T.; Moora, M.; Roosaluste, E.; Zobel, K.; Pärtel, M.; Kõljalg U.; Zobel, M. Monitoring of Biological Diversity: A Common-Ground Approach. *Conserv. Biol.* **2007,** *21,* 313–317.

Tockner, K.; Bunn, S.; Gordon, C.; Naiman, R. J.; Quinn, G. P.; A. S. J. Flood plains: Critically Threatened Ecosystems. In *Aquatic Ecosystems*; Polunin, N. V. C., Ed.;Cambridge University Press: Cambridge, 2008, pp 45–61.

Turner, B. L.; Kasperson, R. E.; Matson, P. A.; Mc Carthy, J. J.; Corell, R. W.; Christensen, L.; … Schiller, A. A Framework for Vulnerability Analysis in Sustainability Science. *Proc. Nat. Acad. Sci.* **2003,** 100, 8074–8079.

Turner, B. L.; Lambin E. F.; Reenberg, A. The Emergence of Land Change Science for Global Environmental Change and Sustainability. *Proc. Acad. Sci. United States Am.* **2007,** *104,* 20666–20671.

UN (United Nations). *The Millennium Development Goals Report* 2011. New York: United Nations: Cambridge, 2011, p 68.

White, P. A.; Goodrich, K.; Cave, S.; Minni, G. Waterways, Swamps and Vegetation of Christchurch in 1856 and Baseflow Discharge in Christchurch City Streams. GNS Science Consultancy Report 2007/103. Taupo, 2007.

CHAPTER 22

Minerals in Forage Consumed by White-Tailed Deer in Northeastern Mexico

ROQUE GONZALO RAMÍREZ LOZANO*

Facultad de Ciencias Biológicas, Dpto. de Alimentos, Universidad Autónoma de Nuevo León

Corresponding author. E-mail: roque.ramirezlz@uanl.edu.mx

ABSTRACT

The present chapter reports mineral contents of diets consumed by white-tailed deer. According to studies of selectivity of the white-tailed deer, in northeastern Mexico, their diets are composed by a mixture of shrubs, grasses, and forbs, with tendency to a predominance of the shrubs. In addition, the occurrence of forbs in the range occurs when there is sufficient humidity that only occurs in the summer and autumn. Therefore, it is not very likely that the deer will manifest symptoms of toxicity caused by an excess in the consumption of forbs with high concentrations of Fe. However, high concentrations of condensed tannins in the plants that consume the deer can decrease the absorption of Fe. Only in summer the shrubs, forbs, and grasses consumed by white-tailed deer in northeastern Mexico contained sufficient amounts of minerals to satisfy metabolic requirements. Results revealed a large variability of mineral contents in forage species consumed by white-tailed deer. Concentrations of Zn during summer were sufficient to satisfy deer requirements. At other seasons, the levels were marginally satisfactory (30 mg/kg).

22.1 INTRODUCTION

The White-tailed deer (*Odocoileus virginianus*) is a mid-sized cervid. White-tailed deer can be found from southern Canada all the way down to South

America (De la Rosa-Reyna et al., 2012). White-tailed deer are herbivores and are considered concentrate selectors. Their diet includes many different types of vegetation and varies greatly with the seasons and the region in which they inhabit. White-tailed deer mostly depend on browse but also feed on forbs, hard and soft mast and grasses (Yarrow, 2009).

In agricultural regions, white-tailed deer may feed heavily upon crops, such as corn, soybeans, and alfalfa, if they are present. During the harsh winters of northern regions white-tailed deer depend on browsing the twigs and buds of woody shrubs and trees while the supply of higher quality feed is scarce (Walter et al., 2009). White-tailed deer are ruminants, so they may consume at a high rate and retreat into safer cover to finish digesting their food. This helps them avoid predation. They also produce a tannin-binding saliva that helps them digest things easier than other herbivores. They may still select for things with lower tannin content (Karns et al., 2011).

Minerals are required for the normal functioning of all essential biochemical processes of the organism. An essential mineral can be defined as that which is required by the deer to support adequate growth, reproduction, and health throughout its normal life cycle, when all other nutrients are in optimal quantities (Grace and Clark, 1991). Based on the identification of one or more metabolic functions, at least 15 minerals (N, P, S, K, Ca, Mg, Na, Cl, Fe, Mn, Cu, Co, I, Mo, and Se) can be classified as Essentials (McDowell et al., 1997). The deficiency of each mineral in the deer results in abnormalities that can only be corrected by the supply of the deficient mineral. The severity of the deficiency will determine the degree and type of abnormality observed. The metabolism and nutrition of minerals are similar in all animal species and therefore observations of one species can be extrapolated to other species (NRC, 2007). The mineral elements are divided into two groups according to the abundance of them in the organism: Macrominerals are elements that are found in abundant form in the organism and have structural functions and microminerals or trace elements that are in the organism in very small amounts and usually perform (Suttle, 2010). This review has the objective to describe the mineral content of the main forages consumed by white-tailed deer in north-eastern Mexico.

22.1.1 *FUNCTIONS OF MINERALS IN DEER*

The minerals carry out diverse functions in deer such as:

1. As structural components of the skeleton, (e.g., Ca, P, and Mg).

2. They intervene in the acid-base balance (pH) of the body fluids (e.g., Na, K, and Cl).
3. They intervene in enzymatic systems as activators (e.g., Zn and Cu).
4. A significant number of them have more than one function (NRC, 2007).

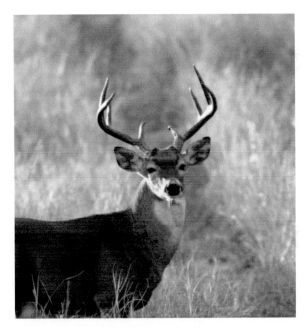

Odocoileus virginianus

However, the alteration in the concentration of the minerals directly affects the health of the deer and, therefore, its productivity, mainly because the food it consumes, has deficiencies or excesses. Mineral deficiencies can lead to disorders in skin, non-infectious abortions, diarrhea, anemia, weight loss, loss of appetite, bone abnormalities, tetany, low fertility, and debilitating diseases, among other clinical signs. In addition, all mineral elements, whether indispensable or not indispensable, can affect the deer adversely, if consumed at excessively high levels (Spears, 1998).

In the ruminal fermentation, the minerals Ca, K, Fe, Zn, and Mn are of great importance for the growth of ruminal bacteria and, therefore, in the digestion of the organic matter that the deer performs (Table 22.1). In addition, P is of utmost importance for the proper metabolism and health of the ruminal microflora (Tomlinson, 2002). P is part of the nucleic acids (DNA and RNA) found in all bacterial cells. In the bacterial cells of the rumen 10.3% of the DNA and 9.6% of the RNA are constituted by this mineral. Most of the RNA from the cells is located in the ribosome and, the ribosomal content in the bacteria is directly related to bacterial growth and, therefore, cellulolytic activity. Zn is essential for all living biological systems. The lack of availability of Zn for bacteria inhibits their multiplication, as well as affecting the ability of cellulolytic bacteria to adhere to the cell wall of plant tissue and actively exert their cellulolytic capacity. In contrast, Mn is required for the growth of most cells and to play an important role in the decarboxylation reactions of the tricarboxylic acid cycle. In addition, it has been shown to stimulate CO_2 binding in the production of succinic acid by rumen bacteria. Therefore, in deer two types of requirements of these minerals should be considered at present: One for the animal and another for the micro-organisms of the rumen (Fuller et al., 2015).

TABLE 22.1   Functions of Minerals in The Rumen of Deer.

Minerals	Functions
P	Energetical processes and of cellular reproduction
Mn, Fe, Zn, Cu, and Mb	Are activators of microbial enzymes
Co	Synthesis of the vitamin cyanocobalamin (B12)
S	Digestion of the cellulose, ingestion of nonprotein nitrogen (NPN) and synthesis of amino acids and vitamins of complex B
Na, Cl, and K	Metabolic processes, regulation of pH y osmotic pressure (NRC, 2007)

22.1.2   AVAILABILITY OF MINERALS IN FORAGE

The main source of minerals is food. However, under certain circumstances, water may contribute significant amounts of the following minerals: Iodine, manganese, iron, sulfur, sodium, chlorine, and magnesium (Hewitt, 2011). Different management practices (grazing pressure) and flooding can cause substantial soil consumption that can provide significant amounts of cobalt, iron, manganese, or selenium to grazing animals. For deer, soil in certain places may be a major source of sodium, especially in the spring. Dry feces are almost pure clay and it is assumed that wild animals consume them to cure.

The best habitat for the deer to develop optimally is the one that contains all the indispensable elements. As are the vegetation cover, water, and space available but the most important is the availability and quality of food.

Habitat conditions have an influence on population size and physical appearance and antler size. The content of the minerals in the forages that the deer consumes changes with the season of the year because the availability of nutrients in the soil and the ability of the root system to absorb them are affected by weather patterns. This variability can produce situations in which the food meets the requirements of deer minerals for some months but fails the rest of the year. Generally, important nutrients, like minerals go parallel to the digestibility of a given fodder (Kammermeyer et al., 2006).

Comparatively little is known about the true availability of the mineral elements of plants. It is speculated, however, that fiber content and lignin can actually promote fecal losses of magnesium, zinc, and iron, either through their binding via cation exchange or by the presence of forms not available in the matrix of the fiber. The cell walls of the forage contain small amounts of nonexchangeable iron and zinc. The silica fraction may be responsible for binding with these two minerals (Moreira et al., 20013). A theoretical explanation of the silicic inhibition of cellulolytic digestion postulates that most of the silica consumed can create trace mineral deficiencies in rumen bacteria.

22.1.3 MACROMINERALS

There are seven main macrominerals that are required by the deer to carry out their vital functions. The functions and symptoms of deficiency (NRC, 2007) are described in Table 22.2.

22.1.3.1 ABSORPTION OF MACROMINERALS

Even though some Ca is absorbed into the rumen, the greater absorption takes place in the small intestine of deer (Dijkstra, 2005). Absorption occurs through passive and active transport the latter aided by vitamin D. When the deer diet is relatively low in Ca, the absorbed proportion increases, on the contrary, when the diet contains more Ca than required, the absorbed proportion decreases (Goff, 2000). Phosphorous absorption from the deer diet occurs mainly in the small intestine, with very little, if any, absorption into the rumen. Phosphate, like nitrogen, is recycled into the rumen through saliva and is thus incorporated into the microbes of the rumen. Recycling of phosphorous in saliva is a characteristic of ruminant animals and is an important factor in the homeostatic control of phosphorus (Iqbal, 2004).

TABLE 22.2 Functions and Symptoms of Deficiency of the Essential Macrominerals for Deer.

Mineral	Functions	Symptoms of deficiency
Calcium	- It is a structural component of the skeleton. - Controls the excitability of nerves and muscles. - It is necessary for blood clotting. - Involved in the ionic movement of sodium and potassium, restricting the movement of potassium.	- Decreased milk production. - Muscle weakness and rumen and heart dysfunction. - Rickets in young deer. - Osteoporosis in adult deer. - Fibrous osteodystrophy. - Tetanic hypocalcemia.
Phosphorous	- It is a component of the skeleton. - It is a component of phospholipids (lecithins). - It acts on energy metabolism as a component of ATP, ADP, and AMP. - It is part of the nucleic acids, RNA and DNA. - It is constituent of several enzymatic systems.	- Decreased food consumption. - Low growth. - Decrease in milk production. - Failure in reproduction and lethargy. - Rickets in young deer. - Osteoporosis in adult deer. - Deprived appetite or pica.
Magnesium	- It is required for normal skeletal development as a bone constituent. - It is necessary for the oxidative phosphorylation of ATP in the mitochondria of the cardiac muscle. - It is needed for the activation of enzymes and enzymatic reactions involving ATP (muscle contraction, synthesis of proteins, nucleic acids, fats and coenzymes and in the use of glucose).	- Tetanic hypomagnesemia. - Decreased activity of magnesium-dependent enzymes.
Potassium	- It is required for the osmotic balance. - It is needed for the base-acid balance (pH). - It is required for various enzymatic reactions. - It facilitates cellular uptake of neutral amino acids. - It influences glucose metabolism.	- It is associated with abnormal electrocardiograms in calves, hens, and pigs, and generally in other species.

TABLE 22.2 *(Continued)*

Mineral	Functions	Symptoms of deficiency
Sodium	• It acts as an extracellular component through an energy-dependent sodium pump. • Together with potassium and magnesium, it is involved in the maintenance of osmotic pressure. • It acts on the base acid maintenance (pH). • Intervenes in the transfer of nerve impulses through the energy potential that is associated with their separation of potassium in the cell membrane.	- Decreased appetite. - Weight reduction. - Decrease in milk production. - Hemoconcentration. - Decrease in plasma volume. - Decrease in the urinary excretion of amino acids. - Abnormal consumption of soil, wood or sweat.
Chloride	- Control of extracellular osmotic pressure. - Maintenance of base acid balance (pH). - It is the main anion of gastric juice where it binds with hydrogen ions to form hydrochloric acid (HCl).	- Decrease in growth rate. - In hens after a sudden noise, they fall forward with their legs extended backward.
Sulfur	- It participates in the biosynthesis of taurine, heparin, and cystine. - As inorganic SO^4 acts on the base acid balance. • Intervenes in the synthesis of proteins forming amino acids. - Involved in the synthesis of lipids as a component of the vitamin biotin. - In the metabolism of carbohydrates as a component of vitamin thiamine. - Involved in energy metabolism as a component of vitamin coenzyme A. - In the metabolism of collagen and connective tissue as a component of mucopolysaccharides. - In blood coagulation as a component of heparin. - It participates in the protection of peroxides from cells as a component of glutathione peroxidase.	- Poor utilization of nitrogenous compounds in the rumen decreasing the synthesis and/or activity of the microbial mass and, therefore, reducing the rate of nitrogen digestion in the rumen. - Decreased production of proteins containing sulfur amino acids

Sodium and Potassium are absorbed mainly in the upper part of the small intestine and, to a lesser extent, in the rumen, abomasum, the lower small intestine and the large intestine (McDowell et al., 1997). Normally the potassium is absorbed from 80% to 95%. Sodium is absorbed in the lower parts of the intestines only if there are metabolic needs. Both elements, but especially the sodium, are recycled through the digestive system, mainly by the secretion in the saliva (Spears, 1998). The high concentrations of condensed tannins found in shrubs consumed by Texas white-tailed deer in northeastern Mexico can reduce sodium uptake and retention (Campbell and Hewitt, 2004). Absorption of magnesium occurs mainly in the rumen and omasum and to a lesser extent in the small and large intestines. The absorption of magnesium is reduced by a high concentration of potassium, probably because the sodium is essential for the transfer of magnesium, through the ruminal wall of the deer, and potassium tends to displace the sodium. Similarly, a sodium deficiency may restrict the absorption of magnesium (Robbins, 2001).

22.1.3.2 COMPOSITION OF MINERALS IN THE DEER

Table 22.3 shows the typical concentrations in the body tissues and antlers and the requirements of the main essential macrominerals of the deer. The total content of the minerals in the deer without the antlers represents only 5.0%, whereas the macrominerals in the antlers comprise between 30% and 35%. And, as shown in Table 22.3, Ca and P constitute almost 95.0% of the antler minerals. To maintain the functioning of microbes in the rumen, homeostasis in the organism, growth, and development of newly weaned fawns and growth and development of adult male antlers, deer should consume a diet containing a mixture of plants with sufficient quantities of macrominerals available (Schults et al., 1994).

22.1.3.3 MACROMINERAL CONTENT IN PLANTS CONSUMED BY DEER

In general, the leaves of the plants contain a higher mineral content than the stems and when they mature, protein increased, and minerals decreased. The forage of native shrub plants growing in northeastern Mexico and being consumed by white-tailed deer contains Ca in sufficient concentrations throughout the year to meet its requirements in all physiological states (Ramirez et al., 1997; Table 22.4). By far the deer consuming either individual or any mixture of these species would most likely not suffer from any of the deficiency symptoms shown in Table 22.2. Native grasses contain higher amounts of Ca than shrubs (Table 22.4) and native forbs (Table 22.4) that grow in northeastern Mexico. In addition, shrubs, grasses, cacti, and flowers and fruits of northern Mexico plants contain levels of Ca to meet the demands of small ruminants in any physiological state (NRC, 2007; Table 22.5).

TABLE 22.3   Typical Concentrations in Body and Requirements of Ca, P, Mg, K, and Na of White-tailed Deer for Growth and Antler Development.

Minerals	Body content, g/kg	Antler content g/kg	Requirements[a]
Calcium	15.0	190.1	4.5
Phosphorous	10.0	101.3	2.8
Magnesium	0.4	10.9	1.0
Potasium	2.0	<1.0	6.0
Sodium	1.6	5.0	1.0

DM, dry matter.
[a]Requirements (g/kg of the diet DM) to satisfy growth, bone, and antlers and development of newborn.

All the shrubs, grasses, and forbs (Table 22.4) consumed by white-tailed deer in northeastern Mexico contain P, throughout the year, in unsatisfactory quantities to meet their needs for growth and development (Ramirez et al., 1997). Therefore, P is a limiting nutrient in northeastern Mexico and southern Texas, USA for optimal growth and development of newly weaned fawns, females in gestation and lactation, and for maximum growth of adult male antlers. However, it has been determined that deer do not show the deficiency symptoms characteristic of P deficiency. This is probably due to deer consuming herbs with a high P content if they are available in the forage. In addition, it is likely that the deer have mechanisms for the conservation and transfer of P from bone tissue to the antlers, similar to those known in Ca. Such mechanisms could enable the deer to select forbs with high content of P in the spring and preserve the P for critical periods (Grasman and Hellgren, 1993).

The excretion of the minerals is done according to the animal species preferably by feces or urine. For example, deer tend to excrete Ca and P through feces while nonruminants do so through urine (Schults et al., 1994; Fig. 22.1).

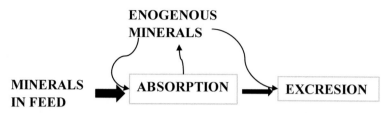

FIGURE 22.1 Deer absorption and excretion of diet and endogenous minerals.

Apparently, the Mg and K contained in shrubs and native grasses growing in northeastern and northern Mexico and southern Texas, USA and consumed by the white-tailed deer (Table 22.4), are not limiting for growth and development of deer, which grow under extensive systems. However, native grasses (Table 22.4) have marginally seasonal (in winter) concentrations of Mg and K. However, this does not represent a pathological problem for deer because native pastures do not represent a quantitatively important component (<1.0%) of their diet (Ramirez, 2003).

Na is the most commonly deficient mineral in temperate climate ecosystems, such as northeastern Mexico and the southeastern USA, and is the only nutrient by which herbivores specifically develop a high appetite (Chiy and Phillips, 1996). Apparently, all shrubs, in all seasons of the year consumed by white-tailed deer in northeastern Mexico and southern Texas, USA, are deficient in Na. The herbs (Table 22.4), however, only in spring and summer, when they are most abundant, contain Na in sufficient quantities to meet the needs of the Texan white-tailed deer. The same tendency is shown by native pastures (Table 22.4), but in autumn, when high precipitation promotes annual pasture growth or perennial regrowth. Therefore, Na is a limiting nutrient for Texas white-tailed deer that develops in the northeastern Mexico and south Texas, USA. However, the apparent deficiencies of deer especially in winter and summer can be covered with the supply of common salt (NaCl), in the "saladeros" commonly used for domestic livestock (Ramirez, 2009).

The temporary shortage of herbaceous vegetation in northeastern Mexico and south Texas requires whitetail deer to consume a rich shrub diet for most of the year (Ramirez, 2003). The deer are likely to seek minerals during periods of high shrub consumption to serve as regulators or precursors to form conjugates in the detoxification of secondary compounds contained in many of the shrub species. Campbell and Hewitt (2004) reported that when fed four male deer with diets consisting of 0, 25, 50, and 75% of *Acacia berlandieri*, they found that the concentration in the diet of Ca, P, and Na decreased with the increase in consumption of *A. berlandieri* while the concentration of Mg did not change. Losses of Ca, P, and Mg occurred mostly through feces, whereas Na losses occurred via urine. The consumption rates of Ca, Mg, and Na in diets consisting of up to 100% of *A. berlandieri* exceeded what was required. During the summer and autumn, the adult male obtained the required P with diets consisting of 100% *A. berlandieri* and obtained during the spring and throughout the year, with diets of <75 and 97% of *A. berlandieri*, respectively. They concluded that supplementary P during periods of low precipitation and high consumption of *A. berlandieri* can reduce the deficit of P in females in the reproductive period (Campbell and Hewitt, 2004).

TABLE 22.4 Seasonal Content de Ca, P, Mg, K, and Na in Native Plants Consumed by Deer in Northeastern Mexico.

Mineral	Winter	Spring	Summer	Fall
Shrubs, g/kg DM basis				
Calcium	27.0	22.0	25.0	27.0
Phosphorous	1.0	1.2	1.2	1.0
Magnesium	6.0	6.0	6.0	5.0
Potassium	13.0	13.0	16.0	13.0
Sodium	0.5	0.4	0.5	0.4
Forbs, g/kg DM basis				
Calcium	29.0	28.0	37.0	31.0
Phosphorous	1.7	1.4	1.7	1.7
Magnesium	4.4	5.3	8.1	5.8
Potassium	20.0	17.0	26.0	24.0
Sodium	0.5	0.5	0.9	0.9
Grasses, g/kg DM basis				
Calcium	6.0	6.0	6.0	6.0
Phosphorous	1.0	1.1	1.3	1.1
Magnesium	1.4	1.3	1.7	1.6
Potassium	10.0	10.0	19.0	13.0
Sodium	0.4	0.4	0.5	0.4

Condensed tannins can strongly chelate mineral elements, which reduces their absorption and increases the endogenous losses via the digestive tract (Perevolotsky et al., 2006) Plants containing either condensed or hydrolyzable tannins may decrease Na content in body of deer. Supplementation with minerals in diets with tannins prevented the drastic reduction of Na and decreased the toxic effects caused by the consumption of tannins (Frutos et al., 2004). Similar effects were obtained when food containing tannins and saponins were provided. Apparently, a triterpene saponin did not cause a drastic decrease of Na. It is known that Na is limiting for some herbivores that frequently exhibit a strong need to consume Na (Lopez-Alonso, 2012). The limitations on Na consumption are closely related to the consumption of tannins and other secondary compounds that are likely to cause a drastic decrease in Na. Supplementation of Na or other minerals provides a mechanism by which plants maintain the carrying capacity of herbivores below levels where they cannot cause severe damage (Shuttle, 2010).

22.1.4   MICROMINERALS

The difference between microminerals and macrominerals is based on the relative amounts that the deer needs from each in the diet for normal functioning. Cobalt, Cu, I, Fe, Mn, Mo, Se, and Zn have been reported to be essential for the normal metabolism of deer (Giżejewska et al., 2017). They generally act as activators of enzyme systems or as components of organic compounds and as such are needed in small amounts (ppm = mg/kg). The functions and symptoms of micromineral deficiency are shown in Table 22.5 (NRC, 2007).

22.1.4.1   ABSORPTION OF MICROMINERALS

Trace elements are absorbed mainly in the small intestine and, to a lesser extent, in the large intestine. In general, the degree of absorption depends on the balance between dietary supply and metabolic demand (Lopez-Alonso, 2012). Absorption in excess is prevented by homeostatic mechanisms. The homeostatic control of the absorption is particularly important in the Fe since the deer has a limited capacity of excretion. Absorption is also influenced by the physiological status of the deer, the chemical form of the ingested element and other components of its diet. During growth, lactation, and pregnancy, there is an increase in demand, particularly for Fe, Mn, and Zn, and, therefore, an increase in the percentage of absorption. In relation to other components of the diet, a high intake of any of the micronutrient cations is likely to interfere with the uptake of others, though not necessarily at all. For example, Mn, Zn, and Cu interfere with Fe absorption, presumably by

TABLE 22.5 Functions y Symptoms of Deficiency of Microminerals for White-tailed Deer.

Mineral	Functions	Symptoms of deficiency
Cobalt	- The only known function is as a component of vitamin B12 (cyanocobalamin)	- It acts as an enzyme in several enzymatic systems, including isomerases and dehydrogenases. - Participates in the biosynthesis of methionine. - Participates in the oxidation of propionic acid. - It is needed as a component of the coenzymes required for the synthesis of methyl groups and their metabolism. - Together with folic acid, they act in the synthesis of nucleoproteins. - Participates in the metabolism of the amino acid leucine.
Copper	- It is needed for the activity of enzymes that are associated with iron metabolism. - Required for elastin production. - It is needed for the production of collagen. - They are required for the production of melanin. - Used for the integrity of the central nervous system. - Prevents oxidation of cells. - Required for the synthesis of ATP	- Gradual copper decline leads to anemia due to association with iron. - Loss of hair pigmentation. - Increased susceptibility to infectious diseases. - It has been found that high consumption of molybdenum and sulfur can form together with copper an insoluble salt that causes poor absorption of copper.
Iodine	- It is part of the proteins that contain iodine and is found in the thyroid, including, mainly, thyroglobulins that produce the hormones triiodothyronine (T3) and tetraiodothyrosine (T4)	- Decrease in the basal metabolic index, due to the control of the oxidation index. In young animals, the disease is called cretinism and in adult myxedema. - Causes Goiter consisting of an enlargement of the cells of the thyroid gland.

TABLE 22.5 (Continued)

Mineral	Functions	Symptoms of deficiency
Iron	- It participates in the transport of electrons as a component of a large number of enzymatic systems including metalloporphyrins. - It helps in the transport and storage of oxygen components of two important proteins, such as hemoglobin and myoglobin.	- The most common symptoms in animal organisms are anemia of the hypochromic microcytic type meaning small and few red cells.
Manganese	- It is indispensable for the formation of chondrioitine sulfate that is a component of the mucopolysaccharides of the organic bone matrix. - It prevents ataxia in animals. - It is a component of several enzymes that act on the metabolism of polysaccharides, glycoproteins, carbohydrates, and lipids.	- Skeletal abnormalities (lameness, shortening, and arching of the legs and increase in joint size) associated with lack of Mn in mucopolysaccharides.
Molybdenum	- It is the component of the enzymes xanthine oxidase, sulfite oxidase, and aldehyde oxidase	- Low levels of xanthine oxidase. - No symptoms of deficiency have been reported.
Selenium	- It is a component of the enzyme glutathione peroxidase, which is involved in the catabolism of peroxides that originate in the oxidation of tissue lipids and, therefore, plays a central role in the integrity of cell membranes. - It is a component of the enzyme diiodotyrosine deiodinase type 1.	- Nutritional muscular dystrophy in ruminants

TABLE 22.5 *(Continued)*

Mineral	Functions	Symptoms of deficiency
Zinc	- It is a constituent of numerous metalloenzymes including carbonic anhydrase, carboxypeptidases a and b, various dehydrogenases, alkaline phosphatase, ribonuclease, and DNA polymerase. - It is needed for normal protein synthesis and for its metabolism. - It is a component of insulin and thus acts on the metabolism of carbohydrates. - It acts on gene expression. - It participates in the stability of the membrane.	- Anorexia in all species. - Thickening or hyperkeratinization of epithelial cells. - Retardation of bone formation. - Hypogonadism occurs in males.

competition for binding sites in the digestive tract and high Fe consumption depresses Cu absorption (Campbell and Hwitt, 2004).

22.1.4.2   CONTENT AND REQUIREMENTS OF DEER MICROMINERALS

Tissue content and requirements of Cu, Mn, Fe, and Zn in white-tailed deer are shown in Table 22.7. The requirements of deer microminerals depend on factors such as sex, age, activity, and the environment where it develops. However, the recommended concentrations include an appreciable margin of safety for the deer not to suffer symptoms of deficiency in their different physiological states including the growth and development of their antlers (Aguilera-Reyes et al., 2013).

22.1.4.3   MICROMINERAL CONTENT IN PLANTS CONSUMED BY DEER

Most of the Cu in the organism of the deer is located stored in the liver (about 80%). However, white-tailed deer requires 8 mg/kg of Cu in the dry matter of its daily diet (Table 22.7). Although the amount required is very small to perform the metabolic functions required by Cu, some shrub species, which are consumed by the white-tailed deer that develops in northeastern Mexico and South Texas (Ramirez, 2003; Table 22.7) have concentrations marginally lower than their Cu requirements. In contrast to a large number of shrub forages containing marginally low levels of Cu, all herbs consumed by white-tailed deer (Table 22.7) contain Cu in concentrations sufficient to meet the requirements of Texas white-tailed deer. Apparently, all native grasses (Table 22.7) that are consumed by white-tailed deer have Cu concentrations in all seasons with insufficient levels to meet the requirements of Texas white-tailed deer (Ramirez, 2009).

The Mn is uniformly distributed throughout the organism of the deer, although with some enrichment in the liver, bone, and digestive tract. The requirements of the deer Mn are 30 mg/kg in the dry matter of their diet. Except for native shrub species, such as *Acacia rigidula, Cercidium macrum, Acacia farnesiana, Porlieria angustifolia, Celtis pallida, Acacia berlandieri, Leucaena leucocephala, Leucophyllum texanum, Acacia greggii, Cordia boissieri, Condalia obovata, Prosopis glandulosa,* and *Opuntia engelmannii,* other 19 plants Table 22.7, have concentrations of Mn to meet the Mn metabolic requirements of white-tailed deer that grows in northeastern Mexico and southern Texas, USA (Ramirez et al., 1997; Barnes et al., 1990).

TABLE 22.6 Body Content and Requirements of Cu, Mn, Fe, and Zn for White-tailed Deer for Growth and Antler Development.

Mineral	Body content, mg/kg[a]	Requirements, mg/kg[a]
Copper	1.0–5.0	8
Manganese	0.2–0.5	30
Iron	20.0–80.0	40
Zinc	10.0–50.0	30

[a]Dry matter basis.

Source: NRC, 2007.

TABLE 22.7 Seasonal Content of Cu, Fe, Mn, Zn in Native Plants from Northeastern Mexico Consumed by White-tailed Deer.

Mineral	Winter	Spring	Summer	Fall
		Shrubs, g/kg DM		
Copper	9	9	10	9
Iron	157	143	160	159
Manganese	84	76	82	71
Zinc	37	38	43	40
		Forbs, g/kg DM		
Copper	12	11	16	15
Iron	189	181	421	275
Manganese	43	51	62	57
Zinc	38	36	65	50
		Grasses, g/kg DM		
Copper	3	4	5	4
Iron	112	132	185	163
Manganese	37	31	44	41
Zinc	40	41	55	45

Apparently native grasses that are selected by whitetail deer in northeastern Mexico and shown in Table 22.7, have sufficient concentrations of Mn, during all seasons of the year, to meet the requirements of white-tailed deer (Ramirez et al., 1996). In addition, the native pastures shown in Table 22.7, which also make up the group of plants that select white-tailed deer in northeastern Mexico, have concentrations of Mn that exceed the metabolic demands of white-tailed deer. *Hilaria belangeri* is a perennial grass native to the flora of the Tamaulipeco Matorral ecosystem, which includes the states of Coahuila, Nuevo León and Tamaulipas and southern Texas, USA, which is consumed by the white-tailed deer, and its foliage is a good source of microminerals including Mn (Ramirez, 2003).

Iron is a mineral found in abundance in all types of plants that select white-tailed deer in northeastern Mexico and southern Texas, USA. All the shrubs that are listed in Table 22.7 have Fe concentrations that cover and in many of them exceed the Fe requirements of the white-tailed deer. Also, the grasses and forbs contain levels of Fe that cover the requirements of the deer (Ramirez, 2003).

22.2 CONCLUSIONS

Only in summer the shrubs, forbs, and grasses consumed by white-tailed deer in northeastern Mexico contained sufficient amounts of minerals to satisfy metabolic requirements. In general, the leaves of the plants contain a higher mineral content than the stems and when they mature, protein increased, and minerals decreased. The excretion of the minerals is done according to the animal species preferably by feces or urine. For example, deer tend to excrete Ca and P through feces while nonruminants do so through urine. The best habitat for the deer to develop optimally is the one that contains all the indispensable elements. As are the vegetation cover, water, and space available but the most important is the availability and quality of food. Habitat conditions have an influence on population size and physical appearance and antler size. The content of the minerals in the forages that the deer consumes changes with the season of the year because the availability of nutrients in the soil and the ability of the root system, to absorb them, are affected by weather patterns.

KEYWORDS

- **white-tailed deer**
- **macrominerals**
- **microminerals**
- **shrubs**
- **forbs**
- **grasses**

REFERENCES

Aguilera, R. U. 1.; Sánchez, C. V.; Ramírez, P. J.; Monroy, Vilchis O.; López, G. I.; Janczur, M. Food Habits of the White-tailed Deer, *Odocoileus virginianus* (Artiodactyla: Cervidae) in Nanchititla Natural Park, Mexico. *Rev. Biol. Trop.* **2013**, *61*, 243–253.

Barnes, T. G.; Varner, L.; Blankenship, L. H.; Fillinger, T. J.; Heinemann, S. C. Macro and Trace Mineral Content of Selected South Texas Deer Forages. *J. Range Manag.* **1990**, *43*, 220–223.

Campbell, T. A.; Hewitt, D. G. Mineral Metabolism by White Tailed Deer Fed Diets of Guajillo. *Southwestern Natur* **2004**, *49*, 367–375.

Chiy, P. C.; Phillips, C. J. C. Sodium Nutrition of Dairy Cows. In Progress in Dairy Science; Phillips, C. J. C., Ed.; CAB International: Wallingford, 1996, 29–44.

Dijkstra, J. *Quantitative Aspects of Ruminant Digestion and Metabolism*; 2nd ed; CABI Publishing: Wallingford, 2005.

Fuller, W. B.; Wang, X.; Johnson, G. A.; Wu G. Select Nutrients and Their Effects on Conceptus Development in Mammals. *Animal Nutr.* **2015**, *1*, 85–95.

Frutos, P.; Hervás, G.; Giráldez, F. J.; Mantecón A. R. Tannins and Ruminant Nutrition a Review. *Spanish J. Agri. Res.* **2004**, *2*, 191–202.

Giżejewska, A.; Szkoda, J.; Nawrocka, A.; Żmudzki, J.; Giżejewski, Z. Can Red Deer Antlers be Used as an Indicator of Environmental and Edible Tissues' Trace Element Contamination? *Environ. Sci. Pollut. Res. Int.* **2017**, *24*, 11630–11638.

Goff, J. P. Pathophysiology of Calcium and Phosphorus Disorders. *Vet. Clin. North Am. Food Pract.* **2000**, *16*, 319–337.

Hewitt, D. G. *"Nutrition" in Biology and Management of White-tailed Deer*; Hewitt, D. G., ed., CRC Press: Boca Raton, F. L., **2011**, pp 75–105.

Iqbal, M. U. Evaluation of Single Superphosphate as a Source of Phosphorus Supplement in Cow Calves Fed on Berseem. M.Sc. (Hons) Thesis, University of Agriculture, Faisalabad–Pakistan, 2004.

Kammermeyer, K. E.; Miller, K. V.; Thomas, L. Quality Food Plots: Your Guide to Better Deer and Better Deer Hunting. Quality Deer Management Association: Bogart, GA, 2006.

Mc Dowell, R. L.; Conrad, J. H.; Hembry, F. G.; Rojas, L. X.; Valle, G.; Velásquez, J. Minerales para rumiantes en pastoreo en regiones tropicales. 2a. edición. Departamento de Zootecnia, Universidad de Florida, Gainesville, Florida, EUA, 1997, 10.

Moreira, L.; Marmo, L.; Vieira, F. de P.; Mendonça, R. A.; Pereira, J. C. A New Approach About the Digestion of Fibers by Ruminants. Revista Brasileira de Saúde e Produção Animal **2013**, *14*, 382–395.

NRC. National Research Council. Nutrient Requirement of Small Ruminant. *Sheep, Goats, Cervids, and New World Camelids*; National Academy Press: Washington, DC, 2007.

Odell, B. L.; Sunde, R. A. Introduction. In *Handbook of Nutritionally Essential Mineral Elements*; Odell, B. L., Sunde, R. A., Eds; Marcel Dekker Inc.: Nueva York, 1997, 1–12.

Perevolotsky, A.; Landau, S.; Slanikove, N.; Provenza, F. *Upgrading Tannin-rich Forages by Supplementing Ruminants with Polyethilene Glycol (PEG). BSAS Publication 34. The Assessment of Intake, Digestibility and the Roles of Secondary Compounds*; Sandoval-Castro, C. A., De, F. D., Hovell, B. D.; Torres-Acosta, J. F. J., Ayala-Burgos A., Eds.; University Press: Nottingham, 2006, pp 221–234.

Ramírez, L. R. G. Nutrición de Rumiantes: Sistemas Extensivos. Editorial Trillas, (En Prensa), 2003, pp 52–74.

Ramírez, L. R. G. Nutrición de Rumiantes: Sistemas Extensivos. Segunda Edición. Editorial Trillas, 2009, pp 52–74.

Ramírez, R. G.; Quintanilla, J. B.; Aranda, J. White-tailed Deer Food Habits in Northeastern Mexico, *Small Ruminant Res.* **1997,** *25,* 141–146.

Robbins, C. T. *Wildlife Feeding and Nutrition. Segunda Edición*; Academic Press: New York, 2001, 13–18.

Schultz, S. R.; Johnson, M. K.; Feagley, S. E.; Southern, L. L.; Ward, T. L. Mineral Content of Louisiana White-tailed Deer. *J. Wildlife Dis.* **1994,** *30,* 77–85.

Spears, J. W. In *Reevaluation of Metabolic Essentiality of Minerals.* Proceedings of New Technologies for the Production of "Next Generation" Feeds and additives. The 8th World Conference on animal Production, Seoul National University, Seoul, Korea, 1998, 68–77.

Suttle, N. F. *Mineral Nutrition of Livestock*; Cabi Publishing: UK, 2010; pp 210–221.

De la Rosa, R. X. F.; Calderón, L. R. D.; Parra, B. G. M.; Sifuentes, R A. M.; De Young, R.W.; León F.; Arellano, V. W. Genetic Diversity and Structure Among Subspecies of White-tailed Deer in Mexico. *J. Mammal.* **2012,** *93,* 1158–1168.

Karns, G. R.; Lancia, R. A.; De Perno, C. S.; Conner, M. C. Investigation of Adult Male White-tailed Deer Excursions Outside Their Home Range. *Southeastern Natur.* **2011,** *10,* 39–52.

Walter, W.; Ver Cauteren, K. C.; Campa, H.; Clark, W. R.; Fischer, J. W.; Hygnstrom, S. E.; Winterstein, S. R. Regional Assessment on Influence of Landscape Configuration and Connectivity on Range Size of White-tailed Deer. *Landscape Ecol.* **2009,** *24,* 1405–1420.

Yarrow, G. White-tailed Deer Biology and Management. Clemson University Cooperative Extension's Forestry & Natural Resources Fact Sheet 34, 2009.

General Conclusions and Research Needs in Bioresource Management

Since ancient times mankind is depending on bioresource (plants/animals) for food, timber, fibers, shelter, honey, medicinal plants, and other daily necessities. Owing to ever-increasing human populations and high demand, bioresources are overexploited leading to a huge number of the species to be endangered. This urges the necessity of sustainable management of bioresources. To meet this demand, significant research inputs have been directed throughout the world on sustainable management of bioresources. This book attempts to put together a few results of various facets of multidisciplinary researches on bioresources undertaken in different countries globally. We represent herein the conclusions on these aspects.

NATURE AND CHANGING CLIMATE MANAGEMENT, ADAPTATION, AND MITIGATION

1 NATURE, CLIMATE CHANGE, AND ADAPTATION

Since remote times nature has intimate relation with well-being of mankind. Dr. Kamjit, an Australian ecological economist recommends ecological service to promote this link. This is a kind of understanding that is required for all of us to connect ourselves with mother nature. The beauty of nature and its surroundings such as blooming flower, chirping birds, sprinkling water fall down the hills, slow moving streams with rhythmic amusing sounds brings heavenly joys to us. We should conserve it and live with its galaxy of beauty.

Impact of climate changes: Climate changes have great impact on the productivity of plant and crops. Increasing global warming owing to constant emission of greenhouse gases (GHGs) associated with abiotic stresses affect the productivity of plants and crops, thereby enhancing poverty. Dr. Mark Arango, Kenya, made a review of climate change in Kenya on agriculture. In Kenya, the increased occurrences of pests and diseases and drought have affected crop and livestock production leading to mortality of livestock, a great concern to the Kenyan populations in rural areas. The climate changes pose a great threat to the agricultural sectors and also the future livelihoods for most Kenyans especially those living in the rural areas. Government has taken measures to mitigate climate changes and increase agricultural productivity. Concerted research inputs need to be directed to alleviate this menace.

Impact of climate changes on boreal trees in Russia: Dr. Natalya S. Ivanova mentioned in his chapter that climatic changes, timber harvesting, and fires affect the structure, functions, and dynamics of forest ecosystems all around the world and as well as the formation of the Ural Mountains in Russia has led to the richness and diversity of natural ecosystems. They are undertaking statistical analysis. The patterns of reforestation after timber harvesting and fires will be revealed (based on regression analysis). Concerted research activities need to be directed to combat these problems.

Impact of climate changes on horticultural productivity: Dr. Debashis Mandal discussed the impact of climate change in productivity of horticulture in northeast Himalayas, India, namely, vegetables, fruits, spices, plantation crops. It focused on physiological aspects like pollination, fruit set, and also an impact over disease and pest incidence and also the strategies for climate resilient horticulture model. Concerted research activities need to be taken up to combat the impact of climate change and development of novel technology to increase the productivity of horticultural crops of great nutritional values.

2   FOREST RESOURCE MANAGEMENT

Since remote times, forest serve the mankind meeting their daily necessities such as food, shelter, timber, medicinal plants, honey, etc., and play very important roles in capture of carbon dioxide and store them as carbon in biomass and timber as a source of energy during the process of photosynthesis and liberation of profuse oxygen for respiration and vital activities. A few research inputs have been directed in this endeavor in the northeast Mexico.

Prosopis being an important woody species of high commercial and economic values, Rahim et al., undertook a comprehensive study on ecological structure and wood volume of *Prosopis* sp. (mesquite) communities in northeast of Mexico. It involves distribution, frequency, wood volumes, and related characteristic in different sites. The average density of shrubs was of 6575 individuals/ha. The relative values of vegetative cover, frequency, density, and importance value of *P. glandulosa* were varied significantly from site to site.

Durability of Prosopis: Carrillo. et al., northeast Mexico, investigated natural durability of *Prosopis laevigata* (mesquite) wood from different regions using a soil bed test (ENpr 807) and a resistance to basidiomycetes test (modified EN 113). In the latter, the durability of extractive-free wood specimens toward basidiomycetes was tested. The growth inhibition caused by ethanol-water extractives at 1000 ppm suspended in a malt-agar medium was 33.3% for *Coniophora puteana*. The results of this study are illuminating, which could be applied in different woods in future.

Researches on native plants and trees: Maiti et al. made a review of research advances on native economic plants and trees and shrubs in Mexico, namely, native crops species, medicinal plants, fiber-yielding plants, and *Cactus* spp. They also made a synthesis of various aspects of applied biology of more than 30 woody plant species of a Tamaulipan thorn scrub, northeastern Mexico on various aspects such as variability in leaf traits, leaf anatomy, plant characteristics, wood anatomy, wood density, phenology, and a few aspects of physiology and biochemistry, namely, leaf pigments, leaf epicuticular wax, trees with high nutritional values, carbon fixation, and nitrogen and protein contents. The results show a large variability of all the morphophysiological traits of the woody species related to the co-existence and adaptation of the woody species in semiarid environment. In view of great importance of these native crop species and other native plants, more research inputs need to be directed for the conservation, sustainable use of these valuable native plants, and development of technologies for efficient uses and increasing productivity.

Water relation of trees and shrubs: Gonzalez Rodriguez reported the physiological adaptation of native trees and shrubs to drought stress in the semiarid ecosystems of northeastern Mexico. The great diversity of native shrub species in northeastern Mexico and their morphophysiological traits reflect the plasticity among these species to cope successfully with a severely adverse environment with dramatic seasonal changes in soil water availability and evaporative demand physiological and morphological adaptations that convey the capacity to maintain a high tissue water status (water potential) have led to the widely spread use of leaf tissue or xylem water potential as a measure of tolerance to water stress under conditions of water deficit. Water relation, water potential determines the drought-resistance capacity of trees and shrubs in semiarid regions, concerted research inputs need to be directed to evaluate and select species resistant to drought.

Chemical composition of woods of trees and shrubs: Gonzalez Rodriguez et al., undertook chemical composition of woods of 37 woody species of northeastern Mexico such as NDF (neutral detergent fiber), ADF (digestible detergent fiber), lignin, cellulose, and hemicellulose. There was a large variability in contents of these components among woods of 37 woody species. The variations in chemical compositions could be related to quality determination and utility of timbers of different woody species. There is a great necessity to evaluate chemical composition of woods of most of the woody species and select species with desirable wood quality for timber and papermaking.

Carbon sequestration: The increased concentration of carbon dioxide owing to the constant emission of carbon dioxide by combustion of fossil fuels from the factories and burning of woods is thus endangering the security of mankind and animals. This has direct effect on climate changes and on enhanced global warming, thereby, reducing crop productivity and aggravating poverty. Maiti et al. undertook carbon sequestration of 44 trees and shrubs, northeast Mexico. Plants contribute a lot in the capture of carbon dioxide load from the atmosphere in the process of photosynthesis, synthesis of carbohydrate, and store carbon in its biomass. Variation in carbon fixation by photosynthesis is related to variation of carbon deposition in plant species. The results show a large variability in carbon sequestration among species studied. It is recommended that the plantation of trees and shrubs with high carbon sequestration have capacity to reduce loads in carbon-polluted area and cities. In the context of the above results it is recommended that in different countries there is a great necessity of selection of native trees with high carbon sequestration capacity 50% or more and shrubs and promote intensive plantation of these in highly carbon polluted area, cities, and factory sites in order to reduce the carbon load in the atmosphere.

Mangrove forest and plantation: Mangroves play an important role in preventing erosion in saline area in sea beaches and offer habitats for birds, animals, and other sea creatures. Pradeep Khanna reported plantation of mangroves in Gujarat, India. This needs to be promoted in coastal areas to check erosions by ocean waves and also reported about the seedling production of forest trees.

Dr. Vilasia Iakovoglou, Greece, developed irrigation techniques for increasing seedling production of forest trees. Mediterranean ecosystems are characterized of a particular ecological importance, but they are facing restoration problems, mainly due to their prevailing semiarid climate. Further, the increased predicted temperatures associated with climate change pose greater obstacles to restoration efforts. Their research directed toward the study the response of *Quercus pubescens* under different irrigation frequencies in order to determine its ability to successfully being restored has revealed the successful transplantation of seedlings and substantial benefit particularly during the summer months exposed to water scarcity.

Seedling production of trees poses a great obstacle. This technique could be utilized for increasing seedling productions of forest trees and shrubs.

3   CROP RESOURCES MANAGEMENT

Management of seed crops: Seeds are of vital importance in agriculture. Dr. Ashok K. Thakur, India, reported in detail the technology of the management of various seed crops for increasing seed productivity. The management of mother crop plays pivotal role in quality of seed produced. Seed production is highly specialized discipline of agriculture. It involves crop and region specific genetic and agronomic principles that need to be precisely practiced to achieve desired quality of seed. In a production system, the good quality seed is when combined with other complementary agro-inputs such as better nutrition, irrigation, plant protection measures, etc., resulted in rapid and substantial increase in productivity. This chapter described the seed quality, its components, and factors affecting seed quality. The genetic, agronomic, legislative mechanisms of seed quality control are described to have better understanding of seed production. However, the major focus remains on the preharvest and postharvest management of seed quality.

Saline soils and saline stresses management in crops: Prof. Cinzia Forni, Rome, Italy, stated that salinity affect greatly agricultural production, causing serious damage to plants and resulting in considerable losses in crop yields. He made an overview and update of the major physiological and biochemical changes occurring in plants exposed to salt stress in crops and to select tolerant genotypes to be used in breeding programs The author makes an excellent review on salt stress on crops starting from agronomic, physiology to molecular levels. In view of the facts that two-third arable lands affect crop productivity in world, there is a great necessity to analyze the gravity of the problem and select species or crop varieties tolerant to salinity.

Biopesticides for sustainable crop protection and improvement: Dr. M. Madhavi et al., reported the use of biopesticides for sustainable crop protection and improvement. This deals with the definition, concepts and importance of sustainable agriculture, impact of conventional pesticides in agriculture, history of biopesticides, classification, preparation, and mode of action.

Indiscriminate use of insecticides to control insects in crop fields affected the quality and increase toxicity of food crops causing hazards and increase soil pollution. Use of bioinsecticides is recommended to combat these hazards.

Morphological characterization of phytopathogenic fungi isolated from seeds of barley plants (Hordeum vulgare): Teresa Romero Cortes and her collaborators in Mexico, described the morphological characterization of phytopathogenic fungi isolated from seeds of barley plants (*Hordeum vulgare*) in Mexico, which helped in proper identification of various fungi. Therefore, performing the morphological characterization of fungal isolates associated with the barley plant in Mexico will allow us to have a more precise idea that microorganisms are present in our country and thus to control those that are harmful to the plant. For that the aim of the research was to isolate and do the morphological characterization of fungi associated with diseased barley plants in Mexico.

Assessment of plant genetic resources of chili germplasm: Chili, *Capsicum* spp. is of high commercial and edible values; there is a great necessity to direct concerted researches on the evaluation, selection, and propagation of this crop. Dr. Biswajit Ghosh, India, discussed centre of origin, (b) global distribution, (c) assessment of germplasms—morphological diversity, chemical diversity (capsinoids and flavonoids), genetic diversity (molecular marker based) and disease diversity (molecular PCR-based viral, bacterial, and fungal diseases), and (d) selection of elite germplasm. Studies on chili germplasm are rare in literature. The results of this research will definitely benefit researchers working on chili to direct their research activities.

Ex-situ conservation of chili germplasm: Dr. Biswajit Ghosh, India, also studied ex-situ conservation of chili germplasm. This includes: (a) field gene bank, (b) greenhouse/polyhouse, (c) seed bank, (d) plant tissue culture, (e) in-vitro conservation, (e) cryopreservation and (f) DNA bank. This novel technique could be utilized by researchers on chili for efficient propagation of chilies. This research has enormous potential in genetic improvement of chili.

Conservation practices may yield sustainable resource: Dr. S. M. Jalil, Bangladesh, mention that conservation practice is a careful preserva-tion and protection of something especially planned management of any resource such as natural resources like vegetation, forests, agri-crops, air, water, minerals, oil, gas, etc., to prevent exploitation, destruction, neglect, or overuse. Lack of awareness, ignorance, negligence, or even unwise use of resource or bioresource have brought down both the resource bases to such a below level in many countries particularly the less developed countries that to produce or regenerate the minimum requirement is very difficult to achieve. Austerity, technology, motivation, cooperation are essential parts of the process of achieving sustainability of resource so developed. In fine, it may be said that at this stage of global biomass status, there is no option other than conservation practices. Effective conservation practices may yield sustainable resources.

Phytochemistry of medicinal plants: Since remote times medicinal plants play important in alleviating diseases in rural and urban areas but the efficacy of these medicinal plants is rarely investigated through analysis of phytochemicals. Dr. Julia Verde Star, Mexico, working on medicinal plants in northeast Mexico worked on phytochemistry of medicinal plants. He describes detailed methodology and techniques. This technique could be utilized to select medicinal species with high phytochemical attributes.

Phytoplankton and toxic threats: Dr. Ahmed Ibrahim, Iraq, studied phytoplankton and toxic threats of marine algae. Microscopic planktonic algae are critical food for filter-feeding bivalve shellfish (oysters, mussels, scallops, and clams) also for the larvae of commercially important crustaceans and finfish. The explosive growths sometimes appear during changes in weather conditions but important contributing causes may be variations in upwellings, temperature, transparency, turbulence, or salinity of the water, the concentration of dissolved nutrients, wind, or surface illumination and contamination. There are many species of planktonic algae that can produce toxins such as paralytic shellfish toxins. Diarrheic shellfish toxins, amnesic shellfish toxins, neurotoxic shellfish toxins, and azaspiracid shellfish toxins showing the effects of bioresource, algae in coastal areas. Here are about 4000 toxic species of phytoplankton reported so far. Its gregarious growth and multiplication affect coastal environments, aesthetics, and human health. The abundance of algal bloom cause anoxic effects causing mortality of marine fish and other organisms in coastal area. Some species they can easily find their way to humans via food chain, also these toxins can cause a variety of gastrointestinal and neurological illnesses and also cause ecological hazards.

4   ANIMAL RESOURCES MANAGEMENT

Shane Orchard, New Zealand, undertook a study on protecting fish spawning habitat after earthquakes. He mentions that dynamic natural resources present particular challenges for management and require methods to account for temporal fluctuations and long-term change. Using the example of fish spawning habitat recovering from a major environmental disturbance, he demonstrates the need to account for spatial variability when determining the boundaries of areas where legal protection mechanisms will apply in important traditional fishery. Using comprehensive field surveys, spawning habitat was found to have shifted following a series of major earthquakes and considerable spatiotemporal variability in the pattern of occupancy was detected. He stresses the widespread need for methods to quantify dynamic resources for protection to ensure that conservation measures can be monitored and their effectiveness guaranteed.

Minerals contents in forage consumed by white-tailed deer in northeastern Mexico: Deer feed on forages grown in forest, Dr. Roque Ramirez, Mexico, undertook a study for the first time on minerals contents in forage consumed by white-tailed deer in northeastern Mexico, of at least 15 minerals (N, P, S, K, Ca, Mg, Na, Cl, Fe, Mn, Cu, Co, I, Mo, and Se). The deficiency of each mineral in the deer results in abnormalities that can only be corrected by the supply of the deficient mineral. The severity of the deficiency will determine the degree and type of abnormality observed. The mineral elements are divided into two groups according to the abundance of them in the organism: macrominerals are elements that are found in abundant form in the organism and have structural functions and microminerals or trace elements that are in the organism in very small amounts and usually perform. The results of mineral nutrition of forages eaten by deers are interesting. There is a necessity to select forage species with high nutritional values and conform their efficacy by experimentation.

—Ratikanta Maiti
Humberto Gonzalez Rodríguez
Ch. Aruna Kumari
Debashis Mandal
Narayan Chandra Sarkar

Index